Hair Loss

Disorders, Restoration and Management

Second Edition

Hair Loss

Disorders, Restoration and Management

— **Second Edition** —

Kabir Sardana MD, DNB, MNAMS

Professor
Department of Dermatology and STDs
PGIMER, Dr Ram Manohar Lohia Hospital
New Delhi

Ananta Khurana MD, DNB, MNAMS

Associate Professor
Department of Dermatology and STDs
PGIMER, Dr Ram Manohar Lohia Hospital
New Delhi

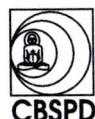

CBSPD

CBS Publishers & Distributors Pvt Ltd

New Delhi • Bengaluru • Chennai • Kochi • Kolkata • Lucknow • Mumbai

Hyderabad • Jharkhand • Nagpur • Patna • Pune • Uttarakhand

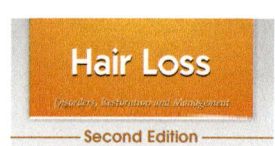

Hair Loss

Disorders, Restoration and Management

—— **Second Edition** ——

ISBN: 978-93-86827-64-7

Copyright © Authors and Publisher

Second Edition: 2018
Reprint: 2025
First Edition: 2016

Published by Satish Kumar Jain and produced by Varun Jain for

CBS Publishers & Distributors Pvt Ltd
4819/XI Prahlad Street, 24 Ansari Road, Daryaganj, New Delhi 110 002, India
Ph: 011-23289259, 23266838   Website: www.cbspd.com
    e-mail: delhi@cbspd.com; cbspubs@airtelmail.in.

Corporate Office: 204 FIE, Industrial Area, Patparganj, Delhi 110 092, India
Ph: 011-4934 4934   Fax: 0114934 4935   e-mail: publishing@cbspd.com; publicity@cbspd.com

Branches

- **Bengaluru:** Seema House 2975, 17th Cross, K.R. Road,
  Banasankari 2nd Stage, Bengaluru 560 070, Karnataka
  Ph: +91-80-26771678/79   Fax: +91-80-26771680   e-mail: bangalore@cbspd.com
- **Chennai:** 18/8B, Subbarayan Street, Shenoy Nagar, Chennai 600 030, Tamil Nadu, India
  Ph: +91-44-42032115, 26681266   e-mail: chennai@cbspd.com
- **Kochi:** 42/1325, 1326, Power House Road, Opposite KSEB, Power House,
  Ernakulum 682 018, Kochi, Kerala, India
  Ph: +91-484-4059061–65, 67   Fax: +91-484-4059065   e-mail: kochi@cbspd.com
- **Kolkata:** 147, Hind Ceramics Compound, 1st Floor, Nilgunj Road,
  Belghoria, Kolkata 700 056, West Bengal, India
  Ph: +91-33-25633055/56   e-mail: kolkata@cbspd.com
- **Lucknow:** Basement, Khushnuma Complex, 7 Meerabai Marg
  (behind Jawahar Bhawan), Lucknow 226 001, UP, India
- **Mumbai:** PWD Shed, Gala No. 25/26, Ramchandra Bhatt Marg, Next JJ Hospital
  Gate No. 2, Opp. Union Bank of India, Noorbaug, Mumbai 400 009, Maharashtra, India
  Ph: +91-22-66661880/89   e-mail: mumbai@cbspd.com

Representatives

- **Hyderabad** 0-9885175004   • **Jharkhand** 0-9811541605   • **Nagpur** 0-8692091830
- **Patna** 0-9334159340   • **Pune** 0-9664372571   • **Uttarakhand** 0-9716462459

Printed at: Print in India

when God leads you to the edge of the cliff,
trust Him fully and let go
only one of two things will happen:
either He'll catch you when you fall,
or He'll teach you how to fly!

to
_____

the people who always stand by me
my wife and fellow dermatologist
Supriya Mahajan
my parents Amba Sardana and Maj Gen KN Sardana
my daughter Zoya
my teachers, colleagues and
students at LHMC, MAMC, RML

Kabir Sardana

my two choicest blessings from God
my daughters Anushka and Ahaana …
my very dynamic husband, Dr Rajat Jain, for always
encouraging me to push barriers and aim high …
my parents Mr SK Khurana and Mrs Suksham Khurana for
giving me all that defines me …
my teachers at UCMS, meeting whose
standards is a constant goal …
and to my seniors, colleagues and
residents at RML hospital …

Ananta Khurana

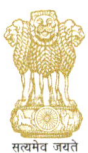

Government of India
Department of Dermatology
Post Graduate Institute of
Medical Education and Research,
Dr Ram Manohar Lohia Hospital
New Delhi

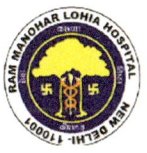

Foreword

The hair is a complex structure whose functional importance other than the cosmetic appearance and beauty in humans, is still to be well understood, although, in other mammals this is better comprehended.

This book is of practical utility as, the emphasis is on the hair diseases seen commonly in dermatology clinics. Besides, it also provides knowledge about some of the newer dermatology practices in hair management. It will also be of great use to those clinicians who have special interest in the field of hair restoration.

The format of the chapters is elegant and has been presented in an easily understandable manner. The book is useful for quick reader, as its contents have been put in very comprehensible clinical perspective.

डॉ. (प्रो.) पी. के. शर्मा, एम.डी.
DR. (PROF.) P. K. SHARMA, M.D.
परामर्शदाता एवं विमागाध्यक्ष, चर्मरोग
Consultant & Head Dept. of Dermatology
डॉ. रा.म.लो. अस्पताल एवं पी जी आई एम ई आर
Dr. R.M.L. Hospital & PGIMER
नई दिल्ली–110001 / New Delhi - 110001

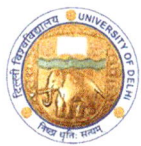
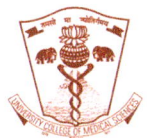

Department of Dermatology and STDs
University College of
Medical Sciences & GTB Hospital
Delhi-110095

Foreword

It is a great pleasure and privilege to write the Foreword to the second edition of the book *Hair Loss: Disorders, Restoration and Management*.

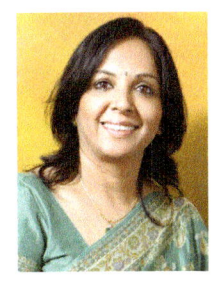

As a girl child, I was always fascinated by the fairy tale of Rapunzel and her beautiful silky long hair. Thick and healthy hairs have always been considered the best accessory for women and men alike. However, like skin, a diversity of environmental, psychological and endogenous/systemic stressors constantly challenge the health of hair. Loss of hair or excess of hair, both are cosmetically unacceptable and can be emotionally detrimental. This book systematically deals with these issues and targets both postgraduate students and practicing dermatologists. The book will provide the readers easy access to the complete and authoritative guidance with respect to the various clinical conditions, their diagnosis and management. The highlights of the book are, inclusions of novel concepts in the etiopathogenesis, utility of upcoming diagnostic tool such as trichoscopy, newer molecules in the medical management and details of surgical intervention from the experts in the respective field. Elegantly drawn diagrams certainly add to the overall lucidity. A chapter dedicated to hair cosmetic and esthetic procedures will fill the lacunae in our knowledge and seems very relevant in today's rapidly changing beauty industry.

Authors of this book Prof Kabir Sardana and Dr Ananta Khurana are both astute academician and have flare for perfection. In this era when there is explosion of information, they certainly deserve hearty congratulations for putting up this much-needed book containing concise and comprehensive information about hair.

Dr Archana Singal
Director Professor
University College of Medical Sciences and GTB Hospital
Head, Department of Dermatology, Faculty of Medical Sciences
University of Delhi (2007–10, 2013–16), Delhi, India

Preface to the Second Edition

"Anyone can be confident with a full head of hair.
But a confident bald man—there's your diamond in the rough."

Larry David

Hair, inspite of the oft stated "dead" state of keratin, is a key to social interaction, notwithstanding the saying by Larry David. How dermatologists manage to treat hair loss with no hair on their head is a feeling that I now understand, when I have greying of hair and patients come for its treatment and give a furtive glance to my own hair! The first edition of this book was targeted at GPs while this targets dermatologists, accounting for the thorough overhaul of each chapter. We have changed the title to include 3 conditions that are crucial for a hair book—hirsutism, hair restoration and trichoscopy. We are fortunate to have some amazingly erudite contributors within the country and outside who have performed excellent work in their fields. This includes researchers who have worked on novel drugs, including some that are soon to be launched. The diagrams have been carefully crafted to make them self explanatory, while the focus remains on therapy. We have not included diagnosis of hair disorders as it is mentioned in relevant sections throughout the text.

The book includes, in addition, chapters on pseudofolliculitis and certain uncommon, and often overlooked, scalp disorders which would be an interesting read for dermatologists. A detailed review of hair disorders in females has been included as a separate chapter. Evidence based treatments have been elucidated wherever possible. A chapter on advanced hair restoration techniques has been included to apprise the reader of the latest in the field. The chapter on seborrheic dermatitis will enlighten the readers with the latest updates on the pathogenesis and treatment of this common disorder. We have included a separate chapter on pediatric hair disorders, covering both inherited and acquired conditions. "Off-label" modalities, which form a bulk of prescriptions for hair loss, have been dealt with, in a rationale and scientific manner, in a separate chapter. Hair aging, with a focus on canities, has also been succinctly presented. The chapter on hair biology has been expanded to include newer concepts related to the hair cycling, including molecular mediators. We hope the book proves to be a ready-reckoner for dermatologists for everything related to hair disorders!

Happy Reading!

Kabir Sardana
Ananta Khurana

Preface to the First Edition

Hair is an inanimate structure but the cosmetic and pharmaceutical industry all over the world depends on it for their sustenance. Though there are numerous books on this topic, some of which I have been mentioned in the bibliography, there are a few books on Indian patients and hair. This book is aimed at the Indian practitioner and thus looks at the common hair problems and their management. We have added two chapters on hair cosmetics and common hair issues as most patients come back with queries on the same.

A book is as good as its contributors and I am fortunate to have contributors who have special interest in their respective topics. The only "tool" in dermatology is the dermatoscope and in hair its extension the trichoscope. We have three masters in this tool, Dr Sidharth Sonthalia, Dr MS Sukesh and Dr Rahul Arora, who have added their experience by way of images in this book. When I was doing my MD, there were posters put up by an MBBS doctor inviting doctors to learn hair transplantation. It was really a vague idea at that time and most of us ignored it. Today we have MD students giving up their training after finishing it from prestigious institutions and just doing hair transplantation! Such is the lure of the art. I am fortunate to have Dr Rajat Gupta, a trained plastic surgeon, who has contributed a chapter on hair transplantation for the book. Dr Khushbu Mahajan my co-author has "tooth-combed" the text in between her holiday breaks and I am always grateful for her inputs.

The book has left out pediatric hair disorders as most of these are genodermatoses, not commonly seen and I dare say difficult to manage. Also I have not covered hirsutism as our topic was hair loss! This book is a part of the series on *Handbooks on Dermatological Disorders* and is not aimed to be a treatise and thus we have purposely left out the verbose pathogenesis and focused on the clinical approach and management concept.

Happy Reading!

Kabir Sardana
Khushbu Mahajan

Acknowledgments

I express my gratitude to God and destiny for giving me the time and opportunity to work on the second edition of the book. The basis of this book is the first edition for which Dr Khushbu Mahajan was a great help, a lot of the basic work is thanks to her. That book needed time, which I got thanks to destiny that gave me a break from work, some of which was contrived by human intervention, a silent thanks to them also! For this edition a big credit goes to the endless energy of the ideally named colleague at RML, Dr Ananta Khurana.

A special thanks to some wonderful people that I rediscovered in the last year—the residents of RML hospital, my old residents at MAMC, my seniors at RML—Dr RK Gautam and Dr PK Sharma, my seniors Dr Archana Singhal, Dr Deepika Pandhi, Dr RP Gupta and Dr SN Bhattacharya, my colleague and friend Dr Rishi Parashar and many more.

I thank all the researchers on hair disorders, who have penned some wonderful books on the topic, which have added so much more interesting data and factoids on the medical science of hair loss.

A big thanks to CBS Publishers & Distributors, Mr SK Jain CMD and Mr YN Arjuna Senior Vice President—Publishing, Editorial and Publicity and their team, Mrs Ritu Chawla Assistant General Manager—Production, Mr Sanjay Chauhan, Mr Vikrant Sharma and Mr Ananda Mohanty; and Mr SK Verma and Mr Sunil Dutt, apart from the great support staff at their easily accessible office.

And at the end, I thank our patients whose hair problems sustain and encourage us to delve deeper into the vagaries of hair loss.

Kabir Sardana
Ananta Khurana

Contributors

Abhinav Kumar MBBS (MAMC), MD (LHMC)
Eugenix Hair and Skin Sciences
Sector 935P, Sector 51, Gurugram
Haryana 122018
Email pradeep@eugenix.in

Anamika Bhattacharyya PhD
Vyome Biosciences Pvt. Ltd.
Plot 465, F.I.E.
Patparganj Industrial Area
Delhi 110092

Ananta Khurana MD, DNB, MNAMS
Associate Professor
Department of Dermatology and STDs
Dr RML Hospital and PGIMER
New Delhi

Arika Bansal MBBS (Gold Medalist), MD (AIIMS), Diplomate of American Board of
Hair Restoration Surgeons
Eugenix Hair and Skin Sciences
Plot 935P, Sector 51, Gurugram
Haryana 122018
Email pradeep@eugenix.in

Chander Grover MD, DNB, MNAMS
Professor
University College of Medical Sciences and GTB Hospital
New Delhi

Deep Dutta MD, DM, DNB (Endocrinology), MNAMS
Specialty Certificate (Endocrinology and Diabetes) (MRCP, UK)
Fellow of American College of Endocrinology (FACE)
Consultant and Head
Department of Endocrinology, Diabetology and Metabolic Disorders
Venkateshwar Hospital, Dwarka
New Delhi

Deepashree Daulatabad MD, DNB, MNAMS
Senior Resident
University College of Medical Sciences and GTB Hospital
New Delhi

Kabir Sardana MD, DNB, MNAMS
Professor
Department of Dermatology and STDs
PGIMER, Dr RML Hospital
New Delhi

Khushbu Mahajan MD
Consultant Dermatologist
Ex-Associate Professor
Hindu Rao Hospital
New Delhi

Masarat Jabeen MD, DNB
Fellow in Aesthetic Medicine (University of Griefswald, Germany)
Consultant Dermatologist
ARV Skin Clinic
Bhatindi, Jammu
Jammu and Kashmir

Pallavi Ailawadi MD, DNB
Senior Resident
Department of Dermatology
Maulana Azad Medical College and Lok Nayak Hospital
New Delhi

Pradeep Sethi MBBS, MD (AIIMS), ISHRS (USA)
Eugenix Hair and Skin Sciences
Plot 935P, Sector 51, Gurugram
Haryana 122018
Email pradeep@eugenix.in

Purnima Malhotra MD
Specialist
Department of Pathology
PGIMER, Dr RML Hospital
New Delhi

Rahul Arora MD, DNB, FISD
Consultant Dermatologist and Trichologist
Max Superspeciality Hospital
Skinmedics Skin and Hair Clinic
New Delhi

Rajat Gupta MS, DNB (Gen. Surg.)
DNB (Plastic Surgery)
Fellow: Instituto de Benito, Spain (Cosmetic Surgery)
Fellow: Hospital Sant Pau (Breast Surgery)
Director: Cosmetic Surgery Skinnovation Clinics, Delhi
Country Head (Hair Restoration and Cosmetic Surgery): Clinic Dermatech

Ramya MN MBBS
Junior Resident (PG, IIIrd Year)
Department of Dermatology and STDs
PGIMER, Dr RML Hospital
New Delhi

Ranjeet Singh Patel MPharm
Vyome Biosciences Pvt. Ltd.
Plot 465, F.I.E.
Patparganj Industrial Area
Delhi 110092

Samipa Samir Mukherjee DDV, DDVL, FRGUHS (Pediatric Dermatologist)
Consultant Pediatric Dermatologist and Dermatotrichologist
Cutis Academy of Cutaneous Sciences
Bengaluru

Selma CH MBBS
Junior Resident (PG, IIIrd Year)
Department of Dermatology and STDs
PGIMER, Dr RML Hospital
New Delhi

Shamik Ghosh
Director
Biology and Pre-clinical Development
Vyome Biosciences Pvt. Ltd.
Plot 465, F.I.E.
Patparganj Industrial Area
Delhi 110092

Sidharth Tandon MD
Senior Resident
Department of Dermatology and STDs
PGIMER, Dr RML Hospital
New Delhi

Sukesh MS MD, DNB (Dermatology)
Consultant, Dermatotrichologist
Fortis Hospital, Rajajinagar, Bengaluru
Citi Hospital, West of Chord Road, Bengaluru
Peoples' Tree Hospital, Peenya, Bengaluru
Mailing Address: No. 246, 6th Main, MS Ramaiah Enclaves, 8th Mile, Nagasandra Post, NH4, Bangalore,
Karnataka, India-560073

Contents

Foreword by PK Sharma   *vii*

Foreword by Archana Singal   *ix*

Preface to the Second Edition   *xi*

Preface to the First Edition   *xiii*

Contributors   *xvii*

1. **Hair Biology and Its Clinical Implications**   1

2. **Trichoscopy in Disorders of Scalp**   14

3. **Male Pattern Hair Loss**   39

4. **Female Pattern Hair Loss**   54

5. **Telogen Effluvium**   70

6. **Pseudofolliculitis Barbae**   94

7. **Alopecia Areata**   105

8. **Cicatricial (Scarring) Alopecias**   140

9. **Pediatric Hair Disorders**   181

10. **Hair Loss in Women**   213

11. **Aging of Hair**   254

12. **Seborrheic Dermatitis**   263

13. **Miscellaneous and Psychogenic Scalp Disorders**   279

14. **Newer and Investigational Drugs for Androgenetic Alopecia**   302

15. **Role of Nutrition and Off-Label Treatments for Hair Loss**   326

16. **Basics of Hair Restoration**   346

17. **Advanced Hair Restoration**   367

18. **Hirsutism**   388

Selected Bibliography   *419*

Index   *421*

1

Hair Biology and Its Clinical Implications

Kabir Sardana, Ananta Khurana

Hair follicles form before the ninth week of fetal life when the hair germ, a solid cylinder of cells, grows obliquely down into the dermis. There it interacts with a cluster of mesenchymal cells (the placode) bulging into the lower part of the hair germ to form the hair papilla. The dermal papilla contains blood vessels bringing nutrients to the hair matrix. The sebaceous gland is an outgrowth at the side of the hair germ, establishing early the two parts of the pilosebaceous unit. Adjacent to the sebaceous gland is the region of insertion of the arrector pili muscle called the **bulge**. This area contains hair follicle **stem cells** which presumably can regenerate the entire hair follicle and sebaceous gland. Damage to this area will cause permanent hair loss. Melanocytes migrate into the matrix and are responsible for the different colours of hair (eumelanin, brown and black; phaeomelanin and trichochromes, red). Grey or white hair is caused by low pigment production, and the filling of the cells in the hair medulla with minute air bubbles that reflect light.

HAIR ANATOMY

The structure of a hair follicle is depicted below. It can be divided into four parts (Fig. 1.1):

1. **Infundibulum**, extending from the follicular orifice to the sebaceous gland.
2. **Isthmus**, extending from the sebaceous gland to insertion of the arrector pili muscle.
3. **Suprabulbar area**, insertion of the arrector pili muscle to matrix.
4. **Bulb**, consisting of the dermal papilla and matrix intermixed with melanocytes.

The hair follicles in mammals are usually clustered in groups of 2–5, referred to as *follicular hair units* (FHU) (Fig. 1.2A and B). In case of androgenetic alopecia, these units decrease with miniaturization of hair, thus 1–2 hair emerge from each unit.

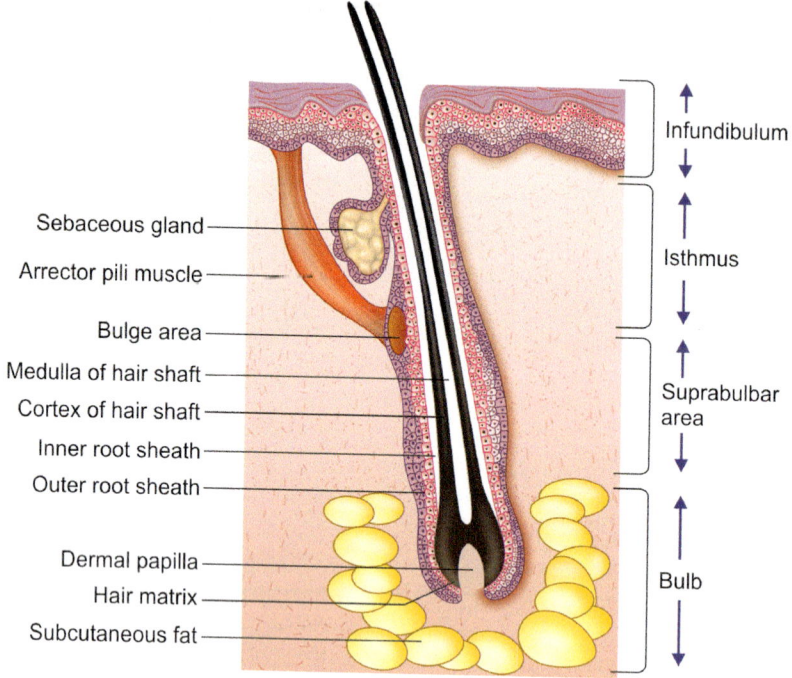

Fig. 1.1: A structural depiction of the parts of a hair follicle

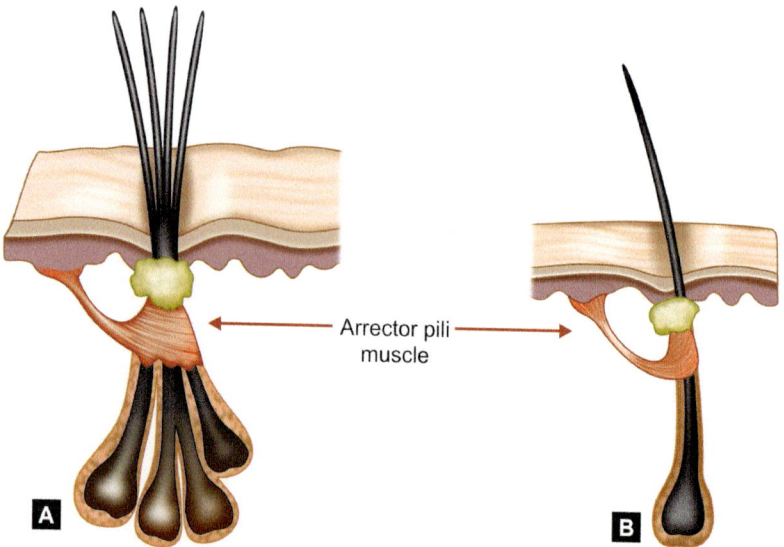

Fig. 1.2A and B: (A) Follicular hair unit on the scalp with multiple hair; (B) FHU on the beard with a single hair

HAIR BASICS

The entire scalp contains around 100,000 pigmented, terminal hair follicles. Hair of people originating from East Asia (China, Korea, and Japan) is usually referred to as oriental or Asian hair. It generally shows the greatest diameter, ranging from 100 to 130 μm.

Hairs are classified into three main types (Fig. 1.3):

1. *Lanugo hairs:* Fine long hairs covering the fetus, but shed about 1 month before birth.
2. *Vellus hairs:* Fine short unmedullated hairs covering much of the body surface. They replace the lanugo hairs just before birth.
3. *Terminal hairs:* Long coarse medullated hairs seen, e.g. in the scalp or pubic regions. Their growth is often influenced by circulating androgen levels.

Terminal hairs convert to vellus hairs (better called vellus like hair) in *male-pattern alopecia*, and vellus to terminal hairs in *hirsutism*. Human vellus hair acts as a very sensitive tactile tool and stimulation of nostril hair triggers sneezing while stimulation of eyelash triggers blinking.

The rate of hair growth is highly variable, but the rates of *scalp* hair growth in humans vary between **0.3** and **0.5 mm per day**, slightly faster in adult women than men but greater in prepubertal boys than girls. Male beard growth has a growth rate of 0.27–0.38 mm/day.

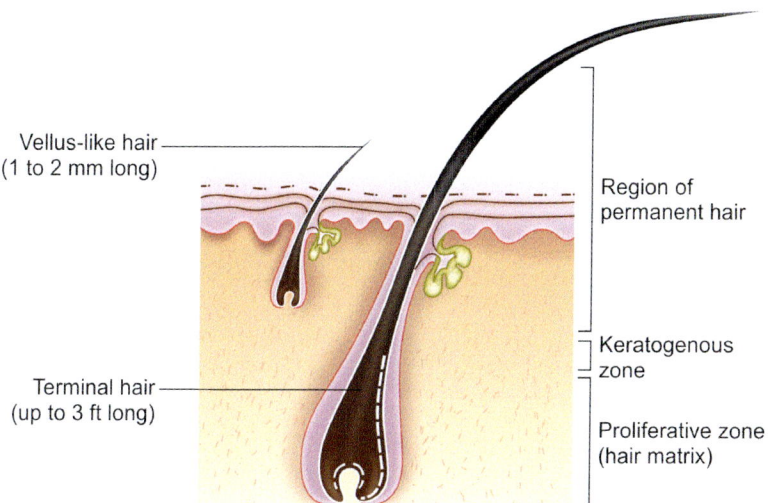

Vellus-like hair (1 to 2 mm long)

Region of permanent hair

Keratogenous zone

Terminal hair (up to 3 ft long)

Proliferative zone (hair matrix)

Fig. 1.3: Vellus-like hairs are less than 0.03 mm in diameter and rarely grow more than 1–2 mm. Terminal hairs are coarse, over 0.06 mm in diameter, and can grow up to 1 m (3 ft)

HAIR CYCLE

Every hair follicle undergoes an individual recurring cycle with growing and resting periods. The growing period **(anagen)** persists for 2–8 years, and the hair grows approximately 1 cm/month or 0.35 mm/day during this time. During the hair cycle, the middle and upper portions of the hair follicle remain stable and thus referred to as the permanent segment, whereas the lower portion undergoes cyclical changes and is non-permanent (Fig. 1.4).

The root (bulb area) of an anagen terminal follicle reaches deep into subcutaneous fat tissue. The anagen phase is followed by a transition period **(catagen)** of 2 weeks, during which the hair follicle undergoes programmed apoptosis. This transitional state is followed by a resting period **(telogen)** that lasts around 3 months. During telogen, the club hair does not grow longer; the shaft is anchored in the mid-deep dermis. It is finally shed through an active process termed **exogen**. This may be followed by a true latent phase of **kenogen**, till the onset of the next anagen phase. Unlike most fur-bearing animals, where the hair cycle is synchronous, on the human scalp there is an asynchronous mixture of hairs actively growing and resting. If many hairs pass into the resting phase (telogen) at the same time, then a correspondingly large number will be shed 2–3 months later (telogen effluvium). Hair follicles in different regions of the skin may also cycle differently. Thus, the duration of anagen on the scalp may last several years, whereas on the eyebrows anagen is very brief.

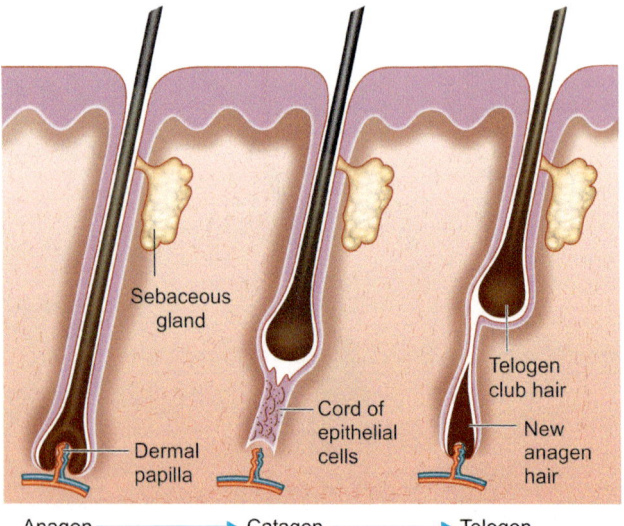

Fig. 1.4: A depiction of the different phases of the hair cycle

The scalp consists of almost **90%** hairs in **anagen,** **1%** in **catagen,** and **10%** in telogen. A normal anagen to telogen ratio for the scalp hair is 9:1, although seasonal variations can be found. The scalp may shed up to **100** telogen hairs per day.

It is useful to examine the hair cycle interchange in detail as some of the factors that play a role in transition can be used clinically for treatments of non-scarring alopecias (Alonso L) (Fig. 1.5).

Anagen

Histologically, anagen follicles are long and very straight, but the follicles are angled to permit the hair coat to lie along the body surface. The proliferating matrix cells have a cell-cycle length of approximately 18 hours. Daughter cells move upwards, adopting one of six lineages of the inner root sheath (IRS) and the hair shaft (HS); from *outermost to innermost,* the layers include Henley, Huxley and cuticle layers of the IRS, and the cuticle, cortex and medulla layers of the HS. As HS cells terminally differentiate, they extrude their organelles and become tightly packed with bundles of 10 nm laments assembled from cysteine-rich hair keratins, which become physically cross-linked to give the hair shaft high tensile strength and flexibility. The IRS also keratinizes so that it can rigidly support and guide the hair shaft during its differentiation process, but its dead cells degenerate as they reach the upper follicle, thereby releasing the HS that continues through the skin surface.

The duration of anagen determines the length of the hair and is dependent upon continued proliferation and differentiation of matrix cells at the follicle base.

Anagen-to-catagen Transition

The matrix cells are referred to as transit-amplifying cells (TAC) because they undergo a limited number of cell divisions before differentiating. As the supply of matrix cells declines, HS and IRS differentiation slow and the follicle enters a destructive phase called catagen.

Molecules that promote the transition to catagen include the growth factors **FGF-5** and **EGF,** neurotrophins such as **BDNF** and possibly the p75-neurotrophin receptor, **p53** and **TGF-β** family pathway members such as TGF-β1 and the BMPRIa (Myung P et al). Factors known to maintain anagen include **SGK-3 and Msx2** (Fig. 1.5).

Catagen

Catagen is the dynamic transition between anagen and telogen. During catagen, the lower 'cycling' portion of each hair follicle regresses entirely in a process that includes apoptosis of epithelial cells in the bulb and outer root sheath (ORS), the outermost epithelial layer. HS

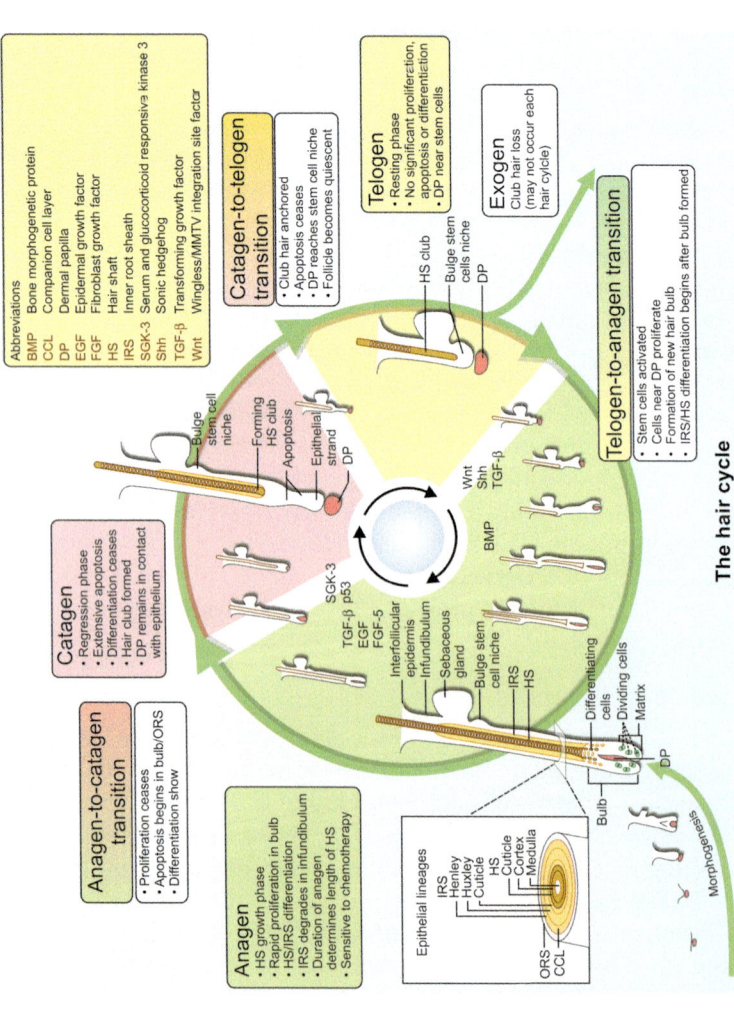

Fig. 1.5: A detailed step-by-step diagram depicting the phases of hair cycle and its mediators

differentiation ceases, and the bottom of the HS seals off into a rounded structure called a club, which moves upward until it reaches the permanent, non-cycling upper follicle, where it remains anchored during telogen. As the lower follicle recedes, a temporary structure forms—the epithelial strand, which is unique to catagen (Fig. 1.3). This connects the dermal papilla (DP) to the upper part of the hair follicle, contains many apoptotic cells and is completely eliminated by the time the DP reaches the cells that surround the remnant club hair.

Telogen

Following catagen, follicles lie dormant in a resting phase (telogen).

The Follicle Stem Cell Compartment

Although no new hair follicles are made postnatally, the lower portion of the hair follicle regenerates in order to produce a new hair. For this purpose, and for the maintenance of the epidermis and sebaceous gland, reservoirs of multipotent epithelial stem cells are set aside during development. These precious cells are found in the lowest permanent portion of the hair follicle—the 'bulge' (Oshima et al, 2001; Taylor et al, 2000). Follicle stem cells are activated at the telogen-to-anagen transition, to initiate a new round of hair growth.

Telogen-to-anagen Transition

The transition from telogen-to-anagen occurs when one or two quiescent stem cells at the base of the telogen follicle, near the DP, are activated to produce a new hair shaft (Blanpain et al, 2004; Tumbar et al, 2004). These cells now begin to proliferate rapidly, and become the **transit-amplifying** daughter cells that are fated to form the new hair follicle.

The new follicle forms adjacent to the old pocket that harbors the club hair, which will eventually be shed (**exogen**). This creates the 'bulge' and adds a layer to the stem cell reservoir. The new hair emerges from the same upper orifice as the old hair. In many ways, the telogen-to-anagen transition resembles the activation of embryonic skin stem cells that are stimulated to make the follicle *de novo*. Signaling by **Wnt** and **Shh** is indispensable for new anagen, whereas BMPs have been implicated in follicle differentiation. The molecular steps involved are likely to hold clues to understanding the activation and specification of stem cells.

FACTORS CONTROLLING HAIR CYCLE AND DISORDERS

The potential trigger factors for hair disorders are many and varied but can be attributed to one or more categories: *Inflammation, genetics, the environment, and hormones*. Different combinations of these can play a role.

Inflammation

The inflammation may be specific for the hair follicle or nonspecific.

For example, skin inflammation associated with **lupus erythematosus** may induce a diffuse alopecia in regions of inflamed skin. Herein, the inflammatory infiltrate is not specifically targeting hair follicles, but because of the general inflammatory effect, hair follicles in the vicinity are adversely affected. Scalp inflammation can be variably associated with androgenetic alopecia (AGA) and may further exacerbate the disease when present.

Alopecia areata is the classical inflammatory disorder wherein there occurs an increase in CD8+ cytotoxic lymphocytes infiltration into the hair follicle, while the CD4+ cells localize around the hair follicle. (Wang E et al). In association with the infiltration is increased expression of MHC class I and II due to a possible loss of IP (immune privilege) supporting factors allowing lymphocyte infiltration (Kang H et al). CD4+ cells promote alopecia areata (AA) by "helping" CD8+ T cells, though the exact antigen is still a matter of speculation.

In **cicatricial alopecias**, classically lichen planopilaris, Langerhans' cells and CD4+ and CD8+ lymphocytes infiltrate the upper permanent follicular epithelium (Hutchens KA). Some hypothesize that a loss of IP in the hair follicle bulge region and, therefore, destruction of bulge stem cells are what lead to the permanent hair loss observed in scarring alopecia (Meyer KC). It is unclear whether the inflammation is the initiating event, causing hair follicle disruption, or a secondary event responding to an unidentified hair follicle abnormality. Additionally, it is unknown whether the inflammatory target antigen is from hair follicle cells or from an external source.

Genetic Influences

Apart from the obvious role in congenital hair disorders, genetics also play a role in some acquired hair conditions. The pathogenesis of alopecia areata entails both genetic and environmental factors for disease initiation. Androgenetic alopecia (AGA) has a strong genetic component. Even with TE, generally accepted as a condition that develops in response to environmental insults, genes may play a role in determining an individual's level of susceptibility to the development of hair loss in response to the insult.

Environment

Hair follicle growth and cycling involve the regulation of stem cell quiescence and activation, transit amplifying cell proliferation, cell-fate choice, cell differentiation, and apoptosis. A variety of extrafollicular agents can modulate the hair cycle. In most instances, this modulation of the hair cycle clock leads to telogen effluvium (TE), either on its own or as part of a larger disorder. When the hair follicle is severely insulted, such as by cytostatic drugs or INH (Sharma PK) it results in anagen effluvium.

An Environment-mediated Hair Loss Disorder: TE

TE is probably the most common cause of diffuse hair loss encountered by dermatologists. A wide variety of potential triggers has been implicated including physiologic or emotional stresses, endocrine imbalances, nutritional deficiencies, severe illness, diet deficiencies, and even changes in medication. Hair follicle cycling can be modulated by classic bioregulators of systemic stress responses (Hadshiew M). A central *stress* response may induce the hair follicle itself to generate stress mediators and to express cognate receptors, which may be directly involved in the modulation of stress responses (Arck PC). Some studies suggest that central stress responses may lead to local *substance P* release from sensory nerve fibers in the skin and this in combination with nerve growth factor, can mediate stress-induced hair growth-inhibitory effects, such as keratinocyte apoptosis, inhibition of proliferation, and premature hair follicle regression.

Seasonal moulting is regulated by the endocrine system under the influence of environmental signals. The most important of these is change in day length (the photoperiod), which in turn, influences the production of melatonin by the pineal gland, which transduces visual signals. Also prolactin secreted by the pituitary, plays a key role in orchestrating endocrine control of seasonal hair growth. Clinical studies have shown that hair loss peaks in **August/September**, when the lowest number of follicles is in anagen, though the diameter of hair is unaffected. The rate of beard growth again varies with the lowest in January/February and increasing steadily from March to July.

The extrafollicular milieu of various stimulatory and inhibitory proteins is responsible for the smooth transition, and in disease states—alteration in the normal hair cycling. Molecular interactions between two key-cell populations in the hair follicle—epithelial stem cells in the outer root sheath and mesenchymal cells in the dermal papilla and dermal sheath are thought to influence intrinsic control of hair cycling. There is a fine balance between the *inhibitory* effect of bone morphogenetic proteins and the *stimulatory* Wnt/β-catenin pathway in regulating stem cell activity during the hair cycle. This is apart from a wide array of other signalling molecules with hair growth *stimulatory* (follistatin, transforming growth factor β2 (TGF-β2), fibroblast growth factors 7, 10 (FGF-7, FGF-10) and *inhibitory* (e.g. Dkk1, FGF-18, 17β-estradiol) effects.

In androgenetic alopecia, genes required for anagen onset (Wnt/β-catenin, TGF-α, TGF-β, stat-3, stat-1), epithelial signal to dermal papilla (PPAR δ, IGF1), hair shaft differentiation (notch, Msx2, KRTs, KAPs), and anagen maintenance (Msx2, activin, IGF-1) are down-regulated, and genes for catagen (BDNF, BMP-2, BMP-7, VDR, IL-1, ER) and telogen induction and maintenance (VDR, RAR) are upregulated.

Hormones

Apart from AGA, which is a classical hormone-mediated disorder, it must be recognized that hair follicles can be sensitive to changes in systemic levels of hormones. Thyroid hormones, glucocorticoids, insulin-like growth factor I, and prolactin can have clinically significant effects on specific aspects of hair growth and systemic imbalances can trigger TE. The most common endocrine triggers of TE include hypothyrosis, hyperthyrosis, hyperprolactinemia, and polycystic ovary syndrome. Prolactin and melatonin regulate winter and summer coat moulting of mammals. Humans may also be receptive to these to some extent, with seasonal shedding observed in some populations or people who suffer from jet lag.

Androgens influence hair growth in several ways. They play a role in the endocrine control of moulting in animals that show seasonal hair growth. In some mammals, androgens stimulate the growth of hair follicles in certain regions of the skin following sexual maturity. Lastly in human androgens are necessary for the development of balding on the scalp.

Growth hormone: It has been seen that growth hormone deficient children are less responsive to androgens. Thus, growth hormone is a synergistic hormone for testosterone, with respect to protein metabolism, growth promotion and androgenicity. This and other pituitary hormones play an important role in hair growth.

Hypothyroidism: The level of thyroid hormone has a profound influence on hair growth. Interestingly both hyper- and hypothyroidism have been linked to diffuse hair loss. Though some studies have noted that up to 10% of women with hair loss have hypothyroidism, a more realistic estimate is probably 1%.

Pregnancy: Postpartum hair loss is probably a common condition and is seen about 2–6 months after delivery. This occurs irrespective of whether the child is breastfed or not. The number of hair in telogen at this stage can be as high as 50% as compared to only 5% in the last trimester of pregnancy.

Malnutrition: The role of nutrition in determining hair strength and cycling is known, especially in studies on animals and specially on the quality of wool in sheep. Whether the same can be extended to humans is debatable. *Iron* levels, specifically ferritin has been shown by some to affect hair loss if the levels are below 10 µg/dl. It has also been shown that the *vitamin D receptor* (VDR) gene may play a role in hair cycling in patients with alopecia areata and pattern alopecia, though the role of vitamin D supplementation is not yet clear.

CONCLUSION

The myriad factors that play a role in regulating hair growth are difficult to encapsulate, but a diagram is depicted in Fig. 1.6.

This can be used by the clinician to organize approaches for treating hair diseases. The basic principle of treatment is to directly or indirectly return an individual's hair follicle size, density, and growth cycles to within normal parameters.

Treatments—current and future—need to be targeted towards one/ more of the following categories:

   a. Modification of the **hair growth cycle** (duration of anagen, duration of telogen, timing of exogen)
   b. Modification of **hair follicle size** (terminal, intermediate, vellus)
   c. Normalization of **hair follicle density** (number of hair follicles per unit area).

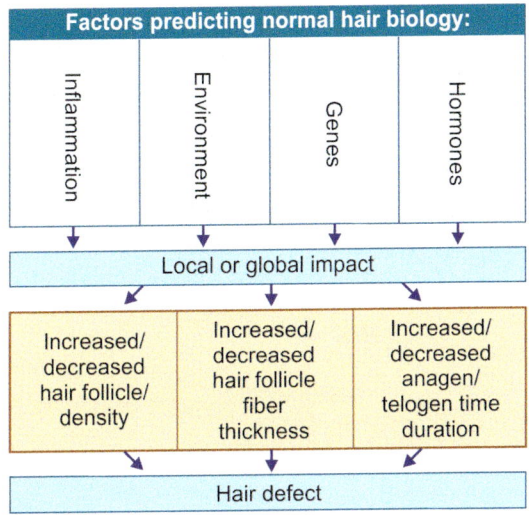

Fig. 1.6: An overview of the main factors that determine hair dynamics

Treatment to remove an initiating event, while not directly acting on the affected hair follicles, may enable the damaged follicles to recover through their inherent regenerative capacity.

Bibliography

1. Alonso L, Fuchs E. The hair cycle. J Cell Sci Feb 1 2006;119(3):391–3.

2. Arck PC, Handjiski B, Hagen E, et al. Indications for a 'brain-hair follicle axis (BHA)': inhibition of keratinocyte proliferation and upregulation of keratinocyte apoptosis in telogen hair follicles by stress and substance P. FASEB J 2001;15:2536–8.

3. Blanpain C, Lowry WE, Geoghegan A Polak L, Fuchs E. Self-renewal, multipotency, and the existence of two-cell populations within an epithelial stem cell niche. Cell 2004;118:635–48.

4. Blume-Peytavi U, Tosti A, Whiting DA, et al. (eds): Hair Growth and Disorders. Berlin, Springer, 2008.

5. Fischer TW, Slominski A, Tobin DJ, et al. Melatonin and the hair follicle. J Pineal Res 2008;44:1–15.

6. Foitzik K, Langan EA, Paus R. Prolactin and the skin: a dermatological perspective on an ancient pleiotropic peptide hormone. J Invest Dermatol 2009;129:1071–87.

7. Hadshiew IM, Foitzik K, Arck PC, et al. Burden of hair loss: Stress and the underestimated psychosocial impact of telogen effluvium and androgenetic alopecia. J Invest Dermatol 2004;123:455–7.

8. Hutchens KA, Balfour EM, Smoller BR. Comparison between Langerhans' cell concentration in lichen planopilaris and traction alopecia with possible immunologic implications. Am J Dermatopathol 2011;33:277–80.

9. Ioannides D, Tosti A (eds): Alopecias—Practical Evaluation and Management. Curr Probl Dermatol. Basel, Karger, 2015.

10. Kang H, Wu WY, Lo BK, et al. Hair follicles from alopecia areata patients exhibit alterations in immune privilege-associated gene expression in advance of hair loss. J Invest Dermatol 2010;130:2677–80.

11. Kligman AM. Pathologic dynamics of human hair loss. I. Telogen effuvium. Arch Dermatol 1961;83:175–98.

12. Meyer KC, Klatte JE, Dinh HV, et al. Evidence that the bulge region is a site of relative immune privilege in human hair follicles. Br J Dermatol 2008;159:1077–85.

13. Myung P, Andl T, Ito M. Defining the hair follicle stem cell (Part I). J Cutan Pathol Sep 2009; 36(9):1031–4.

14. Oshima H, Rochat A, Kedzia C, Kobayashi K Barrandon Y. Morphogenesis and renewal of hair follicles from adult multipotent stem cells. Cell 2001;104:233–45.

15. Rodney Sinclair, Vicky Jolliffe. Fast Facts: Disorders of the Hair and Scalp, 2nd edn, Published in 2013, Health Press.

16. Sharma PK, Gautam RK, Bhardwaj M, Kar HK. Isonicotinic acid hydrazide induced anagen effluvium and associated lichenoid eruption. J Dermatol 2001;Dec;28(12):737–41.

17. Taylor G, Lehrer MS, Jensen PJ, Sun TT, Lavker RM. Involvement of follicular stem cells in forming not only the follicle but also the epidermis. Cell 2000; 102:451–61.

18. Tumbar T, Guasch G, Greco V, Blanpain C, Lowry WE, Rendl M Fuchs E. Defining the epithelial stem cell niche in skin. Science 303:359–63.

19. Wang E, McElwee KJ. Etiopathogenesis of alopecia areata: Why do our patients get it? Dermatol Ther 2011;24:337–47.

2

Trichoscopy in Disorders of Scalp

Rahul Arora, Pallavi Ailawadi

INTRODUCTION

Hair loss is the most common hair problem and a prompt diagnosis of the type of alopecia may sometimes be extremely challenging. Apart from clinical examination, the methods commonly used to investigate the alopecia include invasive (biopsy), semi-invasive (trichogram) or non-invasive (hair count, weighing shed hair and pull test). A recently introduced modality, dermoscopy, also known as epiluminescence microscopy or skin surface microscopy is a non-invasive, *in vivo* technique, most commonly used for viewing pigmented skin lesions. The dermoscopic examination of the hair and scalp is known as trichoscopy. This is a very useful technique for the diagnosis as well as monitoring of treatment of hair disorders.

Normal Scalp

In the healthy scalp, there are evenly spaced groups of a few hair shafts coming out of the same follicular ostium, the number of which varies according to the site (Fig. 2.1A). While the frontal and temporal scalp has mostly single- and double-hair units, the occipital scalp has triple-hair units. The thickness of hair shaft in the frontal scalp is more than the occipital region. The interfollicular region can have both pigmentary and vascular findings. The normal scalp vessels include interfollicular simple red loops structures and arborizing red lines (Fig. 2.1C). The pigmented network comprises a homogenous mosaic of contiguous brown rings in a honeycomb pattern (Fig. 2.1B). Other findings include white dots, related with the acrosyringeal and follicular openings and dirty dots which is accumulated dust and environmental particles in the follicular openings.

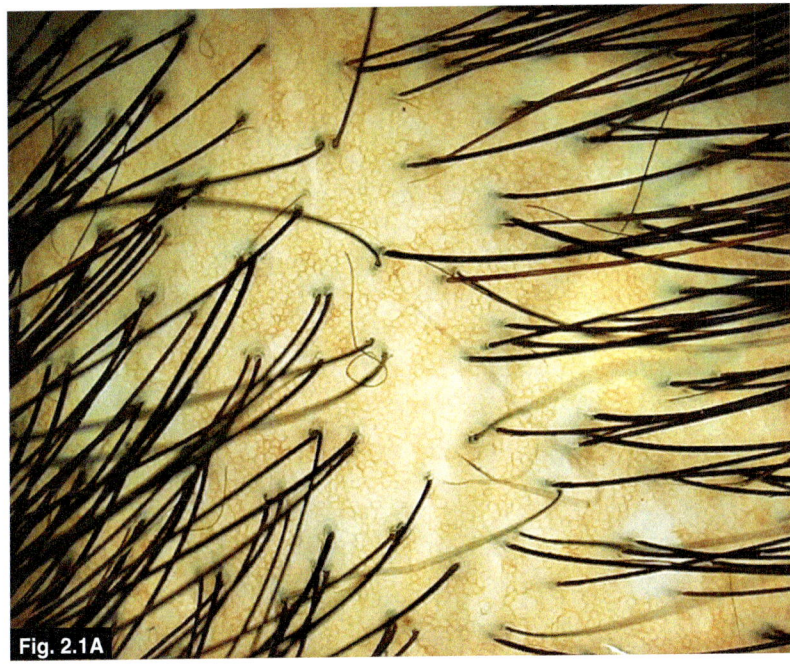

Fig. 2.1A

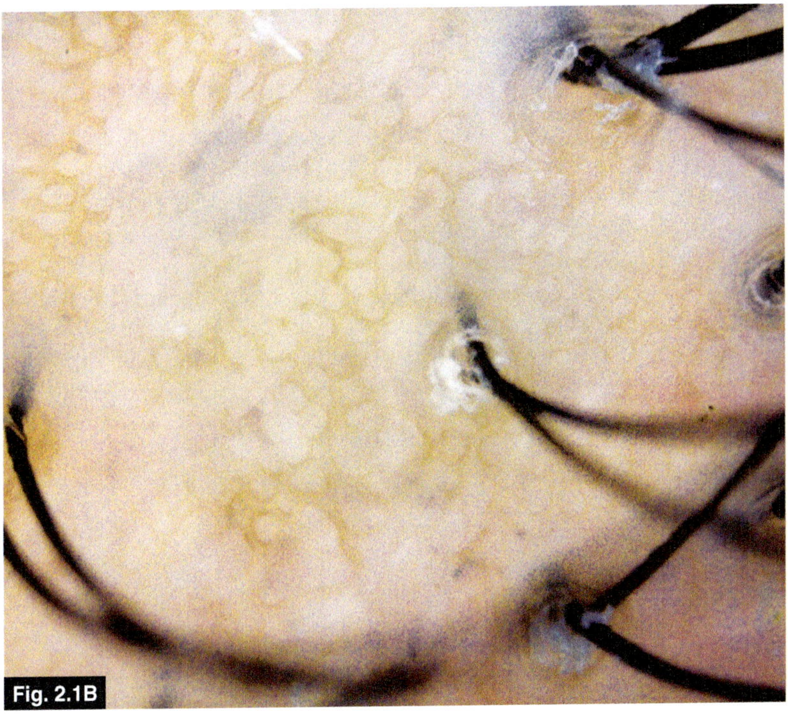

Fig. 2.1B

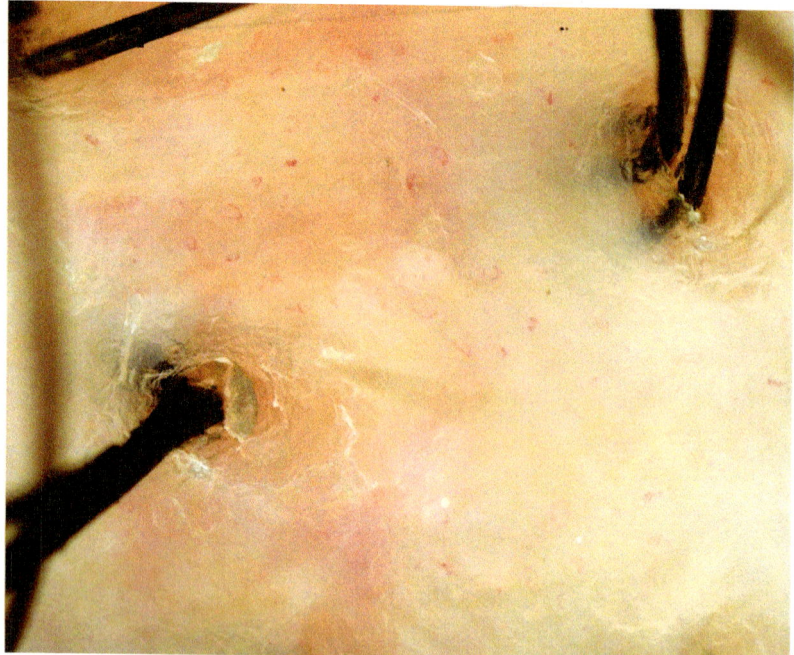

Fig. 2.1A to C: Normal scalp. (A) Follicular pattern; (B) Interfollicular pigment network; (C) Interfollicular vascular pattern

APPROACH TO TRICHOSCOPIC EVALUATION

Trichoscopic evaluation of normal and diseased scalp is based on study of follicular patterns, interfollicular patterns and hair shaft characteristics (Table 2.1). The interfollicular vascular structures and pigmentation patterns are visualized only with a polarizing light source or a polarizing filter. The clinical and pathological correlation of important dermoscopic findings in the common hair and scalp conditions have been summarized in Table 2.2. For beginners, it is always better to visualize the field in low magnification first with both non-polarized and polarized mode followed by a higher magnification in polarized mode.

Table 2.1: Trichoscopic patterns		
Follicular patterns	*Interfollicular patterns*	*Hair shaft characteristics*
White dots (Fig. 2.3D)	Vascular patterns	Specific features of hair shafts, seen in multiple genetic and other disorders
Yellow dots (Fig. 2.2B)	Pigment pattern	
Black dots (Fig. 2.5B)		
Red dots		

Table 2.2: A detailed overview of various patterns and their interpretation

Patterns	Dermoscopic features	Clinical appearance	Pathology	Associated diseases
Follicular	Black dots	Black dots inside follicular openings	Broken hair shaft	Alopecia areata Trichotillomania Timea capitis Dissecting cellulitis
	Yellow dots	Round or polycyclic yellow to yellow-pink dots	Dilated infundibula plugged with sebum and keratin remnants	Alopecia areata Androgenetic alopecia Trichotillomania Dissecting cellulitis Congenital hypotrichosis Kerion
	Blue-gray dots	Target pattern	Melanophages in upper dermis	Discoid lupus erythematosus Lichen planopilaris
	Empty follicles	Skin-colored small depressions without hairs	Empty infundibula	Androgenetic alopecia Telogen effluvium
	Follicular keratotic plugging	Keratotic masses plugging follicular ostia	Hyperkeratosis and plugging of follicular ostia by keratotic material	Discoid lupus erythematosus
	Follicular red dots	0.16–0.47 mm erythematous polygonal, concentric structures in and around follicular ostia	Widened infundibula surrounded by dilated vessels and extravasated erythrocytes	Discoid lupus erythematosus
	Peripilar casts	Concentrically arranged scales encircling emerging hair shaft	Unknown	Lichen planopilaris Frontal fibrosing alopecia Discoid lupus erythematosus

(Contd.)

Table 2.2: A detailed overview of various patterns and their interpretation (*Contd.*)

Patterns	Dermoscopic features	Clinical appearance	Pathology	Associated diseases
	Peripilar sign	Brown halo surrounding follicular opening	Perifollicular inflammation	Androgenetic alopecia
	Peripilar white halo	Gray-white halo surrounding common follicular ostium of 2–3 hair shafts	Concentric fibrosis	Central centrifugal cicatricial alopecia
Interfollicular	Twisted red loops	Multiple red dots at low magnification and polymorphous beaded lines and circles at high magnification	Enlarged dilated capillaries in dermal papillae	Psoriasis Seborrheic dermatitis Folliculitis decalvans
	Arborizing vessels	Branching vessels	Subpapillary vascular plexus	Normal scalp Seborrheic dermatitis
	White patches	Well-demarcated, white patches	Severe tissue fibrosis	Scarring alopecia
Hair shaft	Exclamation mark hairs	Tapered hairs with dark ends	Telogen hairs with broken tip	Alopecia areata
	Circle hairs	Thin, short hairs that form circle	Vellus-like follicles	Androgenetic alopecia Alopecia areata
	Coiled hairs	Broken hairs that curl back	Telogen/catagen	Trichotillomania
	Comma hairs	Short C-shaped hairs	Broken hair shafts with hair ectothrix parasitation	Tinea capitis
	Hair tufting	Tufts of >6 hairs emerging from same ostium	Compound follicular structures (packs of $6 follicles fused by their outer root sheaths)	Folliculitis decalvans Acne keloidalis

Trichoscopic Characteristics

Various follicular and interfollicular patterns in combination with specific features help to form an opinion about the diagnosis. Table 2.3 summarizes the findings in various disorders of hair.

The various clinical scenarios are depicted from Figs 2.2 to 2.11.

Table 2.3: A snapshot of trichoscopic findings of common hair disorders

Non-cicatricial alopecia	Cicatricial alopecia
Presence of empty follicular openings is a common trichoscopy finding	Trichoscopy shows milky-red or ivory-white areas lacking follicular openings in all forms
Female pattern hair loss (FPHL)	**Lichen planopilaris**
The presence of hair with different caliber (anisotrichosis) is typical of FPHL and reflects progressive hair miniaturization due to the disease (Fig. 2.2)	It shows perifollicular inflammation (spare intervening follicles), tubular perifollicular scaling, elongated, concentric blood vessels, and white dots which merge to form white areas (Fig. 2.10)
Androgenetic alopecia (AGA)	**Discoid lupus erythematosus (DLE)**
Anisotrichosis >20% hair multiple thin and vellus hairs, yellow dots, perifollicular brown, and predominance of follicular units with only one hair. These features predominate in the frontal area (Fig. 2.3)	Atrophy, complete follicle paucity, scattered dark-brown discoloration of the skin, large hyperkeratotic follicular, yellow dots and thick large arborizing vessels, and follicular red dots (Fig. 2.11)
Telogen effluvium (TE)	**Frontal fibrosing alopecia (FFA)**
Trichoscopy is largely normal. Frequent but non-specific signs are presence of empty hair follicles over entire scalp, one follicular hair unit dominance and upright short hair regrowth (Fig 2.4)	Mild perifollicular scaling, absence of follicular openings, follicular hyperkeratosis, follicular plugs, and erythema
Alopecia areata (AA)	**Folliculitis decalvans (FD) and tufted folliculitis (TF)**
Uniform black dots and micro-exclamation mark hairs and tapered hairs correlate with disease activity, whereas yellow dots and vellus hairs correlate with disease severity. Pigtail hair and pigmented, upright, regrowing hairs denote regrowth and disease resolution (Fig. 2.5)	Tufted hairs (polytrichia), perifollicular erythema, large follicular pustules with emerging hair shafts and perifollicular starburst pattern hyperplasia (doll hair)

(Contd.)

Table 2.3: A snapshot of trichoscopic findings of common hair disorders (*Contd.*)

Alopecia areata incognita
Numerous diffuse yellow dots of different size and uniform colors within the follicular orifices of both empty and hair-bearing follicles with a large number of re-growing tapered terminal hairs in the entire scalp

Dissecting cellulitis (DC)
Yellow dots imposed over dystrophic hairs; large, yellow amorphous areas, and pinpoint white dots with a whitish halo

Scalp psoriasis
Regularly distributed twisted and lace-like blood vessels (Fig. 2.6)

Pseudopelade of Brocq
Nonspecific. It is seen as white areas with no follicular openings. Also some solitary dystrophic hairs can be seen at the periphery of the lesion

Seborrheic dermatitis
Perifollicular and interfollicular scales. Thin arborizing vessels may be observed (Fig. 2.7)

Trichotillomania (TTM)
Trichoptilosis "longitudinal split ends" and irregular coiled hairs, hair shafts of variable length, coiled fractured hair shafts
Additionally some other findings, include black dots, flame hair, V sign, follicular hemorrhages, tulip hair, and hair powder (Fig. 2.8)

Tinea capitis
Comma shaped, zigzag, corkscrew hairs, black dots, and short broken hairs. Zigzag shaped hairs are the diagnostic trichoscopic features of tinea capitis (Fig. 2.9)

Traction alopecia
It shares some features of TTM with some hair casts, white dots lacking follicular opening, hair thinning, and decreased hair density

Temporal triangular alopecia (TTA)
Normal follicle orifices with vellus hair surrounded by terminal hair

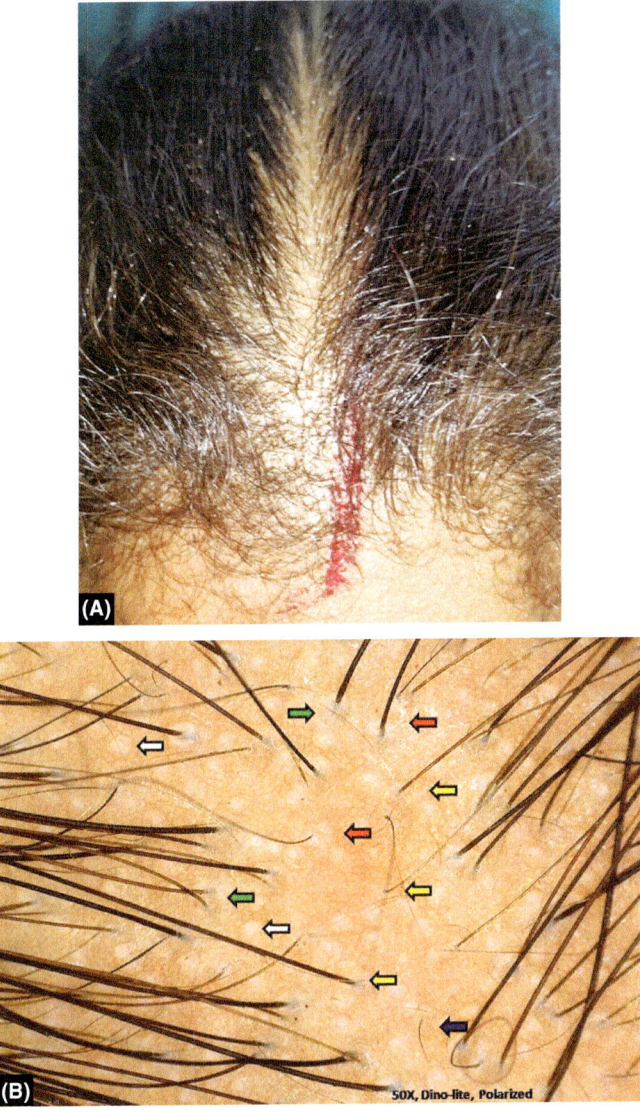

Fig. 2.2A and B: A 26-year-old female presented with complain of diffuse hair loss (A) since 2-year duration. There was a seasonal exacerbation of hair loss along with a decrease in the size of the ponytail. Her hemogram, thyroid function test, serum ferritin, vitamin B_{12} and vitamin D_3 were within normal limits. Her trichoscopic evaluation (B) showed a >20% anisotrichosis, yellow dots (red arrows), white dots (white arrows), peripilar sign (green arrows), vellus hair (blue arrow) and predominance of single hair units (yellow arrows). Based on the trichoscopic findings, a diagnosis of female patterned hair loss was made and minoxidil 2% along with platelet rich plasma therapy was started

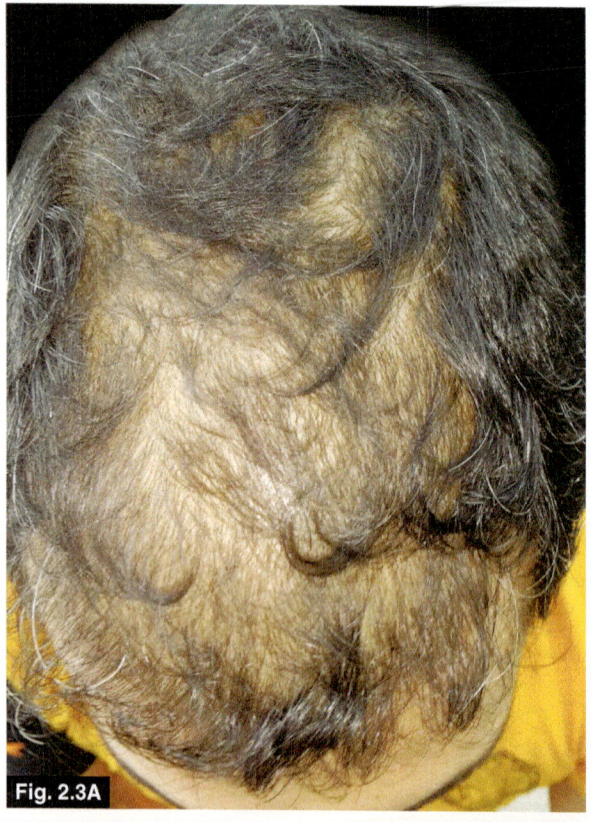

Fig. 2.3A

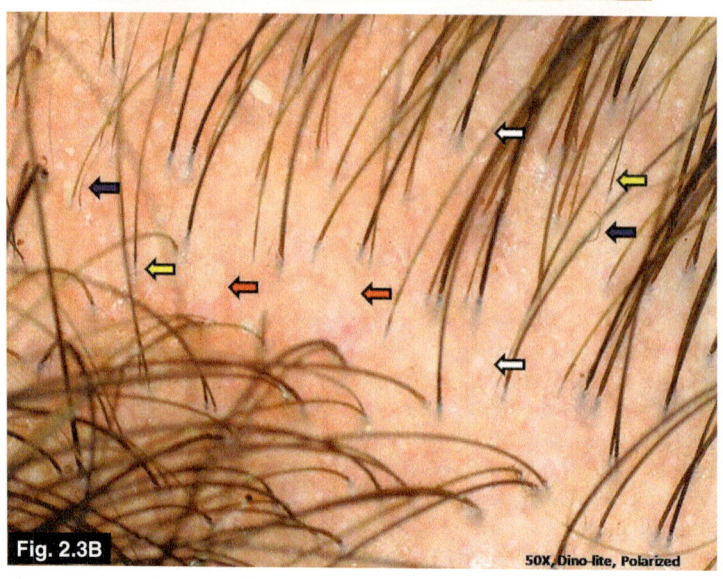

Fig. 2.3B

50X, Dino-lite, Polarized

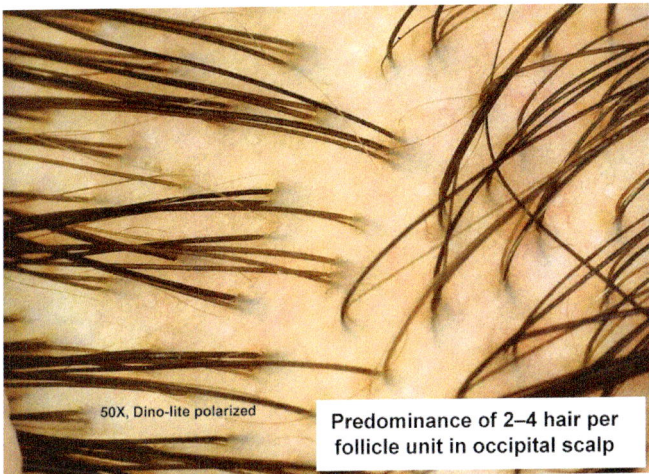

50X, Dino-lite polarized

Predominance of 2–4 hair per follicle unit in occipital scalp

Fig. 2.3A to C: A 28-year-old male presented with thinning of hair in frontal scalp with relatively maintained anterior hairline (A) over past 5 years. There was no family history of androgenetic alopecia. Trichoscopic findings (B) showed presence of >20% variability of diameter as compared to the occipital scalp (C), yellow dots (red arrows), white dots (white arrows), predominance of single hair follicle units (yellow arrows) and vellus hair (blue arrows). Hence, the diagnosis of androgenetic alopecia was made and patient was started on minoxidil 5% in combination with finasteride 1 mg along with platelet rich plasma therapy

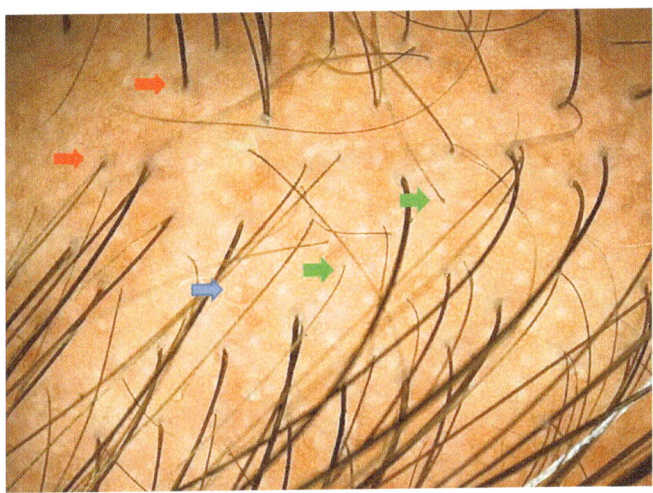

Fig. 2.4: A 22-year-old girl presented with history of diffuse hair loss since 1 year. She was known case of hypothyroidism on thyroxine. On trichoscopy, there was presence of black dots (blue arrow), one follicular hair unit dominance (green arrows) and perifollicular discoloration or peripilar sign (red arrows) suggestive of chronic telogen effluvium

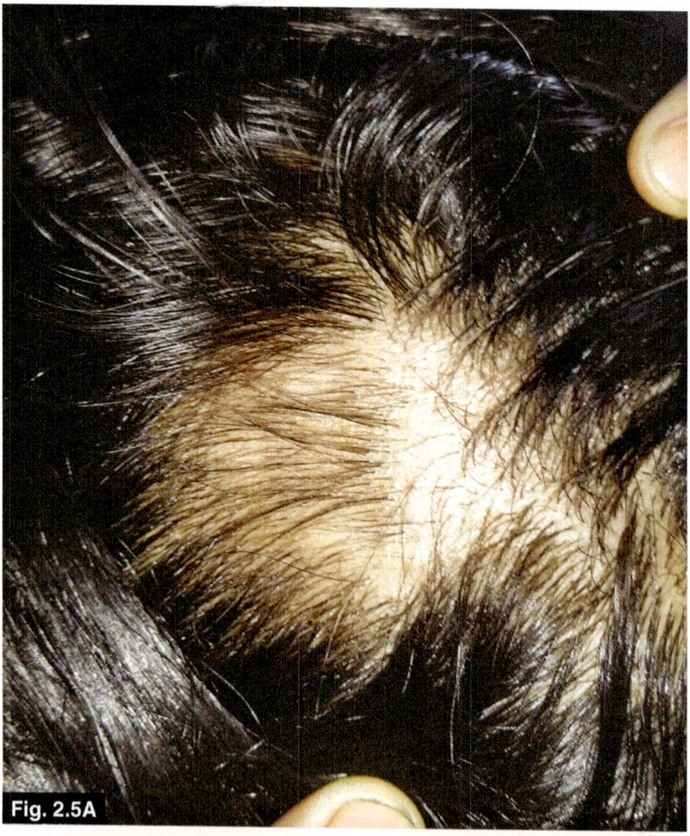

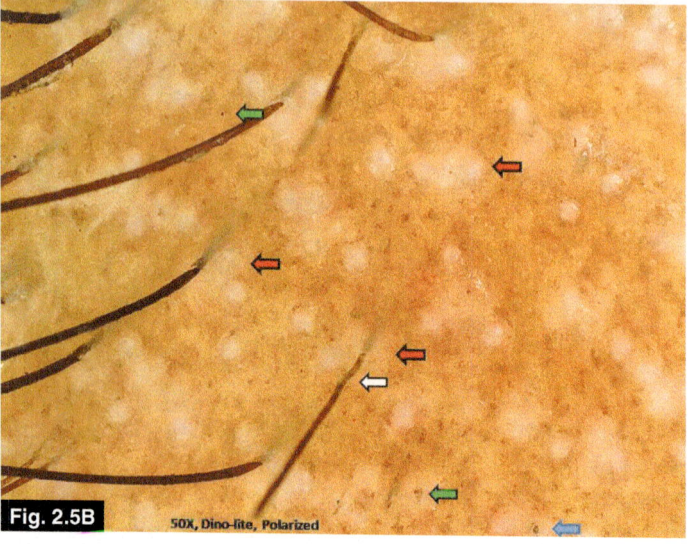

Fig. 2.5A

Fig. 2.5B

50X, Dino-lite, Polarized

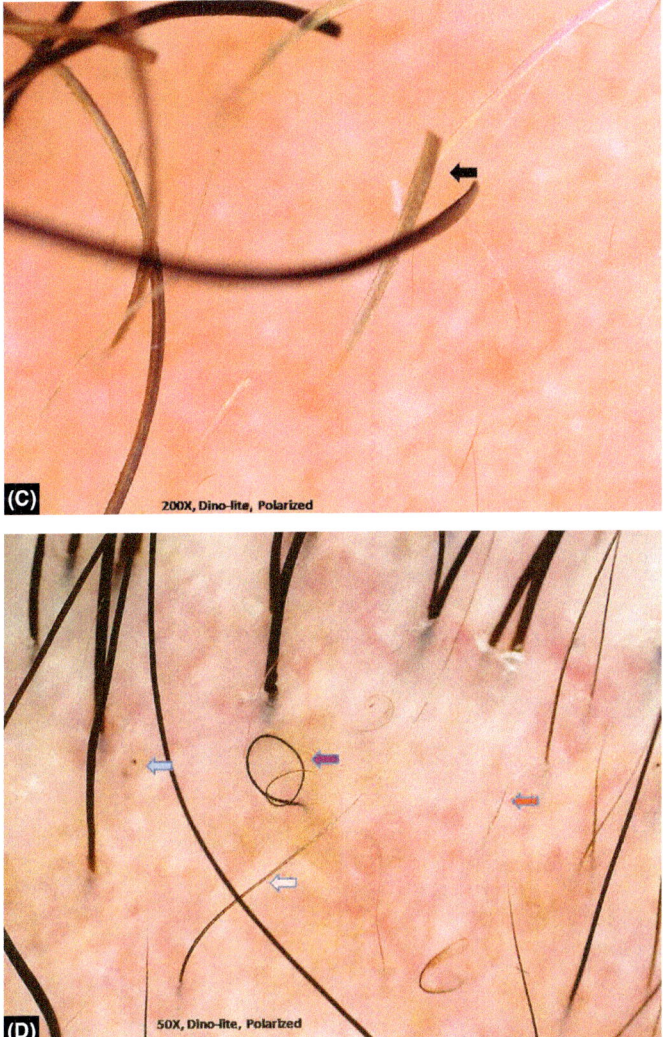

Fig. 2.5A to D: A 22-year-old girl presented with 3 × 4 cm size patch of hair loss (A) on vertex of scalp of 6 months duration. The patch showed partial regrowth in the central area. However, patient complained of increase in the size of the lesion. Trichoscopic findings from the periphery of the lesion (B and C) showed presence of yellow dots (red arrows), black dots (green arrows), cadeveric hair (blue arrow), coudability sign (white arrow) and exclamation mark hair (black arrow) consistent with alopecia areata in active phase whereas the trichoscopy of central area (D) showed pigtail hair (purple arrow), vellus hair (pink arrow) and tapering hair (brown arrow) consistent with alopecia areata in regrowing phase. Hence, patient was given injection triamcinolone acetonide 10 mg/ml only in the margins of the lesion for cessation of disease activity along with topical minoxidil

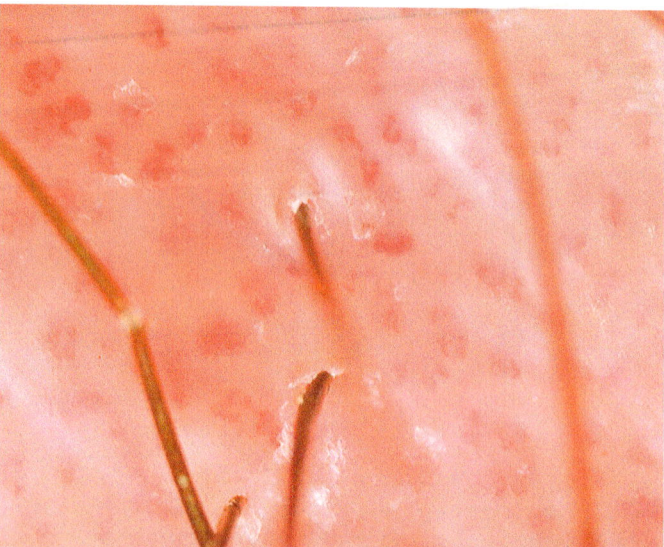

Fig. 2.6: A 36-year-old man presented with multiple itchy scaly plaques on scalp and trunk clinically suggestive of psoriasis. On trichoscopy, there was background dull redness, regularly distributed twisted and loop-like vessels with white colored scales suggestive of psoriasis

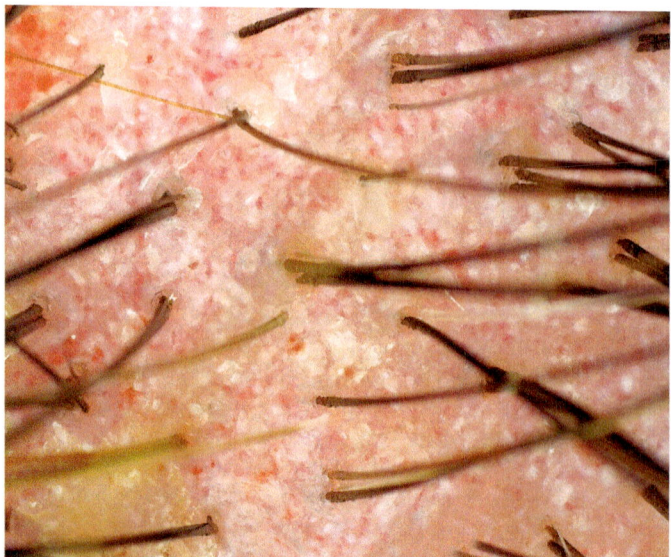

Fig. 2.7: A 25-year-old male presented with itching of scalp along with diffuse hair loss. There was presence of greasy scales all over scalp. On trichoscopic evaluation, greasy perifollicular and interfollicular scales with pinpoint vessels distributed irregularly suggestive of seborrheic dermatitis

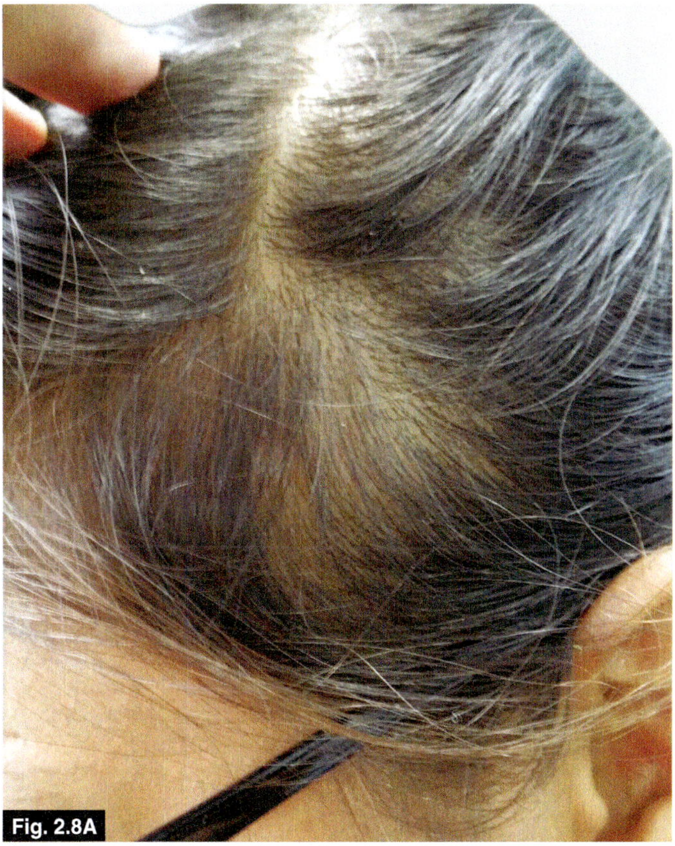

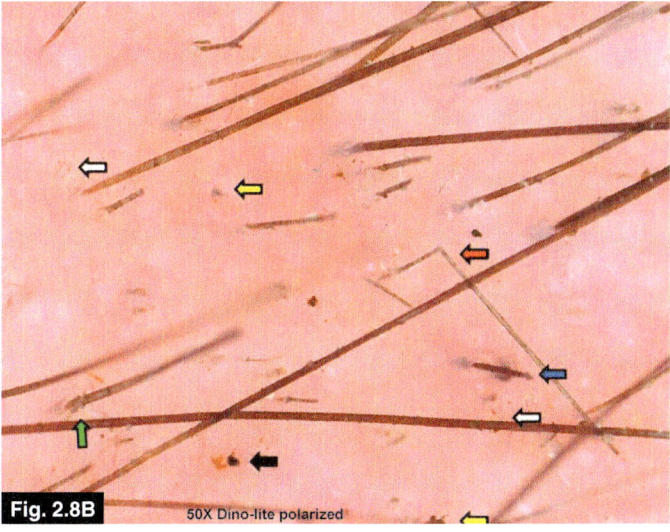

Fig. 2.8A

Fig. 2.8B 50X Dino-lite polarized

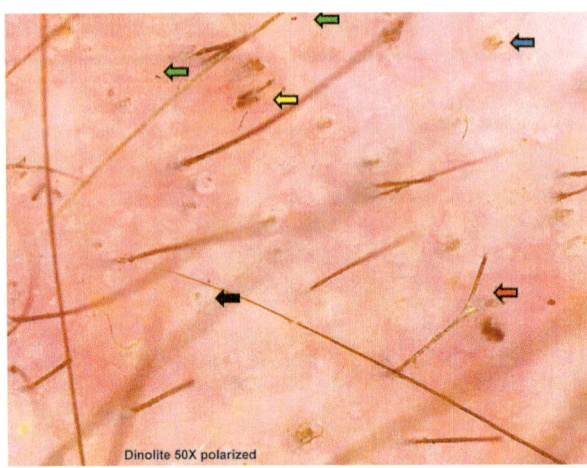

Dinolite 50X polarized

Fig. 2.8A to C: An 18-year-old girl presented with patch of hair loss present on left temporal scalp (A). On examination, the hairs were of unequal length but the patient denied history of pulling of hair. Trichoscopic findings (B) showed unequal length of hair, black dots (yellow arrow), green stick fractured hair (red arrow), V sign (green arrow), tulip hair (blue arrow), hair powder (white arrows) and perifollicular haemorrhage (black arrow). Also, there was presence of (C) longitudinal splitting hair shaft (red arrow), unequal length of hair, black dots (black arrow), V sign (yellow arrow), perifollicular haemorrhage (blue arrow) and hair powder (green arrow). On further questioning, mother complained of irrational behaviour and excessive fights. Histopathology confirmed the diagnosis of trichotillomania and the patient was started on escitalopam and alprazolam combination

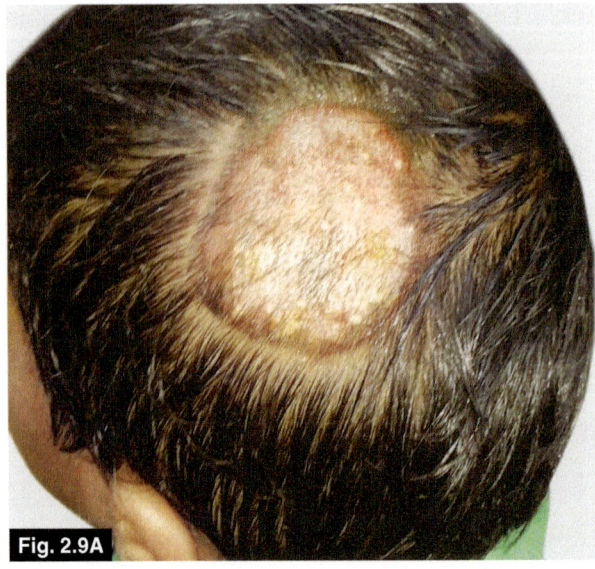

Fig. 2.9A

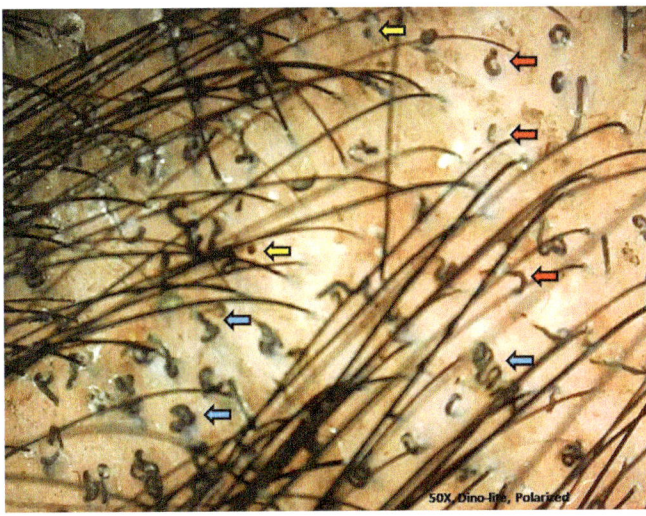

Fig. 2.9A and B: An 8-year-old boy presented with a localized patch of hair loss (A) associated with a painful boggy swelling and cervical lymphadenopathy. Hairs at the margins of the patch were easily pluckable. Trichoscopic evaluation (B) showed presence of black dots (yellow arrow), comma hair (red arrows) and coiled hairs (yellow arrows). KOH evaluation was positive for ectothrix. Patient was started on oral anti-inflammatory and oral griseofulvin with topical ketoconazole lotion

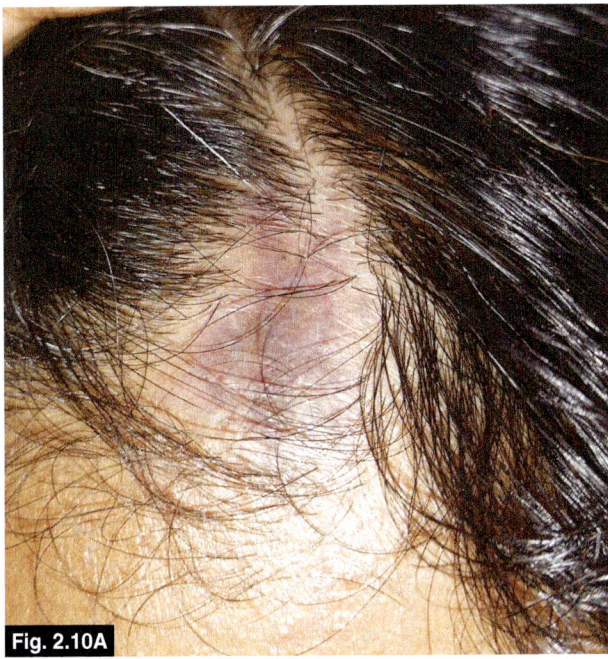

Fig. 2.10A

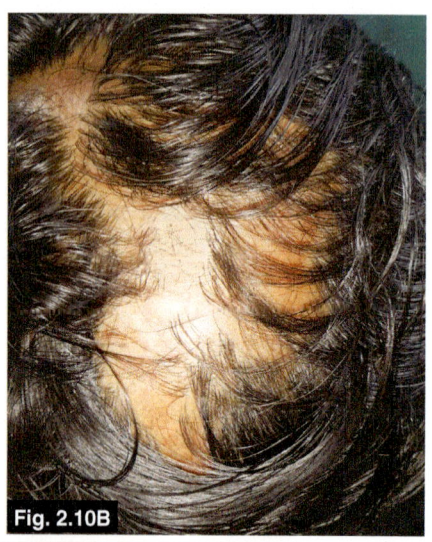

Fig. 2.10B

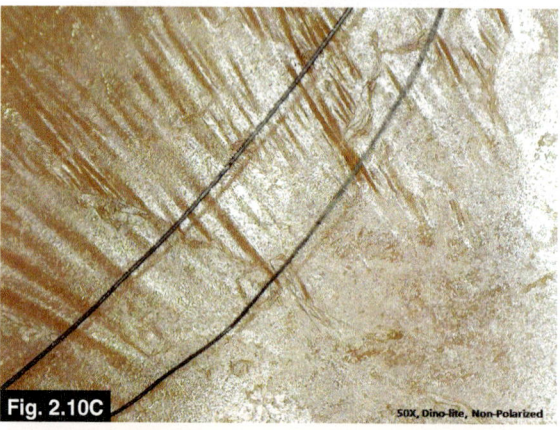

Fig. 2.10C   50X, Dino-lite, Non-Polarized

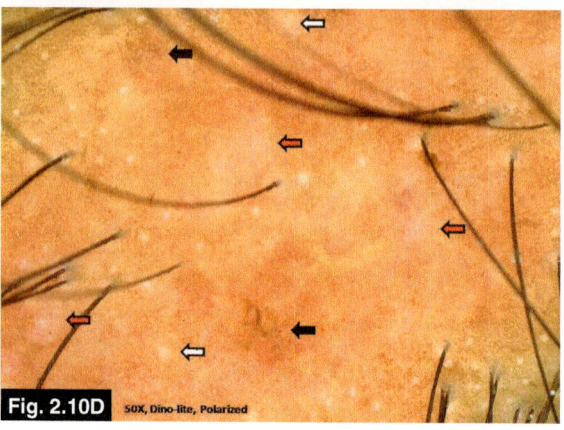

Fig. 2.10D   50X, Dino-lite, Polarized

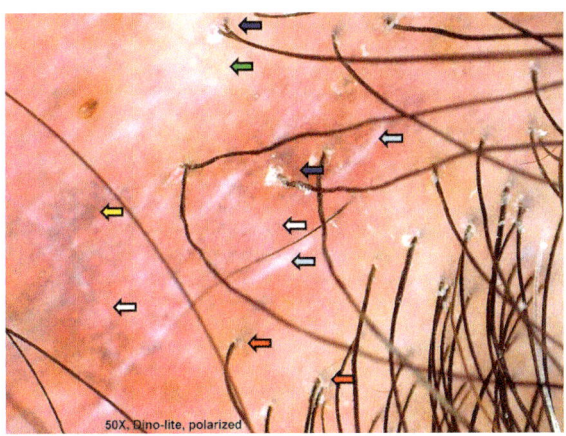

Fig. 2.10A to E: A 30-year-old male presented with multiple patches of scarring alopecia in frontal (A) as well as vertex region (B) of scalp for past 3 years. The patient was unsure about the progression of the lesions in past 1 year. Trichoscopy of the patch present on the vertex region (C) and (D) showed marked atrophy, marked loss of follicular openings, pink-white areas (red arrows), white dots (white arrows), exaggeration of normal pigment network (black dots) absence of blue-grey dots, white dots, and perifollicular casts suggestive of an inactive disease. Whereas trichoscopy of a single 2–3 cm size lesion present on anterior scalp (E) showed presence of blue-gray dots (yellow arrows), perifollicular casts (blue arrows), yellow white areas (green arrows), pink-white areas (white arrows), follicular sinking (red arrows) and Wickham's stria (light blue arrows), which were suggestive of active lichen planopilaris. The findings were further confirmed by biopsy from both the lesions in which the anterior lesion showed lichenoid lymphocytic infiltration at follicular dermoepidermal junction, wedge shaped hypergranulosis and colloid bodies whereas the posterior lesion showed bands of fibrotic scarring with minimal inflammation. Patient was started on oral steroid in combination with methotrexate to control the disease activity

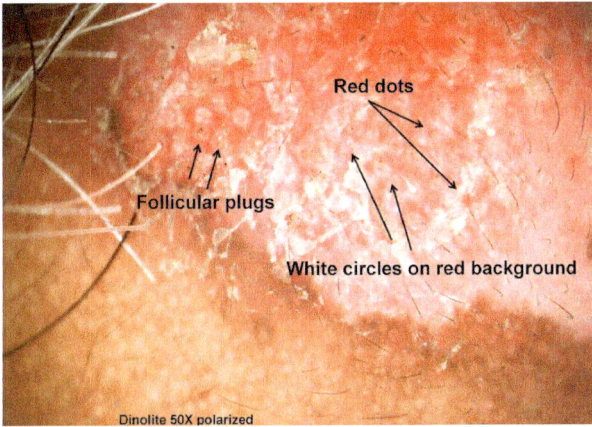

Fig. 2.11: Trichoscopic image of discoid lupus erythematosus

Algorithmic Approach to Trichoscopic Diagnosis

The algorithmic approach towards diagnosis of common hair disorders has been elaborated in Fig. 2.12. The first step is to classify the disease into cicatricial or non-cicatricial disease, for which it is essential to look for follicular orifices. The loss of orifices corresponds to permanent destruction of hair follicles, resulting in fibrosis, and thus a diagnosis of irreversible cicatricial alopecia and, is therefore, of great importance for predicting prognosis. On the contrary, presence of orifices points towards the reversible non-cicatricial alopecias. Further, efforts should be made to look for other findings and dermoscopic patterns which help make the complete diagnosis.

UTILITY OF TRICHOSCOPY IN CLINICAL PRACTICE

The role of dermoscopy in the evaluation of pigmented lesions is largely accepted worldwide, and most dermatologists today use a dermoscope in their daily practice. Trichoscopy has now become a quint essential tool for routine clinical practice even for private practitioners as it helps in:

1. Immediate differentiation between cicatricial and non-cicatricial alopecias
2. Differential diagnosis between telogen effluvium and androgenetic alopecia
3. Diagnosis and information on short-term prognosis of alopecia areata
4. Fast diagnosis of hair-shaft disorders
5. Monitoring of improvement especially after procedures like PRP therapy, intralesional steroids, etc. where clinical improvement may be subtle.

These are just the most common applications; many others are being developed.

1. **Trichoscopy in hair transplant:** Through trichoscopy, a detailed study of the scalps characteristics per square centimetre can be performed such as:
   a. The number, the size and the distances among hair follicles, both for the recipient and for the donor areas.
   b. Assessment of the actual number of hair follicles that can be transplanted, so as to meet the needs of those areas showing hair thinning.
   c. The actual dimensions of the recipient area where hair thinning is still microscopic and may affect the results in future.

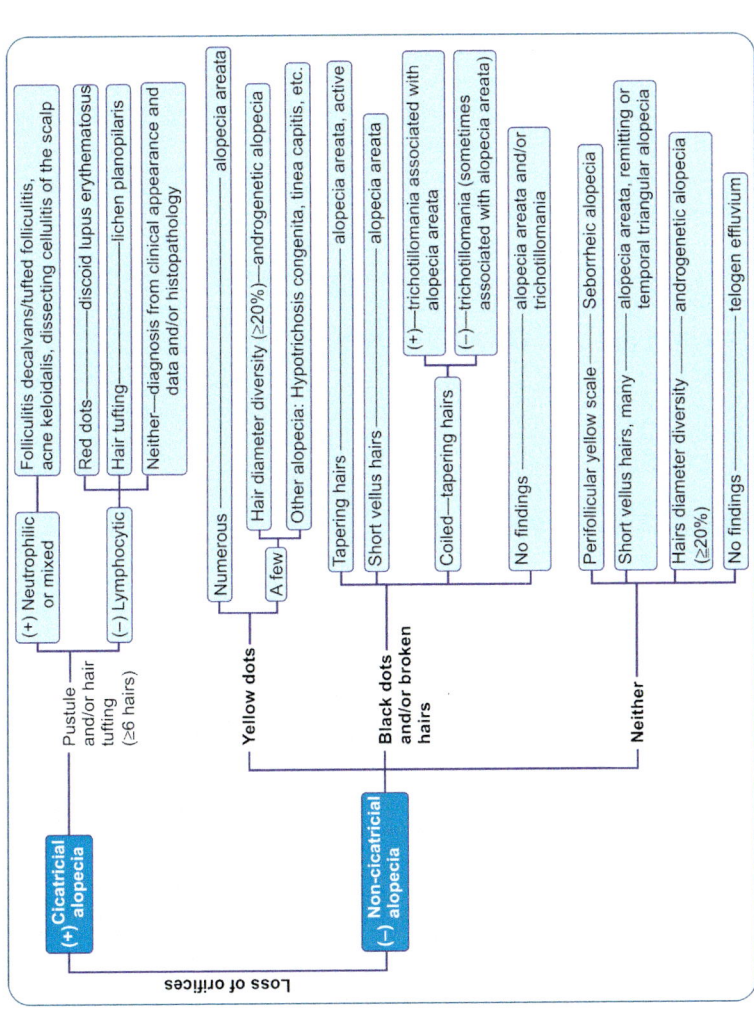

Fig. 2.12: Algorithmic approach to the trichoscopic evaluation for diagnosis of hair and scalp disorders

d. Quality of hair at the areas of hair thinning as well as the donor area which is important for patient expectation alignment.

e. Dimensions of the donor area and the quality and density of hair in it.

f. Quantify the actual number of hair follicles that were transplanted, as well as the number of re-grown hair follicles after transplant.

2. **Trichoscopy in general medicine:** Possible usefulness of trichoscopy beyond dermatology is an interesting area of exploration. This includes possible application of trichoscopy in identifying follicular spicules in multiple myeloma, follicular mucinosis in lymphoproliferative disorders, scalp lesions in Langerhans' histiocytosis or altered interfollicular microvessels in dermatomyositis and scleroderma.

3. **UV-enhanced trichoscopy (UVET):** Newer devices available in the market allow performing trichoscopy with UV light, at a wavelength covering the spectrum of a Wood's lamp. This feature enhances the diagnostic potential of trichoscopy in tinea capitis, pityrosporum folliculitis and various types of porphyrias.

Barriers to its Use in Routine Practice

Barriers to routine use of trichoscopy may include lack of knowledge, necessity of training, costs, and possible disbelief in the technique. Further, many doctors are not familiar with hair and scalp trichoscopy patterns and have a few resources or time to acquire specific training.

Another barrier to broader application is possibly that dermatologists may believe that the cost–benefit ratio of purchasing the instrument and the time for training yields very little to their practice.

Perhaps the best way to dispel this misconception is to state the facts:

1. Trichoscopy does not require expensive tools.
2. Trichoscopy is useful for the evaluation of every patient with hair disorder.
3. Trichoscopy is non-invasive and very well accepted by patients.
4. Its routine use may improve the quality of care for patients with hair and/or scalp conditions and reduce the necessity for invasive procedures such as scalp biopsies.
5. It acts as a USP to the practice whereby the doctor is able to display and discuss both the disease as well as therapeutic response.

HOW TO CHOOSE A TRICHOSCOPE?

Trichoscopy has become an intergral part of routine clinical practice. So choosing a right instrument becomes an important aspect. A number of factors play an important role in deciding the choice of trichoscope.

An *ideal trichoscope* should have:

- Both polarized and non-polarized filters
- Self illumination
- Magnification at least 10X (higher magnification needed for study of interfollicular vasculature)
- Good resolution (in case of videodermoscope)
- Pigment/color enhancement
- Calibration for measurements
- Ability to capture, store images and display images
- Low cost
- Light weight and easy to carry.

Broadly two types of trichoscopes are used in practice:

Hand-held trichoscopes: Provides high resolution and quick examination but have low magnification (10X – 40X), require attachment to a camera for capturing and storing images, require immersion fluid, difficult to project live images, expensive. For example, Dermlite, Heine.

Video dermatoscopes: High magnification (up to 1000X), low-average resolution, requires electronic gadget for display, easy to store and display live images. For example, Fotofinder, Dinolite, etc.

A number of attachments is available which help us to make use of our mobile phone as a trichoscope (e.g. dermalite d3, folliculoscope). Applications like camerafi, mobile scope, etc. help connecting a USB videodermatoscope to our mobile phones obviating the need of a PC / laptop for evaluation.

Overall, according to the authors experience, videotrichoscopes are more useful for beginners as images can be captured instantly and reviewed which helps in overall learning. They suffer from disadvantage of having a poor image quality especially in the low cost instruments. Hand-held trichoscopes have the advantage of a higher resolution and a better image quality. Hence, they are best suited for research and publications. Moreover, they are better suited for a heavy clinical practice for an instant evaluation. The major disadvantage is the necessity of an immersion fluid for a good image quality which makes the evaluation tedious and messy especially on scalp. Also, most good quality hand-held trichoscopes are highly priced. Figure 2.13 compares the trichoscopic image quality in various types of trichoscopes.

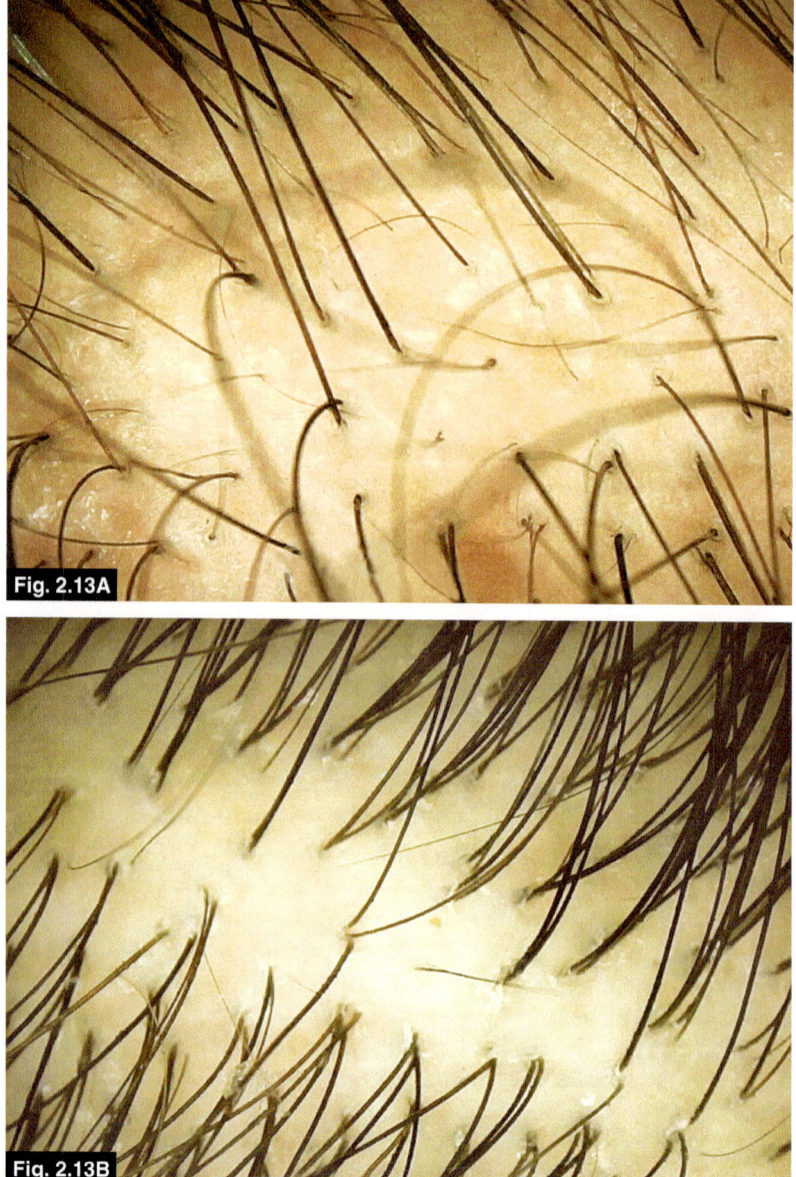

Fig. 2.13A

Fig. 2.13B

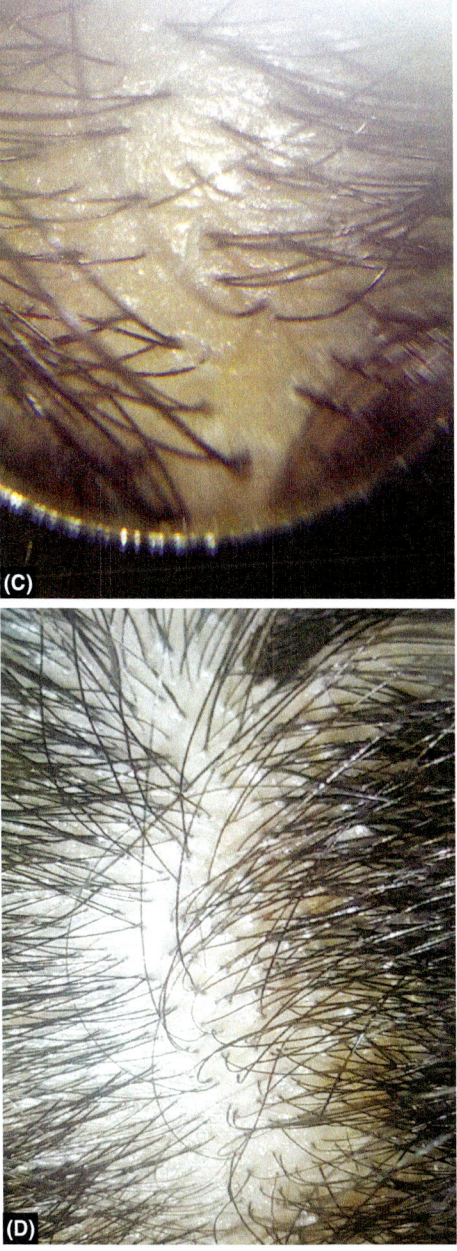

Fig. 2.13A to D: Comparison of trichoscopic images captured using various trichoscopes. (A) Dinolite videodermatoscope; (B) Escope (low cost video dermatoscope); (C) External attachment to mobile phone; (D) Trichoscopy using mobile phone magnification

CONCLUSION

Trichoscopy is a science still under evolution. Therefore, there is a learning curve which can be negotiated by constant reading and correlating it with the literature. An exquisite image capturing and meticulous archiving of the pictures are important aspects for learning it beyond the books. However, integration of trichoscopy to routine clinical practice not only helps the clinician but also helps the patient by averting the necessity of biopsy and convincing the patients about the subtle therapeutic responses which are very slow in most hair disorders, thereby improving the patient's compliance to the treatment.

Bibliography

1. Ebtisam Elghblawi: Frontier in hair loss and trichoscopy: A review. J Surg Dermtol 2016;1(2):80–96.
2. Nilam Jain, Bhavana Doshi, Uday Khopkar. Trichoscopy in alopecias: Diagnosis simplified.

3

Male Pattern Hair Loss

Kabir Sardana,
Khushbu Mahajan, Rahul Arora, Selma CH

Androgenetic alopecia (AGA) or pattern hair loss is by far the most common form of alopecia in men and women. The development and occurrence of AGA depends on genetic predisposition and an interaction of endocrine factors.

Male baldness is a largely genetically determined condition that has an impact on the quality of life, reducing self-esteem and causes stress. Importantly a perception of bald men looking less attractive was found in more than 90% of subjects surveyed. A crucial fact being that, this view was more common in women than non-balding men.

The process starts in the pubertal period with temple recession, and its frequency and severity increases with advancing age. After puberty, hair loss progresses with frontal hairline thinning and recession and / or vertex balding. The evolution and course of this condition is highly variable and in some men there may be diffuse thinning in the parietal area with a retained hairline instead of the classical patterned alopecia.

PATHOPHYSIOLOGY

The main cause is that scalp hair follicles decrease in size and activity during successive hair cycles in what is commonly known as a **'miniaturization'** process. Terminal, thick hair follicles become thinner, shorter and less pigmented until they are finally substituted by vellus hairs. The mean duration of the anagen phase of the hair cycle progressively decreases, whereas the length of telogen remains constant or is prolonged and is driven by the inhibitory follicle response to the potent androgen hormone dihydrotestosterone (DHT) at the level of the dermal papilla cells (Fig. 3.1). DHT is a metabolite formed from testosterone and androstenedione through the action of the enzyme 5α-reductase and has two isoforms; type 1 5α-reductase that is widely distributed in the skin and muscles, while the type 2 isoform is mainly present in the scalp, prostate and epididymis.

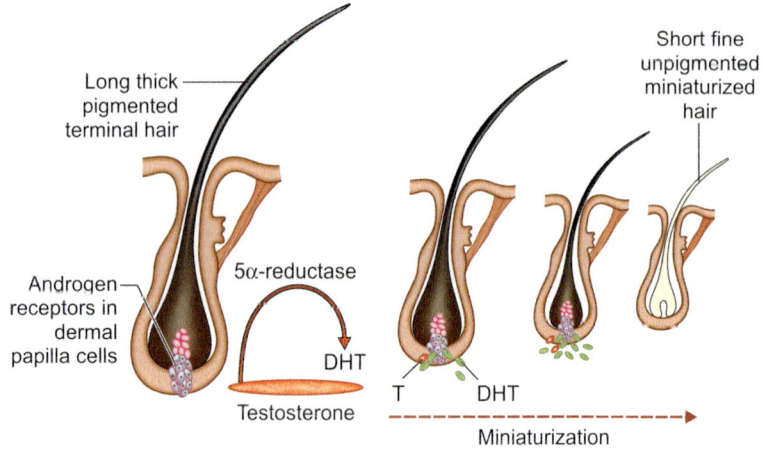

Fig. 3.1: Depiction of the process of miniaturization mediated by the effect of DHT on the dermal papilla cells

The binding of DHT to its receptor in hair follicles leads to the increased production of cytokines, such as transforming growth factors β_1 and β_2, which promotes senescence in the dermal papilla cells. The densities of these receptors are high in the frontoparietal scalp and vertex but low in the occipital area, which is why hair is retained in the latter areas. Genetics also play a role, while the other implicated factors include: Alcohol, sun exposure, nutrition deficiencies and stress.

The accelerated pace of driving hair follicles out of anagen prematurely and the relative lengthening of telogen combine to produce a reduction in the anagen-to-telogen ratio from a normal ratio **12:1** to an aberrant ratio **5:1**, while the proportion of telogen hair increases from the normal 5–10% to 15–20%. The time delay for hair follicles to rotate out of telogen and back to anagen allows for increased exogen shedding and progressive increase in the numbers of empty kenogen hair follicles. An interesting finding is that the number of hair in the **follicular hair unit** (FHU) progressively decrease, due to miniaturization and thus with time the number of hair per FHU are reduced from 2–5 to 1–2, which adds to the overall decrease in density seen on the scalp. It is believed that the arrector pili muscle is crucial in maintaining the hair integrity as hair close to it are lost in the end (Sincliar R) (Fig. 3.2).

A depiction of the clinical appearance of this process is given below Fig. 3.3. Recently, prostaglandin D_2 (PGD$_2$), a known inhibitor of hair growth, has been shown to be elevated in the scalp of men with AGA. Some studies have shown a positive association between male baldness and high risks of coronary heart disease and prostate cancer, specially in the severe types of baldness.

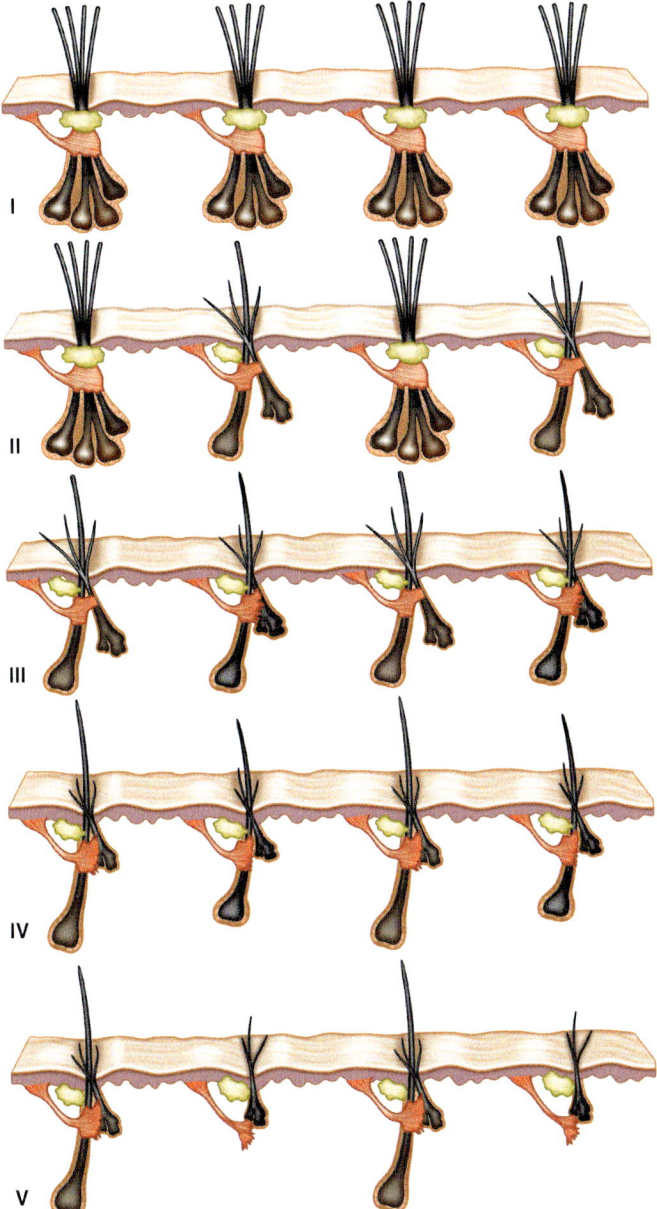

Fig. 3.2: A depiction of the process of hair miniaturization in androgenetic alopecia. The (I) panel shows normal FHU. There is progressive loss of hair in some of the FHUs leading to decreasing density of hair (II–V). Note that the hair closest to the arrector pili muscle is preserved as this is crucial to maintain the stem cell niche in the bulge areas (IV and V) (Sinclair R)

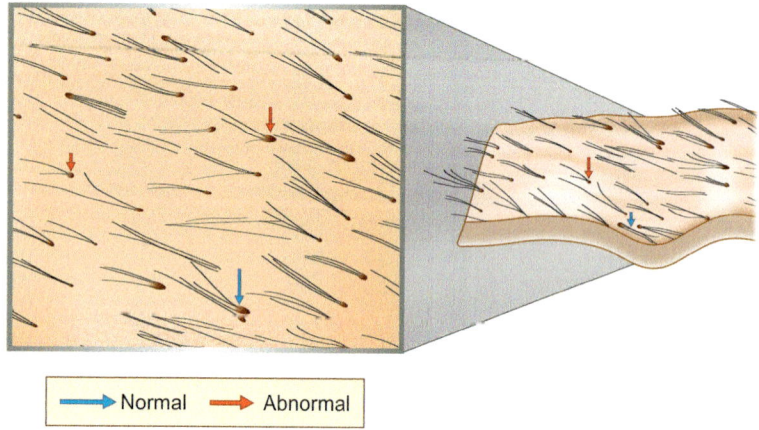

Normal ➡ Abnormal

Fig. 3.3: In a patient with pattern alopecia, there is a progressive reduction in hair density, miniaturization and decrease in the number of hair per hair follicle unit. A normal HFU has 2–5 hairs of uniform diameter (blue arrows). In androgenetic alopecia there is reduction of hair from 3 to 2 or even 1, variable diameter of hair shafts and thinning of hair (red arrows)

Genetics: The concept of a **polygenic** inheritance is more accurate than a single gene model for determining AGA. If the mode of inheritance is regulated by only a single gene, this condition should rarely occur at a frequency greater than 1 in 1000. In AGA, multiple genes are likely involved to determine the age of onset, progression, patterning, and severity of hair loss (Kuster W).

Androgen receptor (AR) expression evaluation in balding scalp suggests mutations in the AR gene and this may be implicated in the causation of AGA (Hibberts NA). Researchers were able to conclude that a restriction fragment length polymorphism in exon 1 of AR was present in 98.1% in young bald men but in only 76.6% of older men without the balding condition (Ellis JA). These data suggest that this particular nonfunctional single nucleotide polymorphism in AR is important for AGA susceptibility.

CLINICAL FEATURES

The clinical diagnosis is fairly simple (trichodynia or scalp pain may accompany AGA). There is decreased hair on various areas of the superior scalp (frontal, temporal, parietal and crown areas) and this is grouped into several stages according to the Norwood-Hamilton classification (Fig. 3.4). Although these grades (Fig. 3.4) are *imprecise measures* of the continuum of hair patterns that are seen in adult males, they are useful as diagnostic aids and in the classification of extent of hair loss in clinical investigations.

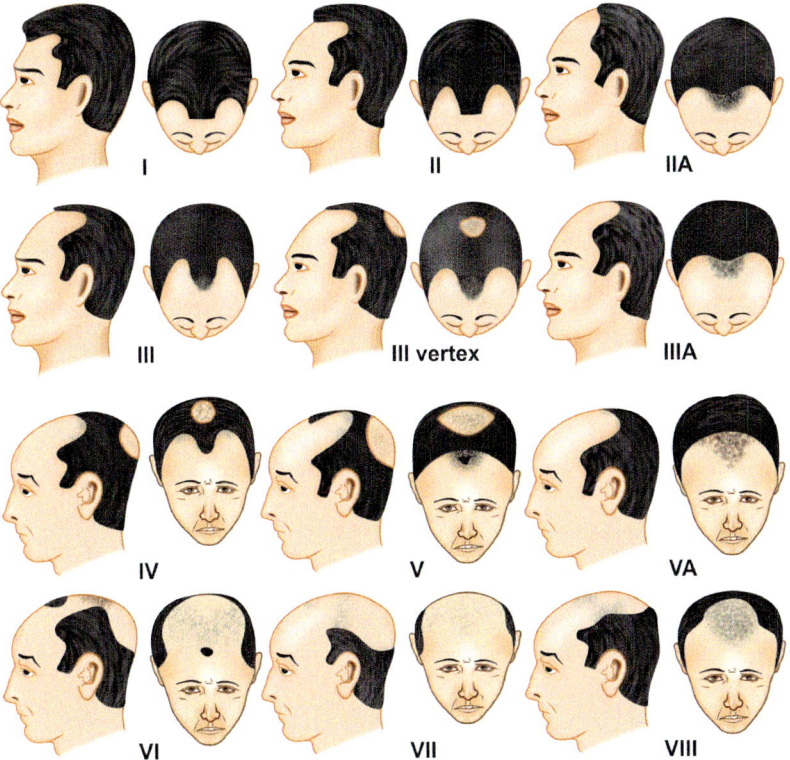

Fig. 3.4: The Norwood-Hamilton classification of male pattern alopecia

The Hamilton scale ranges from types I to VIII. Type I represents the prepubertal scalp with terminal hair growth on the forehead and all over the scalp; types II and III show gradual frontal, mostly M-shaped recession of the hairline; types IV to VI show additional gradual thinning in the vertex area; and types VII and VIII show a confluence of the balding areas and leave hair only around the back and the sides of the head (horseshoe pattern). Some of these patterns are depicted in Figs 3.5 and 3.6.

Some men, especially (Koreans) Asians, might present with a retained hairline and thinning of the hair in the parietal area, similar to female pattern hair loss (Ludwig's classification, Fig. 3.7). An Asian group has proposed a new basic and specific classification to be universally used in men and women (Agarwal S et al).

In the affected areas the hairs are thinner, shorter and less pigmented, and patients commonly complain that the hairs in these areas grow more slowly than those in the rest of the scalp (lateral and occipital areas).

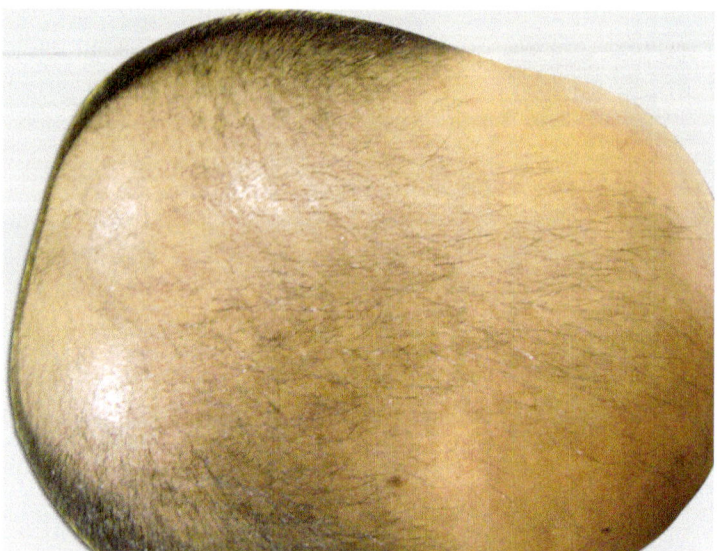

Fig. 3.5: A male patient with Norwood-Hamilton stage V alopecia

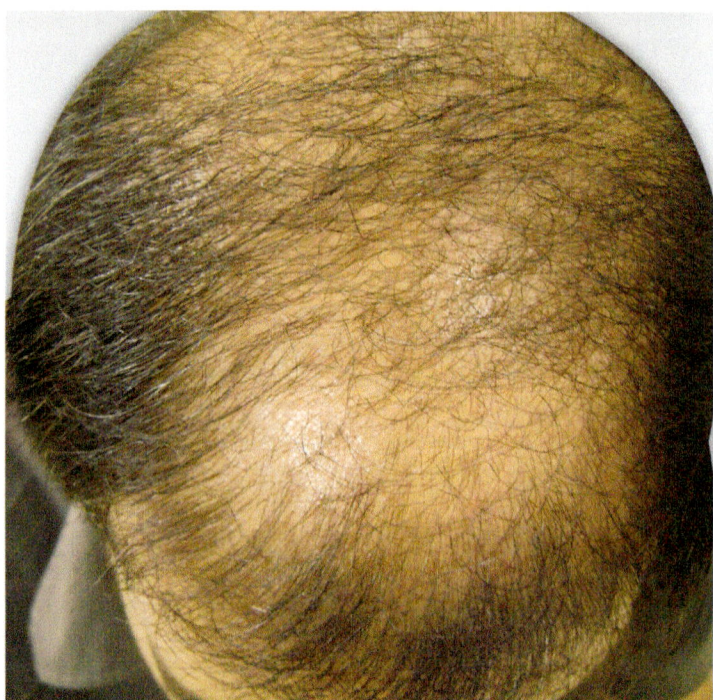

Fig. 3.6: A patient with Norwood-Hamilton stage V with preserved frontal hair margin

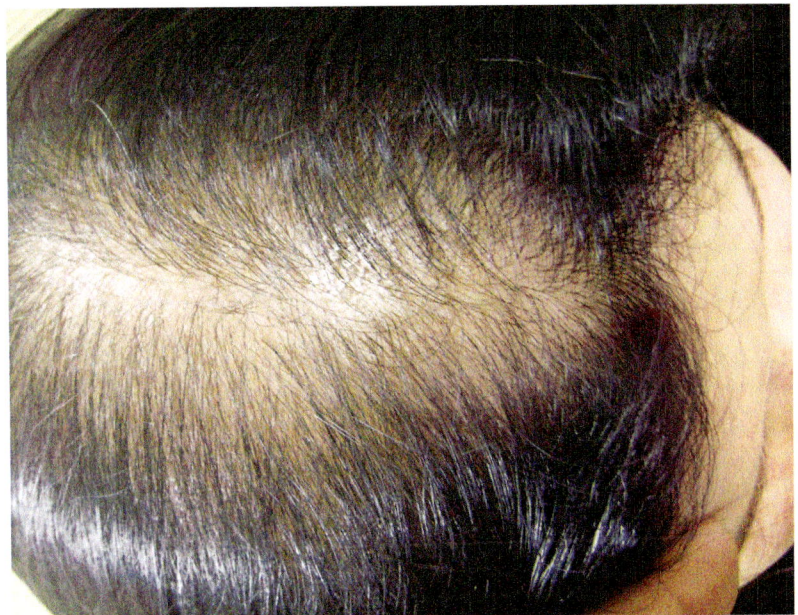

Fig. 3.7: A male patient with Ludwig's type 1 pattern of hair loss with decreased hair in the part width, a pattern normally seen in females

INVESTIGATIONS

Though various invasive methods have been advised including trichogram and biopsy, a **clinical diagnosis** suffices in most patients. **Dermoscopy** is very useful in diagnosing AGA in male patients who do not clinically show classical patterned alopecia (Fig. 3.8A and B). These patients include pediatric patients, young men with the early onset of diffuse parietal hair loss and men who originally had very thick hairs and are complaining of decreased hair density, although it is not obvious clinically.

There is a change in the ratio of **terminal to vellus** hairs from greater than 8:1 to less than 4:1. Also, the anagen-to-telogen hair ratio reduces from 12:1 to 5:1.

On dermoscopy, the characteristic findings include, the *diversity* in hair shaft diameters of greater than 20% in the frontoparietal area (Fig. 3.8A), *peripilar sign* (subtle brown halo reflecting perifollicular inflammation seen in early cases), *yellow dots* (Fig. 3.8B) (sebum and keratin accumulation within dilated follicular infundibula) and an increase in the percentage of *single hair follicular units*.

Histopathology, though not needed, shows a reduction in terminal hairs, an increase in secondary vellus hair (Fig. 3.9) with associated

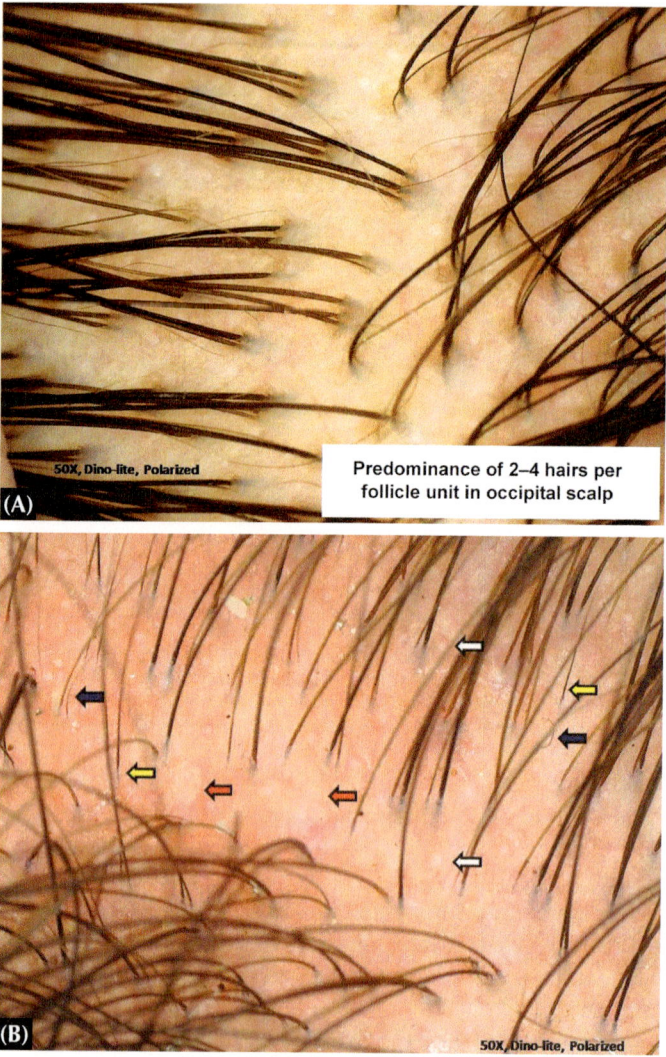

Fig. 3.8A and B: A 28-year-old male presented with thinning of hair in frontal scalp with relatively maintained anterior hairline for past 5 years. There was no family history of androgenetic alopecia. Trichoscopic findings (A) showed presence of >20% variability of diameter as compared to the occipital scalp; (B) Yellow dots (red arrows), white dots (white arrows), predominance of single hair follicle units (yellow arrows) and vellus hair (blue arrows). Hence, the diagnosis of androgenetic alopecia was made and patient was started on minoxidil 5% in combination with finasteride 1 mg along with platelet-rich plasma therapy. Single hair follicular units in the frontal area and increased vellus hairs are also suggestive of early AGA, even when variability is not yet obvious. In males, blood tests are rarely needed, except prostate-specific antigen (PSA) levels if the patient is above 40 years old

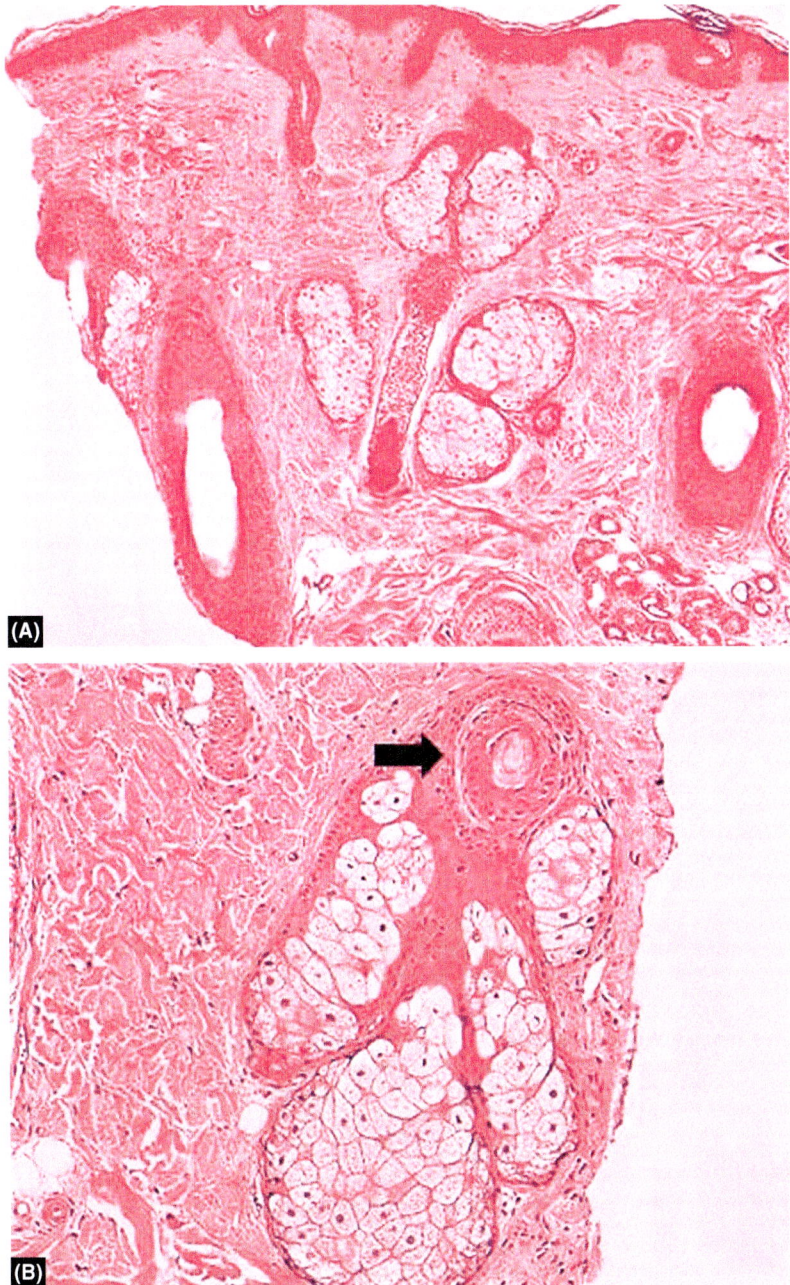

Fig. 3.9A and B: Histopathology from the scalp of a male patient with androgenetic alopecia demonstrates. (A) Hair follicles of varying sizes; (B) A miniaturized follicle (*Courtesy:* Dr Purnima Malhotra)

angiofibrotic streamers, a variable increase in telogen and catagen hairs, and a mild or moderate perifollicular lymphohistiocytic infiltrate, with or without concentric layers of perifollicular collagen deposition.

Although the complete genetic picture is not clear, there is a genetic test (**HairDX**™) that tests for a gene polymorphism and may predict the chances of future AGA development (Randall VA et al). For young patients concerned about hair loss, this test may help to define the value of early treatment initiation. Moreover, a test that predicts responsiveness to treatment with finasteride is also available (Keene S et al).

TREATMENT

Before commencing treatment, counseling about the course of disease and the prolonged duration of therapy for sustained effect is a must. The results obtained with treatment vary and the efficacy is maintained with continuous treatment. If the medications are stopped, the patient will return to baseline in around a year. An algorithm that has been standardized can be used as a tool to decide the intervention for MPHL (Fig. 3.10).

There is extensive research on the topic and a separate **Chapter 14** is devoted to this and possibly in the near future, hair transplantation may not be required in most cases. An overview of the conventional drugs is detailed here.

Topical Therapies

a. Topical Minoxidil

Minoxidil prevents the disease progression and improves hair density and hair thickness in the majority of patients. It is available in 2 or 5% topical solution, foam and gel and the dose is 1 ml twice daily. Though it is generally well tolerated, some patients do have a transient hair shedding when initiating minoxidil application, especially during the first 5 weeks of use, but this might last for up to 3 months. Many patients complain of a worsening in hair quality and texture with product application, and thus, an alternative water vehicle might be used in some cases (gel).

Some might experience itching when they start to use the topical solution, and thus, a patch test might be performed to exclude contact dermatitis, the most common allergen being **propylene glycol**, an alternative to which is a foam vehicle (Price VH). Minoxidil may cause hypotension and thus symptoms like dizziness, headache, hypotension, tachycardia or chest pain may occur occasionally.

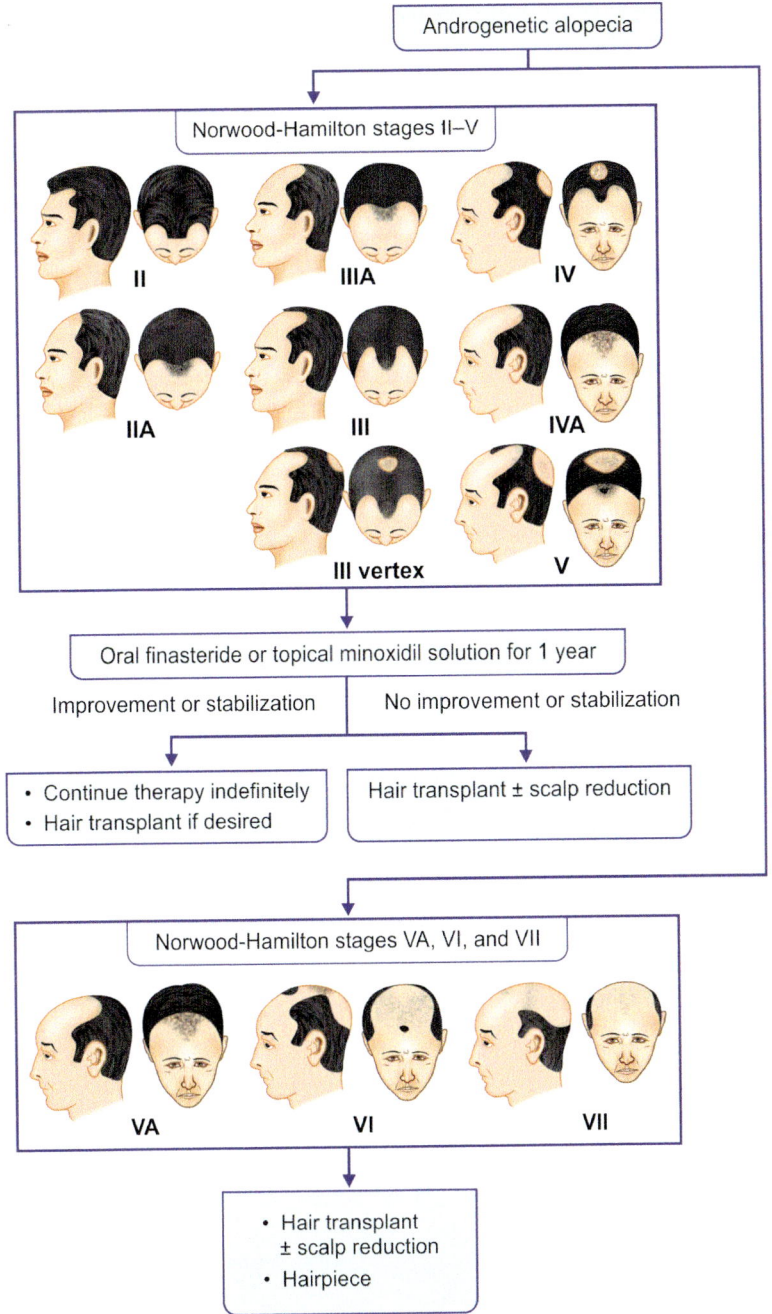

Fig. 3.10: An algorithmic approach to the treatment of male androgenetic alopecia (UCSF-UBC treatment protocol for androgenetic alopecia in men)

Initial clinical studies demonstrated efficacy of minoxidil in vertex thinning, however, subsequent studies confirmed that minoxidil works equally well on **frontal** scalp thinning. Hair regrowth varies, but starts at *3 months,* is obvious by *6 months* and peaks at *2 years* of use. If minoxidil is stopped, acute hair loss might occur within 2–3 months that might last for 3 months. Its positive effects on hair growth are lost after 6 months of stopping treatment.

The best candidates for minoxidil are those in whom the balding process is at an early stage, with a maximum diameter of the bald area less than 10 cm, and in whom the pre-treatment hair density is in excess of 20 hairs/cm^2.

Several products that include minoxidil, combined with other active ingredients such as tretinoin, and even steroids are available but there is no proof that they are superior to minoxidil. Various concentrations of minoxidil are marketed but increasing concentrations only provides a slight increase in efficiency.

b. Miscellaneous

There are various serums and topical peptides that have been proposed to treat male baldness, but there is a lack of sufficient evidence to support their use. These are useful when minoxidil cannot be used and include α-*estradiol, vitamins, mineral and herbal compounds, caffeine, melatonin, retinoids, and ketoconazole* (McElwee KJ).

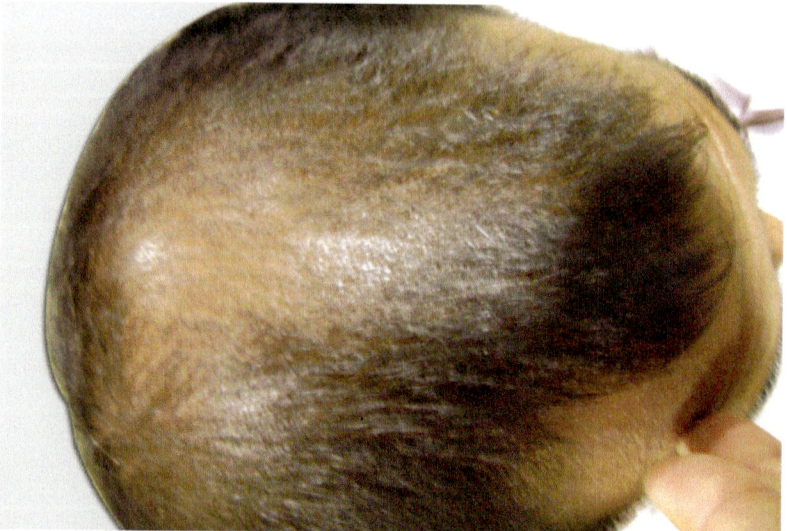

Fig. 3.11: This patient depicted previously in Fig. 3.5, attained a reasonable growth after 6 months of treatment with finasteride 1 mg and minoxidil 5% application

Latanoprost and bimatoprost are prostaglandin F_2 analogs that are being studied as potential new drugs for treating AGA due to their reported effects on eyelashes, though they can be very costly for use on the scalp. Moreover, they are inferior to minoxidil.

Though there is some data on the use of topical finasteride (1% gel or lotion), the evidence for its use as a monotherapy is a matter of individual choice. DCGI had approved a combination with minoxidil and as the data is on file we are unable to comment on its scientific rationale.

Systemic Therapy

a. Finasteride

It remains the most specific and effective oral treatment for male baldness above 18 years of age. It is a selective type II 5α-reductase inhibitor that decreases scalp production of DHT, which is a metabolite of testosterone. The usual dose is 1 mg, to be taken **early morning** at the peak of hormonal conversion. Its absorption occurs independent of food, and it does not interact with any medications. An oral dosage of 1 mg/day reduces scalp DHT by 64% and serum DHT by 68%.

Most patients observe hair regrowth during the first year of treatment. The finasteride-responsive follicles are all activated after **1 year**, and the clinical improvement in scalp coverage results from increase in hair length, diameter and pigmentation. Finasteride reverses the miniaturization procedure and encourages growth of terminal hair. In clinical practice minoxidil is often combined (Fig. 3.11) with topical agents with heartening results. Finasteride therapy has been given up to **5 years** continuously. Finasteride is also effective on the mid-frontal scalp, although the most profound effects are seen on the vertex. It may arrest bitemporal recession but does not reverse it.

Some men might experience sexual side effects which include decreased libido in 1.8% (1.3% in placebo), erectile dysfunction in 1.3% (0.7% placebo), and decreased ejaculate volume in 0.8% (0.4% placebo). Side effects will subside spontaneously in 58% of those who decide to continue the treatment and are reversible within 2 weeks to 3 months on cessation of treatment. Finasteride has no effect on spermatogenesis or semen production.

The package insert recommends a complete blood test with liver function at baseline and then on a regular basis at least every 6 months. In men above 40 years old, it is also recommended that PSA levels are checked prior to the start of therapy.

While giving finasteride in older men, it should be remembered that a 50% reduction in serum prostate-specific antigen levels is likely, thus the value should be doubled to correct for this effect when evaluating for prostate cancer risk.

b. Dutasteride

Dutasteride is a double inhibitor (types 1 and 2 α-reductase) with a potentially strong effect on hair regrowth. It is used off label in select cases, especially in those who do not respond well to finasteride (Olsen EA). Only in **Korea** is dutasteride at a dose of 0.5 mg daily been recently **approved** for the treatment of MPHL.

Its dose may vary from 0.5 to 2.5 mg a day. Due to its long pharmacological half-life (around 5 weeks), some advise once a week or twice a week regimen but the daily regimen is better (Boyapati A).

A recent trial data is detailed in Chapter 14 that comprehensively compares dutasteride with finasteride.

c. Miscellaneous

Some vitamins, minerals and herbal derivatives have been claimed to act as anti-androgens and to promote hair growth. These include *biotin, melatonin, saw palmetto, ketoconazole, black cohosh, dong quai, false unicorn, chaste berry, and red clover* (McElwee KJ).

Laser and Light Therapy

It has become very popular in recent years to use lasers and light devices to treat AGA. There are many devices with different wavelengths and potencies and regimens of use that can be used at home or in the clinic. They are claimed to stimulate hair growth by scalp vasodilatation, but the exact underlying mechanism has not yet been defined (McElwee KJ).

Treatment protocols include 15- to 30-minute treatments on alternating days for 2–4 weeks tapering to one to two treatments per week for 6–12 months, followed by biweekly and once per month maintenance treatments. A change in texture and improvement in hair quality has been reported in patients using laser devices.

Surgery

Some select patients might be recommended to seek a transplant specialist to be evaluated for hair transplant, especially those who cannot undergo clinical treatment for any reason or those who have had poor results with the conventional therapy. Hair restoration surgery is an excellent treatment option for men with AGA Norwood-Hamilton stages III–V. The hair is taken from the occipital area which is usually not affected by the miniaturization process of AGA thus this can be taken and redistributed to the front, parietal area and vertex (*see* **Chapters 16 and 17**).

Other Therapies

Promising therapies include cell-mediated treatments, hair growth factors, platelet-rich plasma and human placenta extract (*see* Chapter 14 page 315).

Wigs and Hairpieces

These may be resorted to when the hair loss exceeds Norwood-Hamilton stage V and progresses to stages VI and VII, where full scalp coverage cannot be achieved with hair restoration surgery, as the donor supply does not equal the demand.

Bibliography

1. Agarwal S, Godse K, Mahajan A, et al. A new classification of pattern hair loss that is universal for men and women: basic and specific (BASP) classification. J Am Acad Dermatol 2007;57:37–46.
2. Boyapati A, Sinclair R. Combination therapy with finasteride and low-dose dutasteride in the treatment of androgenetic alopecia. Australas J Dermatol 2013;54:49–51.
3. Ellis JA, Stebbing M, Harrap SB. Polymorphism of the androgen receptor gene is associated with male pattern baldness. J Invest Dermatol 2001;116:452–5.
4. Hibberts NA, Howell AE, Randall VA. Balding hair follicle dermal papilla cells contain higher levels of androgen receptors than those from non-balding scalp. J Endocrinol 1998;156:59–65.
5. Keene S, Goren A. Therapeutic hotline. Genetic variations in the androgen receptor gene and finasteride response in women with androgenetic alopecia mediated by epigenetics. Dermatol Ther 2011;24(2):296–300.
6. Kuster W, Happle R. The inheritance of common baldness: two B or not two B? J Am Acad Dermatol 1984;11:921–6.
7. McElwee KJ, Shapiro JS. Promising therapies for treating and/or preventing androgenetic alopecia. Skin Therapy Lett 2012;17:1–4.
8. Messenger A. Male androgenetic alopecia; in Blume-Peytavi U, Tosti A, Whiting DA, et al (eds): Hair Growth and Disorders. Berlin, Springer, 2008, 159–68.
9. Olsen EA, Hordinsky M, Whiting D, et al. The importance of dual 5α-reductase inhibition in the treatment of male pattern hair loss: results of a randomized placebo-controlled study of dutasteride versus finasteride. J Am Acad Dermatol 2006;55: 014–23.
10. Price VH, Menefee E, Strauss PC. Changes in hair weight and hair count in men with androgenetic alopecia, after application of 5 and 2% topical minoxidil, placebo or no treatment. J Am Acad Dermatol 1999;41:717–21.
11. Randall VA, Hibberts NA, Hamada K. A comparison of the culture and growth of dermal papilla cells from hair follicles from non-balding and balding (androgenetic alopecia) scalp. Br J Dermatol 1996;134(3):437–44.
12. Sinclair R, Jolliffe V. Fast Facts: Disorders of the Hair and Scalp, 2nd edn, Published 2013, Health Press.

4

Female Pattern Hair Loss

Kabir Sardana, Khushbu Mahajan,
Rahul Arora, Ramya MN

AGA together with telogen effluvium is the most common complaint of women in clinical practice. Though it is believed that the role of genetics and androgens is less pronounced in females, there is evidence that in a proportion of cases, patients have associated features of hyperandrogenemia (HA) and thus FPHL (female pattern hair loss) and FAGA can be used interchangeably. The prevalence of FPHL in women below the age of 50 years ranges between 6 and 12% and increases postmenopausally, suggesting a possible hormonal influence.

PATHOPHYSIOLOGY

While **androgens** have a clear, established role in male androgenetic alopecia (MAGA), their effect on female hair follicles is less clear. Not all females with FPHL have evidence, either clinically or biochemically, of hyperandrogenism, making the role of elevated androgen levels controversial (Rushton DH et al, Schmidt JB et al). Also the circulating testosterone levels may not differ between women with FPHL and controls (Sawaya ME et al).

Contrary to the aforesaid view, there is an another view that FAGA can be related to the excess of androstenedione serum levels of ovarian or adrenal origin and FAGA. M (female androgenetic alopecia with male pattern hair loss) with the increase of dehydroepiandrosterone (DHEA) or DHEAS of adrenal origin. Androstenedione and DHEAS are peripherally transformed into testosterone (T), and this in turn is converted into 4 main metabolites, of which, in alopecia, the most important is 5α-dihydrotestosterone (DHT). This enzymatic conversion is mediated by 5α-reductase (free testosterone to **5α-DHT**).

This conversion of T to DHT requires free T, that highlights the importance of the levels of **SHBG** and the importance of free androgen index (Table 4.1). Once, DHT has been metabolized in the follicular target organ, it is transformed into its metabolite **3α-androstanediol**

Table 4.1: Investigation list in a case of FPHL	
Basic tests	• Full blood count • Serum ferritin, TIBC, transferrin saturation • Serum vitamin B_{12}, vitamin D levels • Thyroid function test (TSH) • Fasting lipids/fasting glucose
Endocrinological tests (if warranted)	• Serum testosterone/ free androgen index • DHEAS • Prolactin • 17-hydroxyprogesterone • AMH (anti-müllerian hormone) • Ovarian ultrasound • Adrenal imaging

glucuronide. Thus, this is probably the *most sensitive* indicator of *peripheral HA*. Prolactin may be also involved in FAGA. It is thought that hyperprolactinemia is associated with an increase in DHEAS as the result of the action of prolactin on the adrenal cortex.

Women have lower levels of 5α-reductase and higher levels of aromatase, which converts testosterone to estradiol and reduces the amount of follicular testosterone that is available for conversion to DHT, in their susceptible hair follicles as compared to men (Sawaya ME et al).

Estrogens may improve hair loss by multiple mechanisms including inhibiting 5α-reductase. This explains the increased prevalence of the condition in postmenopausal women, hair loss that occurs after aromatase inhibitor therapies and prolongation of anagen during pregnancy.

Other proposed parameters that may influence FPHL include insulin resistance, microvascular insufficiency and inflammatory abnormalities.

Genetic predisposition and a polygenic inheritance, have now been confirmed to influence the age of onset, pattern and severity of FPHL (Ellis JA). The speculated genetic link may lie in variations of the AR gene, and is determined by a region of CAG repeats that affects its transcriptional activity. The length of the CAG repeats is associated with the probability of developing FPHL. The newly produced screening test, the hair genetic test, measures the length of the CAG repeats in the AR gene, and shorter lengths are linked to a significant risk of developing FPHL (Schweiger ES).

The diffuse hair loss pattern seen in FPHL is due to a reduction in the *number* of terminal hairs per follicular unit *rather* than *miniaturization* of entire follicular units and thus baldness is a relatively late event in females as compared to males and occurs only when all the hairs within the follicular units are miniaturized.

CLINICAL FEATURES

The classical presentation of FPHL is a gradual thinning of hair, that occurs over a period of years, which results in decreased hair density. Women may present with an episodic or continuous increase in hair shedding *without* any noticeable reduction in hair volume, increased hair shedding with loss of hair volume over the crown, or *diffuse thinning* over the crown with no history of hair shedding. The first pattern mimics chronic telogen effluvium and is treated likewise for many years before the clinical picture becomes obvious. The most informative question to ask balding women is about the change in the thickness of their ponytail.

The clinical morphology is characterized by a diffuse rarefaction of scalp hair over the mid-frontal scalp and a more-or-less intact frontal hairline without any signs of inflammation or scarring (Fig. 4.1). However, there are patients with increased temporal and/or vertex involvement, which resembles the male pattern hair loss. In the early stages of the disease, the widening of the area of hair loss is mostly seen when the hair is parted at the midline, which, when it involves part of the frontal hairline, resembles a 'Christmas tree' pattern, with its base at the frontal hairline (Fig. 4.2). Bitemporal recession occurs in 13% of premenopausal women and 37% of postmenopausal women. Needless to say, women with FPHL are affected socially and are more psychologically distressed than men, as hair plays a central role in their femininity and beauty.

In 1977, Ludwig first described 3 patterns that represent the stages of FPHL, and these stages have traditionally been used as a classification system (Fig. 4.2). Stage I is characterized by perceivable mild thinning of the hair over the anterior part of the crown, with a wide midline part. In stage II, hair thinning on the crown is more pronounced, and decreased hair density over the frontal and vertex regions becomes evident (Fig. 4.3). Stage III is encountered in postmenopausal women and is characterized by a severe decrease in hair density over the crown and prominent diffuse rarefaction. A composite classification is depicted in Fig. 4.2 and clinical cases are represented in Figs 4.1 and 4.3.

Most women who present with hair loss have no other evidence of virilization. Certain features though point towards an underlying hyperandrogenism, such as sudden and advanced hair loss, menstrual disturbances, hirsutism or recrudescence of acne.

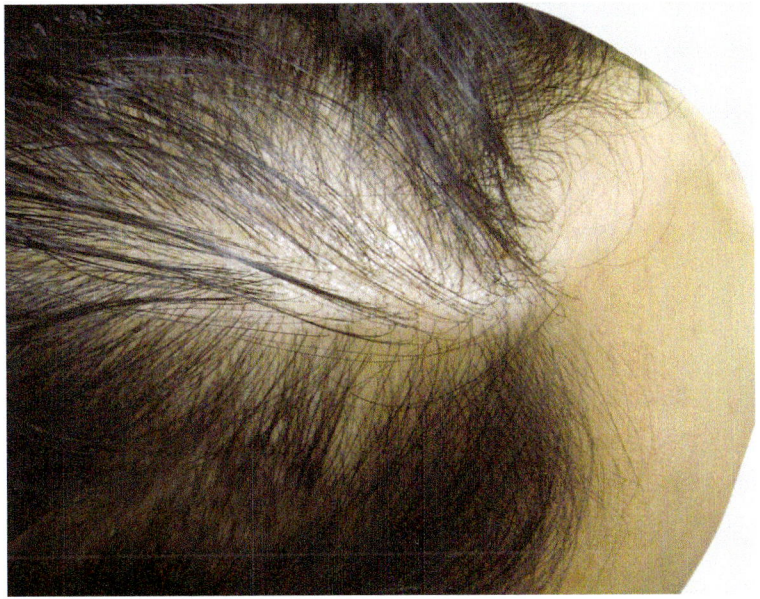

Fig. 4.1: Early stage of female pattern alopecia with reduced hair in the frontal area of the scalp

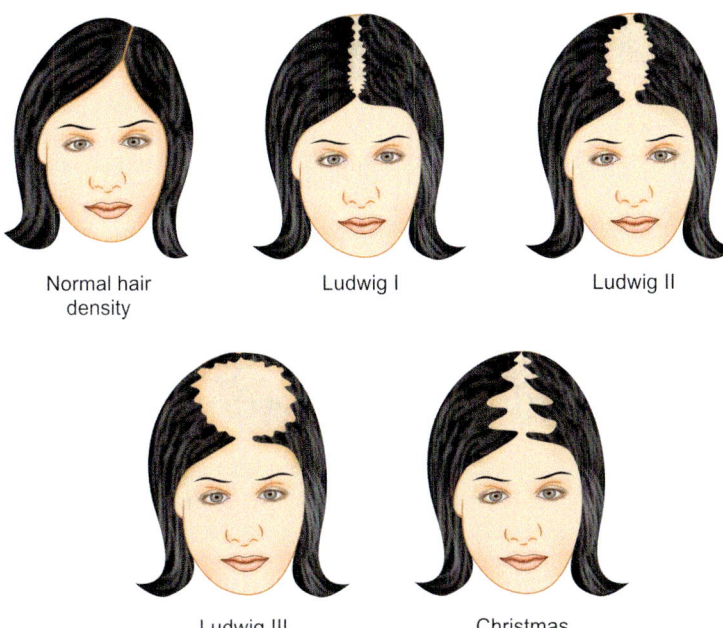

Normal hair density   Ludwig I   Ludwig II

Ludwig III   Christmas tree pattern

Fig. 4.2: A depiction of various stages of alopecia in females

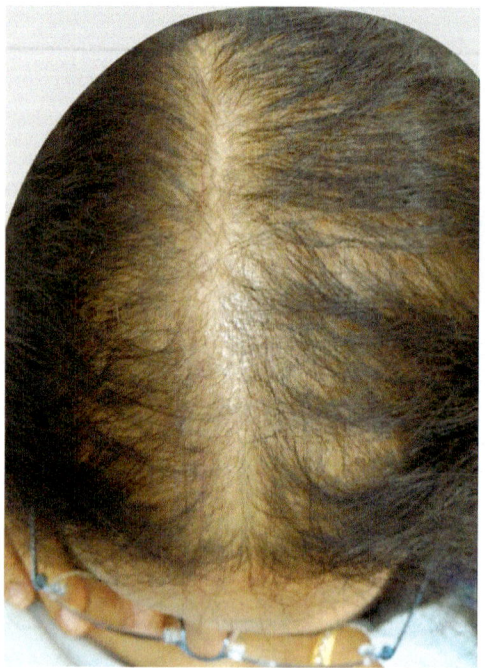

Fig. 4.3: A case of Ludwig stage II alopecia

Studies have shown association of FPHL with hyperaldosteronism, hypertension, hyperandrogenism, polycystic ovary disease, elevated cholesterol and an increased risk of late-onset diabetes, thus these may need to be excluded in appropriate clinical setting.

DIAGNOSIS

The diagnosis is *clinical*, but there are cases that mimic CTE, in fact CTE may unmask FPHL. Hair evaluation methods may be non-invasive, semi-invasive and invasive and include hair pull testing, trichoscopy, trichogram, laboratory tests and skin biopsy. Practically in the clinic, trichoscopy and in select cases biochemical investigations are the most practical.

Scalp *dermoscopy* (Fig. 4.4) in the early stages of female pattern hair loss reveals contrasting hair density between the mid-frontal and occipital scalp. Thus, over the occipital area—two or three terminal hairs of equal fibre diameter are seen per infundibulum. In comparison, the number of terminal hairs per infundibulum is reduced to one or two over the mid-frontal scalp. When two hairs emerge from a single infundibulum on the mid-frontal scalp, one is often noticeably thinner than the normal hairs indicating miniaturization of the follicle. This

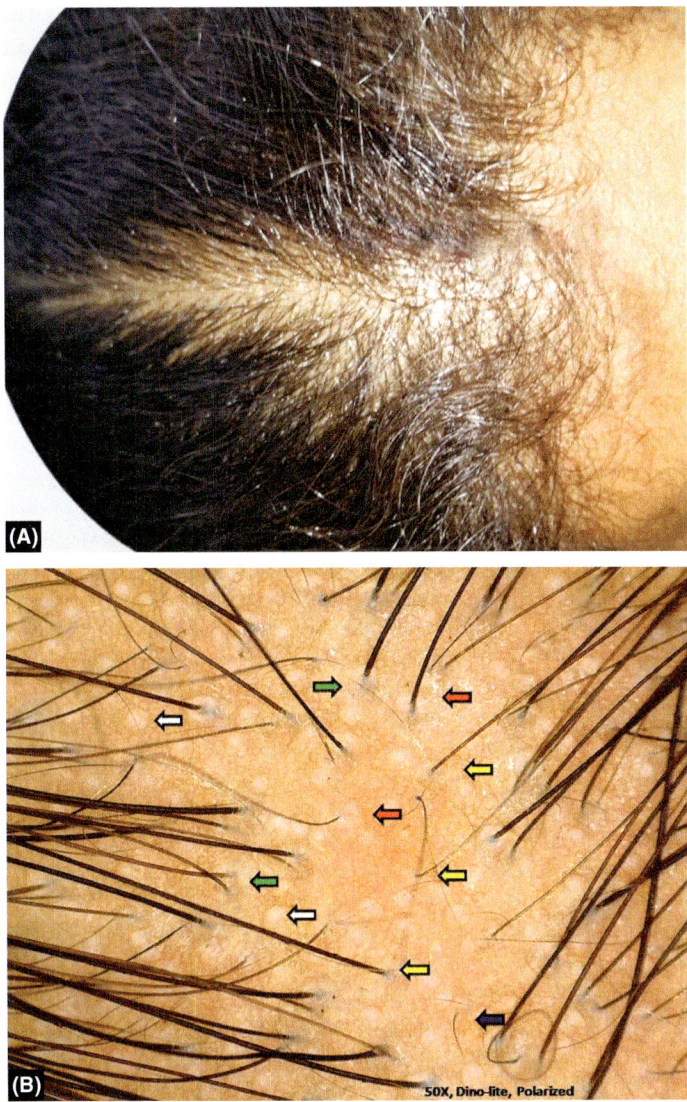

Fig. 4.4A and B: (A) A 26-year-old female presented with complain of diffuse hair loss since 2-year duration. There was a seasonal exacerbation of hair loss along with a decrease in the size of the ponytail. Her hemogram, thyroid function test, serum ferritin, vitamin B_{12} and vitamin D_3 were within normal limits. Her trichoscopic evaluation; (B) Showed a >20% anisotrichosis, yellow dots (red arrows), white dots (white arrows), peripilar sign (green arrows), vellus hair (blue arrow) and predominance of single hair units (yellow arrows). Based on the trichoscopic findings, a diagnosis of female patterned hair loss was made and minoxidil 2% along with platelet-rich plasma therapy was started

has been described as hair diameter diversity or anisotrichosis. Another dermoscopic sign that is suggestive of FPHL is the peripilar sign that corresponds to perifollicular inflammation.

Histopathological features are similar to that of male AGA. The ratio of terminal to vellus hairs on a horizontally sectioned 4 mm punch biopsy may help to differentiate FPHL from CTE—a ratio of <4:1 is diagnostic of FPHL, whereas a ratio of >8:1 is indicative of chronic telogen effluvium.

The *biochemical investigations* (Table 4.1) are usually performed as it is often difficult to distinguish FPHL from telogen effluvium and in some they may overlap. Thus, laboratory tests for thyroid-stimulating hormone (TSH) and ferritin are advisable as deranged levels of both these can trigger telogen effluvium that may mimic AGA. Tests for vitamin D, vitamin B$_{12}$, selenium and zinc are sometimes recommended.

In the absence of clinical evidence of hyperandrogenism, extensive work-up is not routinely necessary (Futterweit W et al). Women with a history of menstrual disturbance, impaired fertility or signs of *androgen excess* should be investigated for hyperandrogenism (e.g. polycystic ovary syndrome, androgen secreting tumour). Considering the potential associations, screening for hypertension, hypercholesterolaemia and late-onset diabetes are warranted.

The basic tests and the advanced tests, the latter of which are needed only in suspected cases of hyperandrogenism or if the patient does not respond appropriately to minoxidil.

DIFFERENTIAL DIAGNOSIS

In women, the challenge is to distinguish FPHL from chronic telogen effluvium (CTE). Some pointers to CTE include, *diffuse* loss of hair, *bitemporal* recession, *no widening* of central part width, similar *density* in frontal and occipital area and *trichodynia*. Though some claim that the hair pull test is positive in telogen effluvium, and may be normal in pattern hair loss, this is not always true as there is an increase in easily extracted telogen hairs in active pattern hair loss.

TREATMENT

The aim of therapy is to reduce hair loss and promote hair regrowth. Early initiation of treatment and the combination of various modalities seems to be more efficacious than monotherapy (Fig. 4.5). An overview is given here and more details are covered in the Chapter 10, Hair Loss in Women.

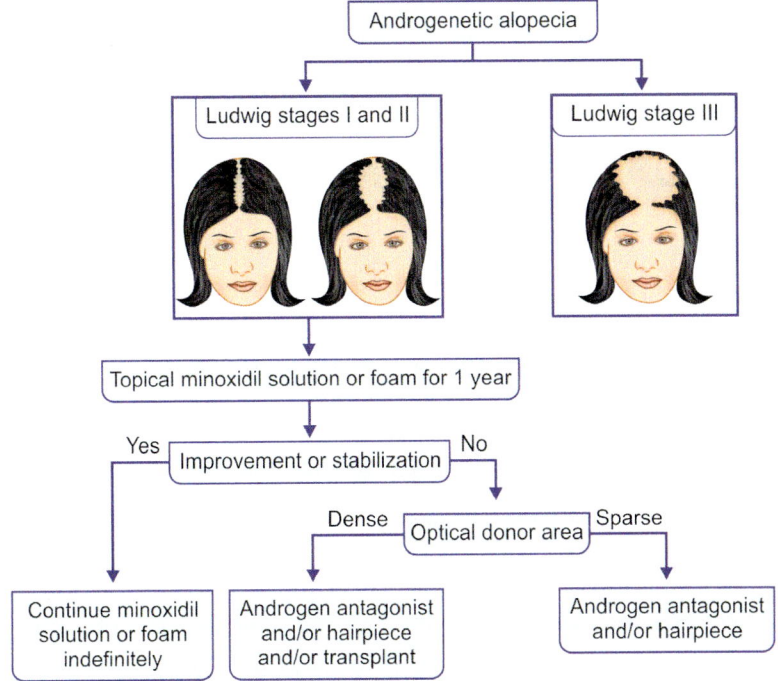

Fig. 4.5: A protocol for teatment of female pattern hair loss

Topical Agents

1. Topical Minoxidil

Only two pharmaceutical treatments have been approved by the FDA for the therapy of FPHL: 2% minoxidil solution, and recently, 5% minoxidil foam. Its use is indicated in women older than 18 years with mild to moderate hair loss (Ludwig stage I or II). Topical minoxidil arrests hair loss or induces mild to moderate hair regrowth in approximately 60% of women with FPHL. With twice daily application, higher concentrations (5%) seem to be superior to the 2% formulations, but with more treatment-related local side effects, such as facial hypertrichosis (it disappears within 4 months after discontinuation of therapy and frequently decreases even with continuous use after 1 year) and contact dermatitis with scalp pruritus and irritation. The 5% foam administered *once daily* has been shown to be clinically as effective but with less undesirable side effects. Minoxidil is applied onto the **dry scalp**, 25 drops (or 1 ml) twice a day, on the frontoparietal and vertex area. Studies have shown *75% of absorption* in the first **4 hours** after application; therefore, the scalp and hair should not be washed for at least **4–6 hours** after application.

2. Topical Prostaglandin Analogs

Latanoprost, travoprost and bimatoprost, when used topically for the treatment of glaucoma, promote eyelash growth, and bimatoprost is an FDA-approved therapy of eyelash hypotrichosis. Preliminary results on the use of these agents for MAGA and FPHL treatment have shown some results but they do not compare remotely with the results of minoxidil.

3. Topical Ketoconazole

The use of ketoconazole shampoo results in the stimulation of hair growth, especially when combined with finasteride and possibly through androgen-dependent pathways.

4. CG210™

CG210™ is a novel topical botanical hair lotion whose safety and efficacy have been demonstrated in more than 400 male and female volunteers with MAGA and FPHL (Cucé L). The proposed mechanism of action includes a regulation of apoptosis through normalization of the level of the intracellular antiapoptotic Bcl-2 protein, the reduction of inflammation and the increase in collagen content.

5. Stemoxydine®

The induction of **hypoxia signaling** may have an important role in maintaining hair follicle stem cell function and the ability of stem cells to respond to external signals and generate new hair (Bernard BA). A new compound, pyridine 2,4-dicarboxylic acid diethyl ester (stemoxydine), has been identified as a competitive inhibitor of hypoxia inducible transcription factor 1 (HIF1) and is functionally able to induce hypoxia-like signaling *in vitro*, thus acting as a hair kenogen phase shortener, leading to an increase in hair density.

6. Finasteride

A topical finasteride 0.05% gel formulation has been used for the treatment of pattern hair loss and has shown promising results (Hajheydari Z).

Systemic Therapy (Antiandrogens)

Antiandrogens are frequently prescribed as an off label indication and it must be emphasized that proper birth control measures should be taken during their use, specially with 5α-reductase inhibitors, as these agents are known teratogens and may cause hypospadias in the male fetus. The choice of anti-androgens vary across the globe and also depend on the prevailing approvals, thus *spironolactone* is preferred in **Australia** and **USA**, while *finasteride* is used off label in other parts of the world.

The treatment of hyperandrogenic women with their different possibilities of androgen origin and normoandrogenic women with FPHL is based on the same principles that is used in other dermatological hyperandrogenic diseases, such as hirsutism. Though details have been covered in another chapter, a few **principles of therapy** are enshrined below. These revolve around an understanding that a large majority of females of FPHL are actually FAGA and manifest varying degrees of the SAHA syndrome (Orfanos CE), which is hindered by the lack of extensive hormonal profiling.

1. It must be understood that HA is a continuum with an overlap of acne, hair loss and hirsutism. Different drugs have varying effects on different components and every clinician has to arrive at his own choice. This is compounded by the receptor variability in women.

2. For **adrenal SAHA** associated FAGA, **CPA** is the ideal drug, though most would prefer the combination of an antiandrogen and OCP.

3. For **ovarian SAHA**, **OCPs** are the ideal choice. Some gynecologists have been using finasteride from doses varying from 2.5 mg for ovarian SAHA to 5 mg for overt PCOS. With this, hirsutism and acne have responded remarkably, though hair loss may not achieve the same effect.

4. Androgen sensitivity in the cell is determined by the number of cytosine-adenine-guanine repeats in the androgen receptor gene. Lower CAG repeats have been associated in previous studies with androgenic conditions such as acne, hirsutism and hair loss in men and women. Thus, the dose of finasteride may need to be varied based on CAG repeats.

5. **Finasteride** doses vary from 2.5 mg (premenopausal women) to 5 mg in postmenopausal women.

6. **Dutasteride** (0.5 mg) should be used ideally in postmenopausal women, in premenopausal women finasteride is preferred and, wherever possible, with an OCP.

7. The effects of antiandrogens takes time with visible improvement by 6–12 months.

An overview of various drugs used is given below and is based on classification of androgenic defect based on the various sources of androgens, manifesting as SAHA (seborrhea, acne, hirsutism, androgenetic alopecia) (Table 4.2).

Table 4.2: Systemic therapy of FAGA based on the source of the androgen imbalance (SAHA)

SAHA	Drug class site	Drug	Dose
Adrenal SAHA	Adrenal suppression	Dexamethasone Prednisone Deflazacort	**Dexamethasone** 0.5 mg every night for 3 months and then alternate nights for another 3 months
	Antiandrogens	Central antiandrogens	Cyproterone acetate Spironolactone Flutamide Drospirenone	**CPA:** Hammerstein schedule **Spironolactone** 50–200 mg daily for 6 months **Flutamide** 250 to 375 mg daily for 6 months 3 mg/d of **drospirenone** given with 30 μg of ethinyl estradiol is considered the treatment of SAHA
		Peripheral antiandrogens	Finasteride Dutasteride	Finasteride 2.5–5 mg/d along with OCP (drospirenone and ethinyl estradiol) Dutasteride[2] 0.25 to 0.5 mg/d

FPHL in adrenal hyperandrogenism
FPHL in postmenopausal hyper- or normoandrogenic women

(Contd.)

Table 4.2: Systemic therapy of FAGA based on the source of the androgen imbalance (SAHA) (Contd.)

SAHA	Drug class site	Drug	Dose
Ovarian SAHA	FPHL in ovarian hyperandrogenism FPHL in normoandrogenic postmenopausal women	Ovarian suppression	OCP	EE + DRSP (21/7 schedule) Medroxyprogesterone 5 mg daily or twice a day
	Gonadotropin-releasing hormone agonists (GnRH-a)			Only for associated severe HAIRAN syndrome
	Antiandrogens			Ovarian SAHA with 2.5 mg/d finasteride and PCOS with 2.5 to 5 mg/d of finasteride and 0.5 mg/d dutasteride
		PCOS		Endocrinologist or gynecologist treatment
Pituitary SAHA	Hyperprolactinemic SAHA		Bromocriptine	2.5 to 7.5 mg/day
	Pituitary hyperandrogenism		Cabergoline	0.5 mg/week

Hammerstein schedule: 50 to 100 mg/d of CPA from 5th to 15th day of the menstrual cycle for a 6-month period, which is the time of the glucocorticosteroid suppression.
- Doses of 5 mg are used in **normoandrogenic women** as these patients have excessive activity of 5α-reductase enzyme.
- Dutasteride is preferred to be given in **postmenopausal** women.
- OCP: This is the first-line therapy for hair loss and acne in women with ovarian SAHA syndrome and PCOS.

a. Peripheral Antiandrogens

Finasteride: It is a specific inhibitor of 5α-reductase type II and blocks the conversion of testosterone to DHT. Though approved in males, it does not seem to be as efficacious in women, specially in postmenopausal women over a 1-year treatment period (Price VH, 2000). There are other studies that have shown its efficacy in postmenopausal women with or without features of hyperandrogenism (**2.5–5 mg/d × 6–12 months**) which goes to show that there must be an inter-individual receptor variability that determine the action of finasteride. Similarly, its use in premenopausal women has shown conflicting results with various doses recommended (**2.5–5 mg/day**) (Shum K et al, Yeon JH et al) (Fig. 4.6A and B).

Dutasteride: It is a more potent 5α-reductase types I and II inhibitor that has not currently been approved for the treatment of pattern hair loss. It can lower serum DHT levels by more than 90% and in females it has been reported to be successful at doses ranging from **0.25 to 0.5 mg/day** for up to 6–9 months (Olszewska M). Mesotherapy with a dutasteride-containing preparation was found to augment hair growth in women after 18 weeks of treatment.

b. Androgen Receptor Antagonists

Spironolactone: This drug reduces total testosterone levels and blocks the androgen receptor (AR) in target tissues. The standard dose is 100–200 mg daily, but treatment is usually initiated with a dose of 50 mg daily. Drug absorption is increased by **food**. Spironolactone is metabolized in the liver and excreted in urine and bile. The maximum androgen suppression is reached after 4–12 months but with dosages of **200 mg** daily. A combination of spironolactone and minoxidil 5% has also been tried, with good results (Hoedemaker C).

There are two issues with this drug. Firstly, at doses of 200 mg, there are menstrual problems, hence lowering the dose (50–75 mg) or adding OCP may be needed. Another problem is that spironolactone may reduce hair shedding in individuals with hyperandrogenism, but it does not consistently demonstrate significant hair regrowth (Price VH).

Cyproterone acetate: Cyproterone acetate exerts its antiandrogen properties by competing with DHT for AR binding and by inhibiting the gonadotropin-releasing hormone. It has only been approved in Europe and Canada for the treatment of hirsutism and acne, and is best used in combination with an oral contraceptive. The existing data support a role of cyproterone acetate in FPHL, alone (25–50 mg/day on days 1–10 of the menstrual cycle) or in combination (2 mg/day) with ethinyl estradiol or spironolactone, especially in cases of hyperandrogenism.

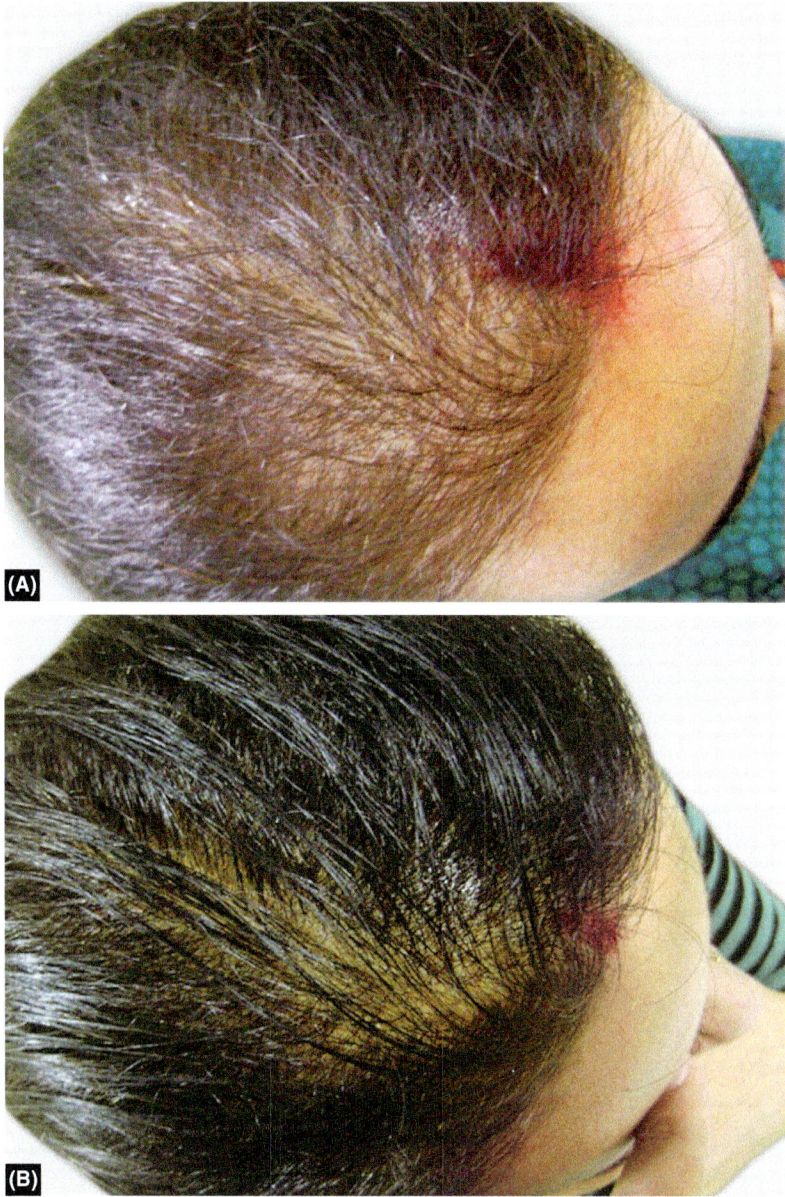

Fig. 4.6A and B: This female patient had failed all conventional approved medications. She had a history of menstrual irregularities but no overt PCOS. The patient had been treated also, as a case of diffuse AA and psychogenic telogen effluvium. She was initiated on finasteride 5 mg with EE/DRSP (24/4), the latter as she was obese and the (21/7) OCP has higher estrogen and can cause weight gain. After 9 months visible improvement is noted

Flutamide: It inhibits the binding of androgens to their receptors and has been found to be an effective treatment for FPHL, with yearly reducing doses of 250, 125 and 62.5 mg/day; a maximum response is seen at 2 years with a long-term maintenance of results (Paradisi R). There is a risk of dose-dependent hepatic dysfunction.

Platelet-rich Plasma Therapy

Platelet-rich plasma therapy represents a concentrated source of autologous platelets from a patient's own plasma and, when injected, releases different growth factors and other cytokines that promote hair regrowth. Preliminary data have shown beneficial results (Takikawa M) that have to be confirmed by larger scale trials.

Future Therapies

Botulinum toxin (150 units) injections have been used for the treatment of FPHL (Freund B) and may work by improving blood flow to the hair follicle **(*See* Chapter 14)**.

Hair Transplantation

Hair transplantation is another treatment option for women with FPHL which will be discussed in detail in another Chapters (*see* Chapters 16 and 17). Hair follicles are taken from the occipital scalp and implanted into the area of thinning. Optimal candidates for hair transplantation are those with high donor hair density and frontal accentuation of hair loss. Most importantly, in women, underlying causes for telogen effluvium should be ruled out, as this can spoil the final results. Overlapping of AGA and alopecia areata can occur, with 1.7% of patients with AGA having had, or having chances of developing, alopecia areata. If an AGA patient has a previous recent or remote history of alopecia areata, he or she must be warned that it could recur after surgery.

Bibliography

1. Bernard BA. The human hair follicle, a bistable organ. Exp Dermatol 2012; 21:401–3.
2. Cucé L, Consuelo JR, Régia CRP. Cellium® GC: Evaluation of a new natural active ingredient in 210 mg/ml topical solution, through scalp biopsy. Surg Cosmet Dermatol 2011;3:123–8.
3. Ellis JA, Harrap SB. The genetics of androgenetic alopecia. Clin Dermatol 2001;19:149–54.
4. Freund B, Schwartz M. Treatment of male pattern baldness with botulinum toxin: a pilot study. Plast Reconstr Surg 2010;126:246e–8.

5. Futterweit W, Dunaif A, Yeh HC, Kingsley P. The prevalence of hyperandrogenism in 109 consecutive female patients with diffuse alopecia. J Am Acad Dermatol 1988;19:831–6.

6. Hajheydari Z, Akbari J, Saeedi M, Shokoohi L. Comparing the therapeutic effects of finasteride gel and tablet in treatment of the androgenetic alopecia. Indian J Dermatol Venereol Leprol 2009;75:47–51.

7. Hoedemaker C, van Egmond S, Sinclair R. Treatment of female pattern hair loss with a combination of spironolactone and minoxidil. Australas J Dermatol 2007;48:43–5.

8. Olszewska M, Rudnicka L. Effective treatment of female androgenetic alopecia with dutasteride. J Drugs Dermatol 2005;4:637–40.

9. Orfanos CE, Adler YD, Zouboulis CC. The SAHA syndrome. Horm Res 2000; 54(5–6):251–8.

10. Paradisi R, Porcu E, Fabbri R, Seracchioli R, Battaglia C, Venturoli S. Prospective cohort study on the effects and tolerability of flutamide in patients with female pattern hair loss. Ann Pharmacother 2011;45:469–575.

11. Price VH. Treatment of hair loss. New Engl J Med 1999;341(13):964–73.

12. Price VH, Savin R, Bergfeld W, et al. Lack of efficacy of finasteride in postmenopausal women with androgenetic alopecia. J Am Acad Dermatol 2000;43:768–76.

13. Rushton DH, Ramsay ID, James KC, Norris MJ, Gilkes JJ. Biochemical and trichological characterization of diffuse alopecia in women. Br J Dermatol 1990; 123:187–97.

14. Sawaya ME, Price VH. Different levels of 5α-reductase types I and II, aromatase, and androgen receptor in hair follicles of women and men with androgenetic alopecia. J Invest Dermatol 1997;109:296–300.

15. Schmidt JB, Lindmaier A, Trenz A, Schurz B, Spona J. Hormone studies in females with androgenic hair loss. Gynecol Obstet Invest 1991;31:235–9.

16. Schweiger ES, Boychenko O, Bernstein RM. Update on the pathogenesis, genetics and medical treatment of patterned hair loss. J Drugs Dermatol 2010;9:1412–9.

17. Shum K, Cullen D, Messenger A. Hair loss in women with hyperandrogenism: four cases responding to finasteride. J Am Acad Dermatol 2002;47:733–9.

18. Singal A, Sonthalia S, Verma P. Female pattern hair loss. Indian J Dermatol Venereol Leprol 2013;79:626–40.

19. Takikawa M, Nakamura S, Nakamura S, et al. Enhanced effect of platelet-rich plasma containing a new carrier on hair growth. Dermatol Surg 2011; 37:1721–9.

20. Yeon JH, Jung JY, Choi JW, Kim BJ, Youn SW, Park KC, Huh CH. 5 mg/day finasteride treatment for normoandrogenic Asian women with female pattern hair loss. J Eur Acad Dermatol Venereol 2011;25:211–4.

5

Telogen Effluvium

Kabir Sardana, Chander Grover,
Ananta Khurana, MS Sukesh

INTRODUCTION

Telogen effluvium (TE) is a form of diffuse, nonscarring hair loss characterized by loss of predominantly telogen hair. This can present as an acute onset hair loss (**acute TE**) or could be a more chronic loss of hair. The **chronic** diffuse loss of telogen hair can be an *idiopathic* pattern (**chronic TE**) or it may be *secondary* to identifiable causes (chronic diffuse telogen hair loss or **CDTHL**). The loss of hair in TE occurs primarily as a result of an abnormal shift in follicular cycling, which leads to a premature entry of hair into telogen and their subsequent shedding (Grover C et al).

EPIDEMIOLOGY

Acute TE may occur at any age, including infants and children. For reasons unknown, women are more likely to present for evaluation of acute TE than men. Chronic TE is much less common than the acute variant, and is most frequently diagnosed in women between the ages of 30 and 60 years (Grover C et al).

PATHOGENESIS

In infancy, follicular cycling is synchronous. Neighbouring hairs grow together, involute together and are shed together. Synchronous shedding produces a moult wave. Such synchronous shedding with moult wave persists indefinitely in many mammals but in humans this disappears in childhood and the hair cycle of individual hairs tend to become asynchronous. An adult human tends to lose up to 100 hairs each day, from different parts of the scalp.

Scalp hair pluck test reveals that an average of 86% of plucked hairs are in anagen, 1% in catagen and 13% are in telogen. However, if we analyze horizontal scalp biopsies, these figures are 93% of follicles in anagen and 7% in telogen (Whiting DA). This roughly means that if the average number of scalp hairs is 100,000, then 7,000 hairs should be in telogen at any one time. As the approximate duration of telogen is 100 days, about 70 hairs should be shed each day.

Telogen effluvium reflects a disturbance of the hair cycle. The shedding results in a diffuse loss over the scalp, though it may be more accentuated in the *central, frontal*, and *temporal* areas.

The hair cycle consists of distinct growth phases. The first is the anagen in which the follicle actively grows. The duration of this phase of growth is highly variable from one individual to another, depending on multiple factors including age, sex, and anatomical region. Subsequently, hair enters the catagen phase of acute irreversible follicular involution. The last phase is the telogen or resting phase, characterized by the involution of the bulb and subsequent shedding. Depending on the type of hair being shed, and the underlying mechanisms involved, we can characterize at least five functional types of effluvium:

Type I: **Immediate anagen release (premature ending of the anagen phase):** This common form of telogen effluvium starts quickly, within 3–5 weeks, and is caused by *drugs, high fever, or psychological stress*.

Type II: **Delayed anagen release:** The preceeding anagen phase is unusually **long**; this phenomenon underlies TE in the *post-partum period*.

Type III: The **short anagen phase** syndrome is characterized by a distinct but prolonged effluvium. Hair loss becomes clinically apparent only after a decrease of at least 50% of the duration of the anagen phase. This presents as *CTE* and is also seen in *androgenetic alopecia* where TE commonly precedes visible balding of the scalp.

Type IV: **Immediate telogen release:** Follicles in the telogen phase eliminate mature hair prematurely. This premature removal could be triggered by an extrinsic factor, such as a drug. It seems that such a phenomenon is triggered by local application of **minoxidil**.

Type V: **Delayed telogen release:** Extension of the telogen phase. This phenomenon allows the elimination of winter coats in some animals. It is triggered by the increased exposure to light and can be observed in a modified form in humans.

ETIOLOGICAL APPROACH TO DIAGNOSIS OF TE

The causes of TE are listed in Table 5.1. In the normal scalp, approximately 90% of the follicles will be in the anagen phase, whereas the remainder (10%) are in the telogen phase; just a few hairs will be found in the transition phase (catagen: around 50–80 hairs shed daily).

Table 5.1: A summary of etiological causes of TE

Physical and/or emotional stress	• Postpartum (physiologic) • Shedding by newborn • Post-surgical • Psychological stress • Crash dieting • Seasonal variation • UV induced
Disease	• Severe infection • High fever
Endocrine causes	Thyroid disorders
Drugs	• Acitretin • Amitriptyline • Anticholesterol—statins • β-interferon • β blockers—propranolol • Carbamazepine • Cidofovir • Danazol • Discontinuation of contraceptives • Dopamine • Heparin • Heavy metals: Thallium, arsenic, lead • Isotretinoin • Lamotrigine • Lithium • Methimazole • Minoxidil • Omeprazole • Paroxetine • Anticonvulsants: Phenytoin, valproic acid • Terbinafine
Dermatitis	ACD to hair dyes
Alopecia areata with slow progression	
Androgenetic alopecia	In a proportion of patients chronic TE may overlap with FAGA
Psychogenic pseudoeffluvium	
Other causes	HIV, CRF, cancer

The biologic clock determining the end of the anagen phase and the beginning of the catagen/telogen phase is a complex phenomenon in which multiple proteins, such as **BMP-2, BMP-4, Dkk-1, Sfrp-4, follistatin, Wnt, Wnt/β-catenin, and TGF-β,** among others, participate (Fig. 5.1). Various metabolic and physiologic changes are capable of adjusting this biologic clock within the hair follicles, and it is possible for abnormally large number of hair entering the telogen phase simultaneously, causing profound hair loss. This begins approximately 3 or 4 months after a physical or emotional event. In the case of infection or drugs, hair loss can start earlier (Table 5.1).

The most common causes of TE are **physiologic postpartum or post-surgical processes, infections, and drugs** (Table 5.1). Other causes

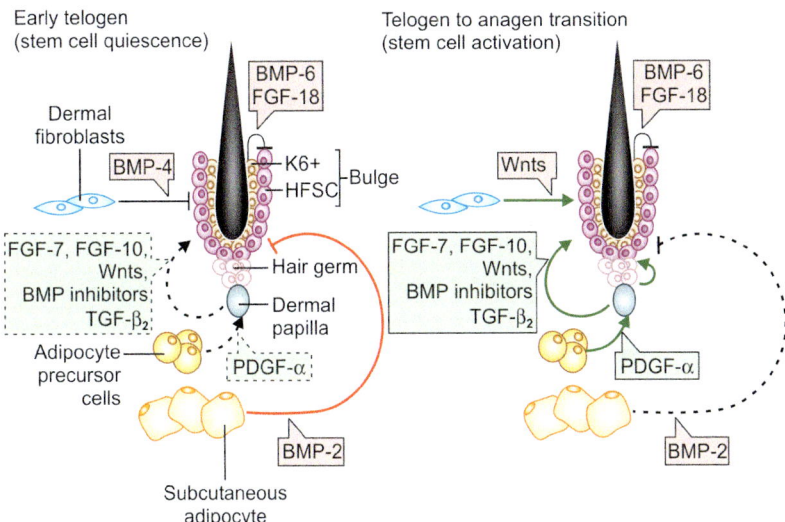

Fig. 5.1: Hair follicle stem cells (HFSCs) reside in the outer bulge layer. Keratin 6 expressing (K6+) inner bulge cells are downstream progeny of HFSCs and express high levels of bone morphogenic protein 6 (BMP-6) and fibroblast growth factor 18 (FGF-18), which are quiescence inducing factors for HFSCs. During telogen, subcutaneous adipocytes express BMP-2 and dermal fibroblasts express BMP-4. Near the end of the resting phase, the dermal papilla produces HFSC-activating factors, including FGF-7 and FGF-10, BMP inhibitors and transforming growth factor β_2 (TGF-β_2) to counteract the inhibitory effects on the niche. TMEFF-1 (transmembrane protein with EGF-like and follistatin-like domains 1) is induced in hair germ cells by TGF-β_2 to dampen the suppressive effects of BMPs. In addition, adipocyte precursor cells secrete platelet derived growth factor-β (PDGF-β) to induce the expression of as-yet-unidentified activating factors in the dermal papilla. The macroenvironment of the underlying dermis also participates, progressing to a BMP low and Wnt high state

include UV radiation on the hair; seasonal changes (e.g. peak incidence from July to October); crash diets; iron deficiency; and triggers like contact sensitizers, such as hair dyes, which lead to lipid, keratin, melanin damage, promoting apoptosis, and hair loss.

CLINICAL FEATURES

The diagnosis of TE is based on the clinical presentation and the confirmation of excess telogen hair loss. The specific time of onset is important to establish the diagnosis.

TE can start **2 weeks** after a trigger but **peaks** between **6 and 8 weeks** and then tapers off in about **6–8 weeks** if the trigger is removed or treated.

The onset and history of hair loss should be determined; abrupt onset of TE is generally associated with a specific factor. However, a more *gradual* onset may reflect **short anagen phase syndrome** and one should rule out other conditions like alopecia areata, androgenic alopecia, and diffuse scarring alopecia.

The hair and scalp surface should be inspected carefully. Normally, the hair diameter is uniform, and less than 10% of hair are of a reduced diameter. This helps differentiate it from androgenetic alopecia.

Acute TE (ATE)

The trigger factor for acute TE generally precedes the excessive loss of hair by **2–4 months**. The sudden baldness predominant on the *temples* (Fig. 5.2) is reversible over the next **4–6 months** (Fiedler VC, Gray AC). The functional mechanism of shedding in these cases is *immediate anagen release*. Hair loss is usually less than 50% of scalp hair. The diffuse hair loss from the scalp may produce thinning of hair all over the scalp, but frequently manifests with a *symmetrical bitemporal thinning*.

The **main causes** for ATE are:

- An important **psychological stress** (a serious accident, death, divorce, etc.). There is no evidence to suggest that the stresses of everyday life are sufficient to induce diffuse hair loss.
- **Dietary inadequacies,** especially if a "healthy balanced diet" is not being taken.
- Acute hemorrhage, shock, or acute iron deficiency.
- Childbirth, miscarriage, or termination of breastfeeding (restoration of the normal cycling pattern may not occur in some).

   Telogen gravidarum/postpartum TE refers to this telogen hair loss seen 2–3 months after childbirth and is an example of delayed anagen release. It is universal but variable in severity and is often

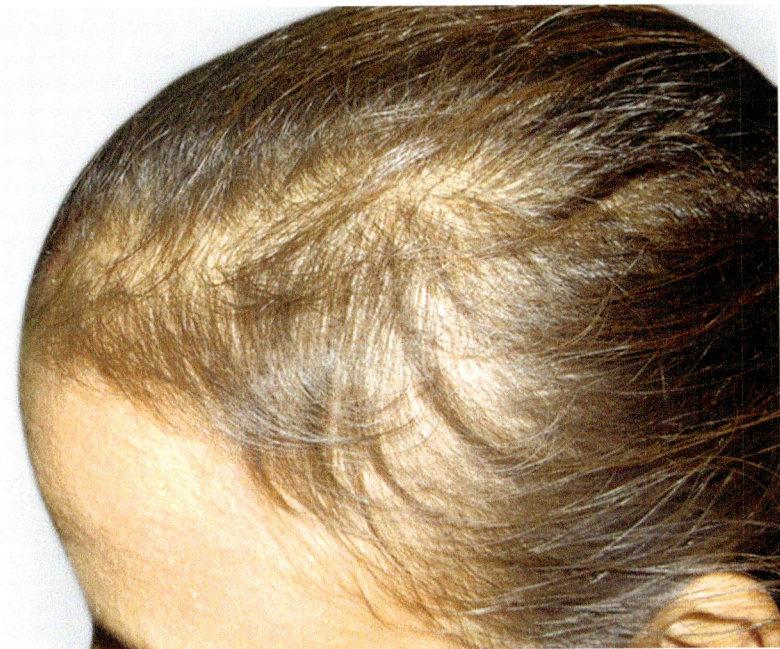

Fig. 5.2: A young girl with ATE. There was history of markedly increased hair shedding for the past two months. The frontal and temporal recession is marked in this case

subclinical. Recent literature has however cast a doubt on the existence and incidence of this disorder (Reborah 2016, Gizlenti 2014, Marallas 2016), claiming lack of scientific evidence (Lynfield 1960). The cause may be the synchronization of hair growth in pregnancy. Most women will return to their usual hair growth cycle between **6 to 12 months** after birth. Postpartum hair loss usually returns the hair to pre-pregnancy thickness, unless it leads to female androgenetic alopecia.

Persistent postpartum effluvium (>12 months postpartum), refers to an excessive hair loss which may be caused by common conditions, such as female androgenetic alopecia, iron deficiency, or hypothyroidism. Lesser common conditions include persistent hyperprolactinemia (Chiari–Frommel syndrome) and postpartum hypopituitarism (Sheehan syndrome) caused by pituitary necrosis due to blood loss and hypovolemic shock during childbirth.

- **Seasonal hair loss:** On the basis of changes seen in different phases of the hair cycle; Headington had proposed a delayed telogen—release type of telogen effluvium, in which hair follicles remain in prolonged telogen rather than being shed and recycled into anagen.

When teloptosis finally sets in, the clinical sign of increased shedding of club hairs is observed. This process underlies moulting in mammals and probably also seasonal shedding of hairs in humans or mild TE following travel from low-daylight to high-daylight conditions.

A comprehensive study by Kunz et al, otherwise healthy women with TE seen over a period of 6 years, demonstrated the existence of an overall annual periodicity in the growth and shedding of hair, manifested by a maximal proportion of *telogen* hairs being seen in **July**. Assuming a telogen phase duration of approximately 100 days, one would expect shedding of these hairs by autumn (Fig. 5.3). In **India,** it is our observation that a marked hair fall occurs in the monsoon period (August/September), not in October as would be predicted by the maximum telogen levels in July. A second peak of telogen hair loss seems to exist, although less pronounced, in the month of April.

From an evolutionary point of view, the maintenance of the low winter level of hair shedding and the postponement of hair fall until the end of summer might, perhaps, be postulated as having a selective advantage with respect to isolation of the head against the cold in winter and protection of the scalp against the midday sun in summer.

- Camacho et al reported a peculiar type of TE following **sunburn of the scalp,** after 3 to 4 months, with hairstyles that left areas of scalp

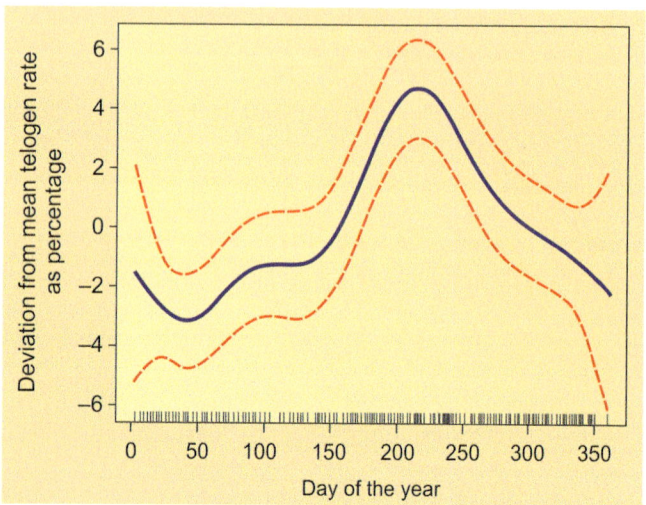

Fig. 5.3: Fluctuations in frontal telogen rates in a 823 patients in relation to the day of the year (Kunz et al, 2009)

uncovered during prolonged sun exposure. The clinical features were increased frontovertical hair shedding along with a trichogram that revealed an increase of telogen hairs and dystrophic hairs. In women, the hairs on the frontal region appeared unruly and the frontovertical alopecia showed loss of the frontal hair implantation line.

The pathomechanisms of this type of TE is not clear. It has been proposed that the columns of the cells in the hair shaft act as an efficient fiberoptic-type system, transmitting UV light downward into the hair follicle. Morphologically, the keratinocytes within the hair shaft are arranged in compressed linear columns that resemble the coaxial bundles of commercial fiberoptic strands. Thus, hair follicular melanocytes located in the region of the hair matrix may function as UV biosensors and respond to photonic inputs. Depending on the quantity of UVR exposure, it is conceivable that photodamage may occur at this site, resulting in TE (Camacho et al).

- **Contact allergic dermatitis:** ATE may be induced by allergic contact dermatitis to hair dyes, particularly to paraphenylenediamine. In these cases, patch testing will reveal the culprit.
- Recent medical illness with hyperthermia greater than **39.5°C** is associated with ATE.
- Recent **surgery** under general anesthesia.
- Recent **hair transplant surgery**.
- **Food alopecia** may be related to the ingestion of various kinds of plants containing cytostatic ingredients or antimetabolites (such as **cashews**).
- Alopecia due to occupational **poisoning** has been reported with drugs such as thallium (used in rat poison), borax (detergents), chloroprene (rubber), or arsenic.
- **Drugs:** There is a marked individual susceptibility to drug induced hair loss. If a particular drug is suspected, testing involves stopping it for at least **3 months**. Regrowth following discontinuation and recurrence on re-exposure to the drug supports the conclusion that the drug caused the alopecia. Dose-related diffuse telogen hair loss is common with acitretin but less common with isotretinoin. This class of drugs appears to cause a telogen anchorage defect and reduce the duration of anagen. *Importantly*, patients who complain of continued retinoid-induced TE, *long* after the retinoid has been *stopped*, often have coincidental **androgenetic alopecia**.
- Radiotherapy is responsible for a reversible or permanent alopecia depending on the dose delivered.

Chronic Diffuse Telogen Hair Loss (CDTHL)

Chronic diffuse telogen hair loss (CDTHL) (Messenger AG et al) refers to telogen hair shedding persisting for longer than 6 months. It is secondary to a variety of causes and may co-exist with female pattern hair loss. When no triggering/underlying cause of chronic telogen loss is found, it is labeled as CTE. Chronic diffuse alopecia can derive from persistence of acute alopecia, or have a general endocrine or metabolic cause (Whiting DA,1999). Please remember that in a case of chronic telogen loss where *no other cause* is found a very likely cause could be the coexistence of *androgenetic alopecia*.

The typical patient is a vigorous otherwise healthy woman between 30 and 60 with a full, thick head of hair (Fig. 5.4). On examination, there is some bitemporal thinning and a positive hair pull test, equally over the vertex and occiput. There is no widening of the central part, as is common in androgenetic alopecia. The patients are remarkably distressed and may bring large balls of hair for inspection. There is a marked seasonal periodicity in the growth and shedding of hair with maximal proportion of telogen hair loss at the end of summer and the beginning of autumn.

The mechanisms implicated include synchronization phenomena of the hair cycle, shortening of the anagen phase, or premature teloptosis.

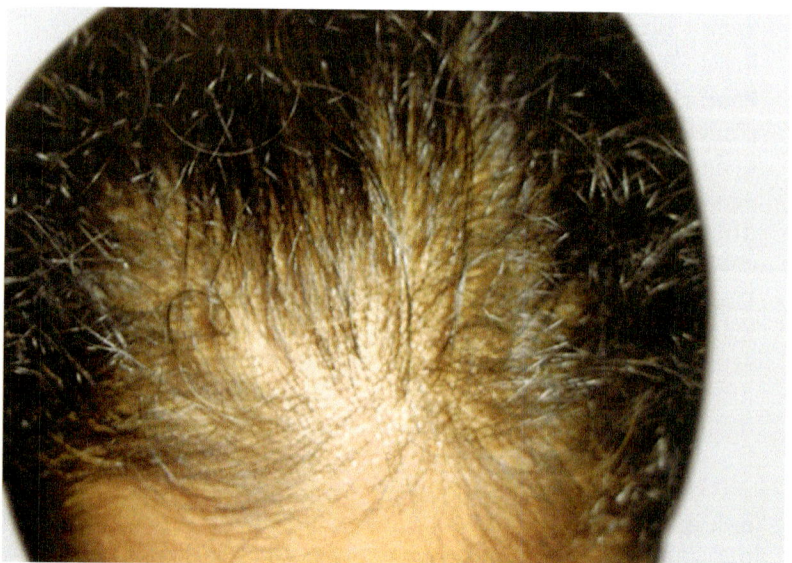

Fig. 5.4: A 40-year-old lady with history of increased hair shedding over the past one year. The patient had CTE unmasking a marked thinning of frontal hair, due to coexistent female androgenetic alopecia

Endocrine Causes

Hair cycle is dependent on many endocrinological factors:
- *Hyperthyroidism:* Hair is thin and brittle, appearing silky.
- *Hypothyroidism:* Diffuse alopecia sometimes along with eyebrow loss, axillary and pubic hair loss, and nail brittleness.
- *Hypoparathyroidism:* Hair is fine and the nails opaque, lined, and brittle.
- *Hypopituitarism:* The skin is pale and associated with fine and dry hair.
- *Hyperadrenocorticism:* There is associated hirsutism in women.
- Uncontrolled diabetes
- Cushing syndrome
- Acromegaly
- *Hyperprolactinemia*
- Perimenopausal hormone changes. There are a large number of middle aged females who complain of hair loss. A possible reason could be that the inherent hormonal fluctuations alter the circadian control genes leading to hair loss (Mirmirani P).

Metabolic and Nutritional Causes

These cause the hair to become thin, brittle, and dull. Though there is a differing view on the role of nutritional levels and TE, a recent study by Cheung EJ et al opined that **vitamin D, ferritin**, and **zinc deficiencies** may have a role to play in hair loss.
- Iron deficiency is best studied by the serum levels of ferritin rather than by determining serum iron. Serum ferritin levels less than 30 µg/L can precipitate a telogen hair loss. Profound iron deficiency anemia can cause a diffuse telogen hair loss that is corrected by iron replacement. The relationship between iron deficiency with no anemia or only mild anemia and chronic diffuse hair loss is, however, more complex and controversial (Rushton DH, Sinclair R, 2002, Hard S). If and how iron deficiency without anemia predisposes to hair loss has been a controversial topic being researched for decades, but without a fool proof answer yet. Some authors have persistently stated its role (Rushton et al, 1990, 1992, 2002, 2003), while others have refuted these claims (Sinclair 2001, Olsen 2010). Depending on how it is defined, low iron stores are a common finding in women of child-bearing age. Bregy and Trueb evaluated the relationship between serum ferritin levels and hair loss activity determined by trichograms, in a retrospective case study of 181 women with hair loss (2008) undergoing biochemical investigations and trichograms. 61.9% had a ferritin level >**30 µg/L**, 30.4% between 10 and **30 µg/L**, and 7.7% ≤**10 µg/L**, and *no*

correlation was found between ferritin levels >**10 µg/ml** and telogen rates. A summary of the cut-off levels of ferritin and the parameters for diagnosing iron deficiency anemia are given below to help diagnose overt anemia in patients (Table 5.2). Normal serum ferritin levels are taken to be 18–270 µg/L in men and 18–160 µg/L in women.

- Folate deficiency or vitamin B$_{12}$ deficiency.
- Vitamin D deficiency.
- Zinc deficiency (acrodermatitis enteropathica).
- Nutritional deficiencies associated with dieting, malabsorption syndromes, parenteral nutrition.
- Kidney failure, liver failure.

Rare Causes

- Systemic lupus erythematosus causes frontal, non-scarring hair loss and thinning, known as lupus hair.
- Secondary syphilis causes "patchy" alopecia that differs from other alopecias. It has many bald patches scattered from 1 to 3 cm in diameter, like a "clumsy scissors" cut on the temporoparietal regions.
- External or traumatic causes (frequent brushings, hairstyles that involve the hair being pulled backwards, or chemicals (dyes and repeated "perm" styling).
- Psychological causes (emotional stress, bereavement) can take over from organic causes.

Table 5.2: Diagnosis of iron depletion*				
Age	Serum ferritin (µg/L)	% of serum ferritin values below cut-off	% of transferrin receptor values above cut-off	Interpretation
5 years of age or older	<15			
5 years of age or older	<15	Lower than 20%	Lower than 10%	Iron deficiency is *not* prevalent
		Lower than 20%	10% or higher	Iron deficiency is *prevalent* Inflammation is prevalent
		20% or higher	Lower than 10%	Iron deficiency is *prevalent*

*Modified: WHO/NMH/NHD/MNM/11.2: Serum ferritin concentrations for the assessment of iron status and iron deficiency in populations.

Idiopathic

Diffuse alopecia without obvious cause **(idiopathic)** has been reported in **5–40%** of cases in various series.

Chronic Telogen Effluvium

Chronic telogen effluvium (CTE) is an idiopathic and sometimes self-limiting condition affecting middle-aged women that is distinct from androgenetic hair loss and chronic diffuse TE secondary to organic causes (CDTHL) (Whiting DA, 1996). Women describe this as a sudden onset of increased hair shedding persisting for at least 6 months.

There is *no* associated visible widening of the central parting line, nor is there any miniaturization of hair follicles on scalp biopsy. CTE contrasts with the acute form of TE by its prolonged fluctuating course. It occurs mainly in **women** aged between 30 and 50 years. Hair shedding is much less obvious in males with short hair, and for unknown reasons, few males with long hair present with increased hair shedding (Thai KE). Although some cases of CTE follow an ATE with an identified trigger, such as pregnancy or systemic illness, in most cases **no trigger** can be identified. Any of the functional types of TE could account for CTE but it is believed to be related to a reduction in the variation of anagen duration without any reduction in the mean duration of the anagen phase of the hair cycle (Gilmore S).

Trichodynia or scalp dysaesthesia may accompany CTE although it is not specific to this condition. The mechanism is unknown. Treatment is difficult, but many cases respond to measures to reduce hair shedding such as minoxidil.

INVESTIGATIONS

Telogen effluvium is a clinical diagnosis. However, the clinical suspicion needs to be confirmed in some cases, especially if other causes of hairloss, especially patterned hairloss, are coexisting.

1. Hair Pull Test (Shrivastava SB)

Hair pull test aids in the recognition of active hair shedding. Approximately 30–60 hairs are grasped between the thumb, index and middle fingers from the base of the hairs near the scalp and firmly, but not forcefully, tugged away from the scalp. If more than 10% hairs are pulled away from the scalp, this constitutes a positive pull test and implies active hair shedding. The patient must not shampoo for at least a day prior to the pull test. The pull test has to be performed in several areas of the scalp (Fig. 5.5).

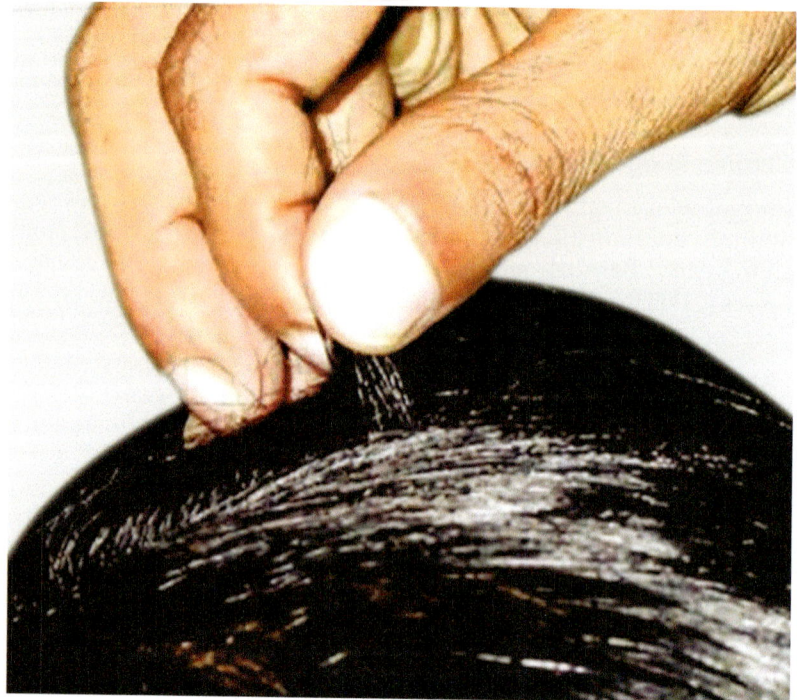

Fig. 5.5: Pull test: Approximately 60 hairs are grasped from the proximal portion of the scalp and tugged from the proximal to the distal end

Examination of the hair shafts under a light microscope or trichoscope (trichoscopic trichogram) is then used to confirm that the shed hairs are telogen hairs. Increased telogen hair, both in occipital and mid-scalp areas, is suggestive of TE (Fig. 5.6).

Of note, a false-negative hair pull test can occur if the patient has shampooed or vigorously groomed the hair on the day of examination. Conversely, a false-positive hair pull test may be noted if the patient has not shampooed or combed the hair for several days.

2. Hair Counts (Shrivastava SB)

Hair count is a very subjective although easy to perform and inexpensive test. It is neither standardized nor diagnostic. No clinical study or standardized method has validated the acceptable physiological hair loss per day (although 100 hairs are taken arbitrarily). However, hair counts are useful to the physician to help quantify how much the patient is losing and make sure that this is not more than the physiologic hair loss. It also helps to monitor and assess treatment response.

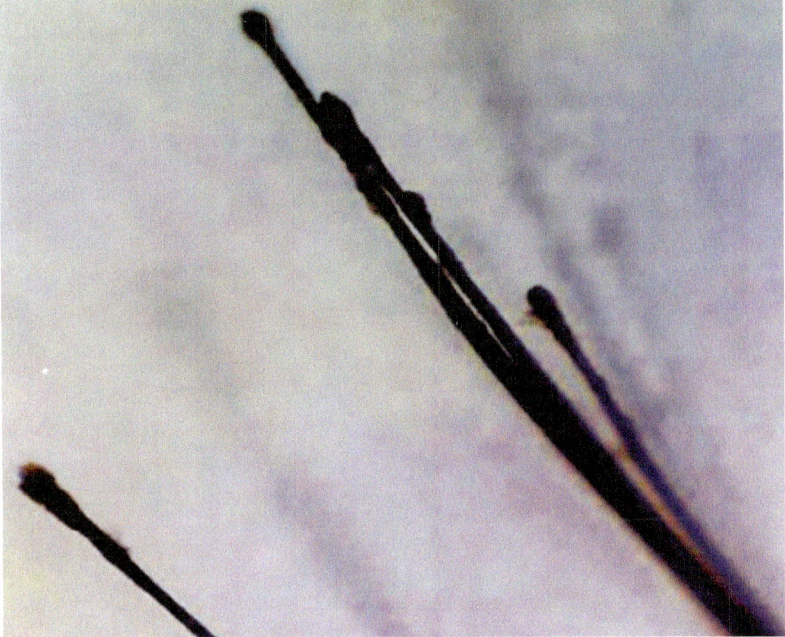

Fig. 5.6: Trichoscopic trichogram: Increased telogen hair, both in occipital and mid-scalp areas, is suggestive of TE

Daily Hair Count

Patients are instructed to collect hairs shed in one day, count them and place them in plastic bags. All shed hairs in the shower or sink or on the brush are collected. Daily hair counts for at least 7 days are maintained (Fig. 5.7). It is expected to lose more hairs on shampoo days. If the patient is losing more than 100 hairs per day, the hair should be examined microscopically to detect the pathology in hair bulb and hair shaft abnormalities. Appearance of the hair bulb can distinguish between TE, anagen effluvium and active diffuse alopecia areata.

Standardized Wash Test

The patient refrains from shampooing for 5 days and then he/she shampoos and rinses the hair in the basin with the hole covered by gauze. The hairs remaining in the water and the gauze are collected, counted and examined. Shedding of more than 100 hair with <10% shed hair being <3 cm suggests CTE. Shedding of >100 hair with >10% being 3 cm or shorter suggest co-existence of CTE and FPHL.

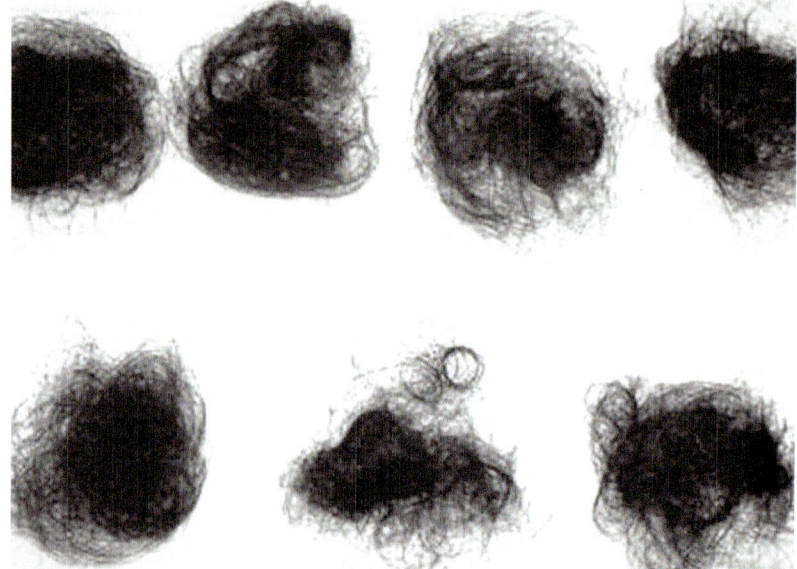

Fig. 5.7: Daily hair count: Collected hairs of 7 days

60-Second Hair Count

Before shampooing, the patient is instructed to comb hair for one minute over a pillow or sheet of color contrasting to that of the hair, starting with the comb at the back top of the scalp and moving the comb forward to the front of the scalp. The procedure is repeated on next 3 alternate days, using the same comb or brush. The number of hairs in the comb or brush and on the pillow are counted and recorded. The above procedure can be repeated monthly for monitoring purposes.

3. Trichoscopy

This may be a helpful test for a better diagnosis of the etiology. In cases with TE, no characteristic findings are seen on trichoscopic examination. A decrease in hair density and empty follicles can be seen (Fig. 5.8). Numerous regrowing hair can often be visualized. Nevertheless, the importance of trichoscopic examination is in ruling out androgenetic alopecia (AGA) (typically shows hair diameter diversity) (Fig. 5.9) and alopecia areata incognito (shows characteristic findings of alopecia areata) (Miteva M at el). It may also help in identifying other possible causes of hair loss, e.g. mild seborrheic dermatitis which may not be evident to naked eye.

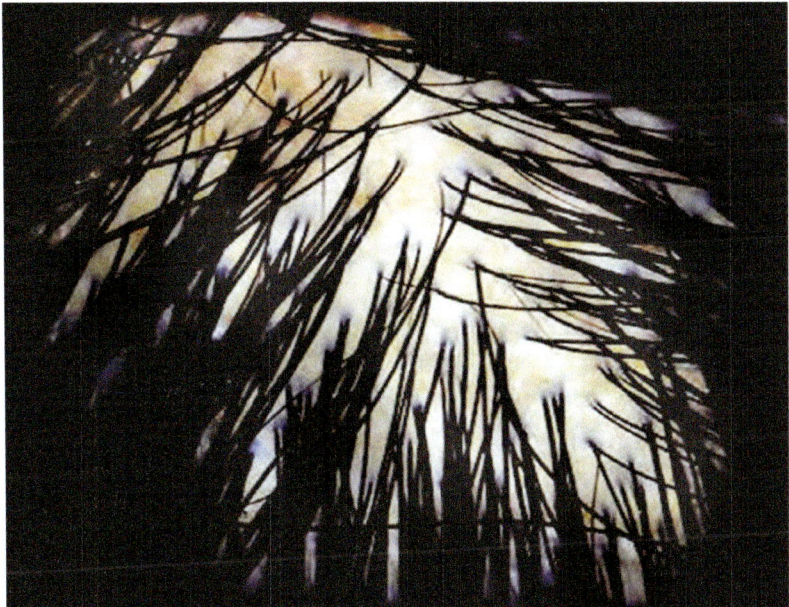

Fig. 5.8: Trichoscopy shows decrease in density of hair. However, the hairs are of normal thickness and there is no diversity of hair diameter

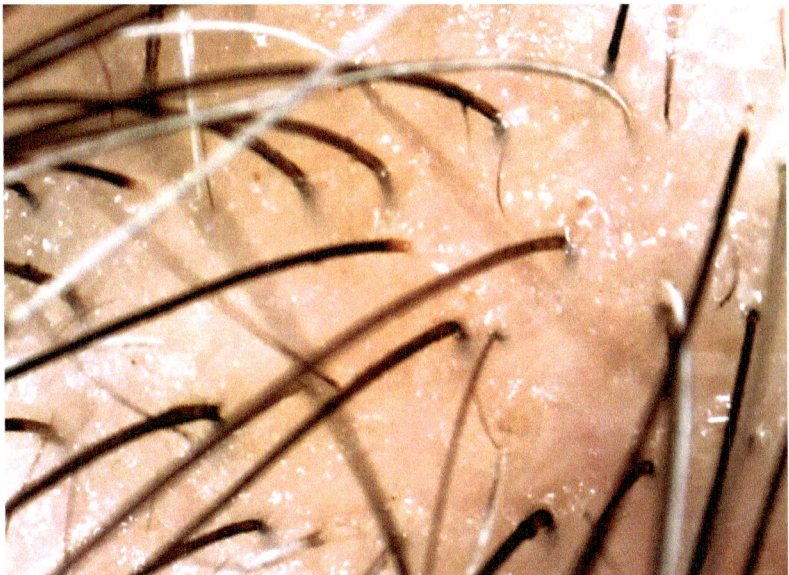

Fig. 5.9: Trichoscopy of the temporal area in a patient with chronic diffuse telogen hair loss. There is reduced hair density with some regrowing hair. The hair shaft diameter variability suggests androgenetic hair loss as well

4. Trichogram

This test is used to detail hair loss and indicate its intensity. Although, it can help confirm TE, it is rarely perfomed clinically (Figs 5.10 and 5.11).

A digital phototrichogram can be used; it is useful to assess changes in hair density as well. The presence of numerous dystrophic anagen hairs suggests a diagnosis of anagen effluvium.

5. Scalp Biopsy

It is indicated when the diameter of the hair is reduced (possible androgenetic alopecia) or when there is doubt about the presence of an inflammatory alopecia (alopecia areata).

Scalp biopsy is usually not needed or done for TE, but is the most definitive way to diagnose it. Two biopsies, one for horizontal sectioning and one for vertical sectioning are preferably taken. An increased proportion of telogen follicles is the key histopathological finding. Proportion of telogen follicles more than 15% suggests TE but more than 25% is a definitive feature. Scalp biopsy also helps to rule out FPHL and alopecia areata. Unlike AGA, the proportion of vellus hair follicles is not increased in TE. A biopsy of chronic TE will show an anagen–telogen ratio (A:T) of 8:1 compared with 14:1 from normal scalp (Headington JT). However, by the time a biopsy is done

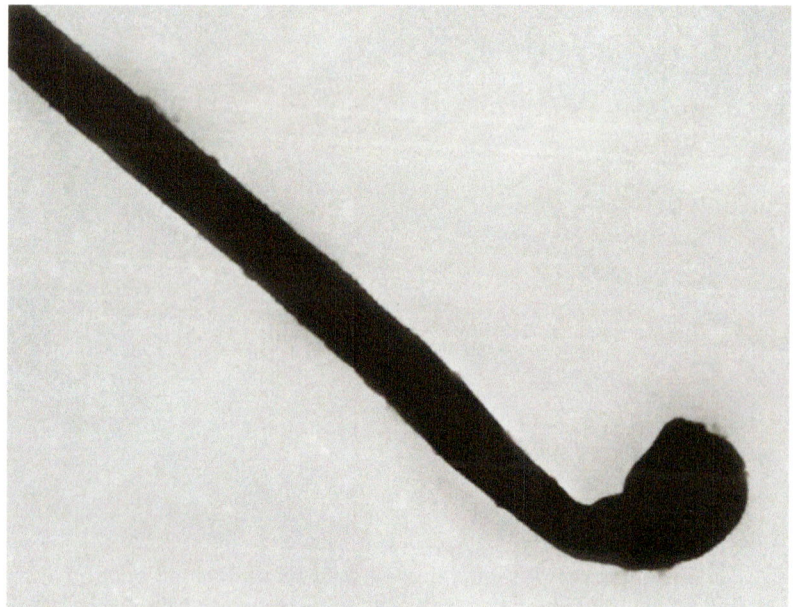

Fig. 5.10: Trichogram showing an anagen hair bulb

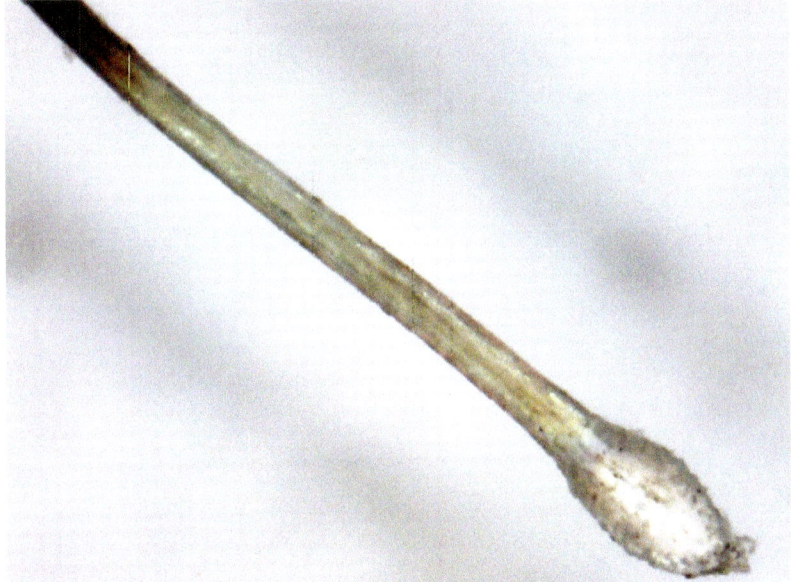

Fig. 5.11: Trichogram showing a telogen hair bulb

in ATE, there may be an increased proportion of follicles in the anagen phase as the telogen hair may have already been shed. Such a finding may thus be misleading.

Scalp biopsies from patients with TE do not demonstrate inflammation, unless it is incited by an inflammatory condition, where it demonstrates histopathological findings consistent with that of the inciting disorder (Headington JT).

6. Other Laboratory Tests

A detailed history and clinical examination help detect the cause of TE in most cases. However, in most cases, a minimum battery of laboratory tests should be performed. The commonly performed tests are listed in Table 5.3. Hormonal tests may be needed to rule out hyperandrogenemia which may cause FAGA/FPHL which frequently overlaps with CTE.

DIFFERENTIAL DIAGNOSIS

AGA: A characteristic patterned hair loss and presence of miniaturized hairs on clinical examination suggests this diagnosis. It can be further confirmed by documenting hair shaft diameter diversity on trichoscopic examination. A biopsy can be useful for differentiating between these diagnoses in difficult cases. Histological differentiation

Table 5.3: A simplified approach to investigate a hair loss patient

Increased hair shedding

Serum ferritin (and C-reactive protein)		<10–30 µg/L** (abnormal)
Transferrin		
Vitamin B$_{12}$ (ng/L) 300–1000		<200, >1,500
Folic acid (nmol/L) 5–40		>45 (abnormal)
Thyroid-stimulating hormone		Hypothyroidism

Diffuse hair loss

Free androgen index	>5	HA
Prolactin	25–200 ng/ml	>100 ng/ml
AMH*	2–7	Abnormal >4.5: PCOS
USG*	Transvaginal	PCOS, tumors

*Associated acne/hirsutism; HA: Hyperandrogenemia** Please *see* text (Page 79)

is possible on the basis of follicular miniaturization, the hallmark of AGA. A Terminal: Vellus ratio of less than 4:1 is considered pathognomonic of AGA, whereas a ratio greater than 8:1 indicates CTE. Also, the two conditions may coexist, and telogen hair shedding can occur early in the course of AGA.

Diffuse alopecia areata: In these cases, hair pull test (revealing dystrophic anagen hairs and telogen hairs) can help. Trichoscopic examination shows classical features and when in doubt, a scalp biopsy can reliably differentiate it from TE.

Anagen effluvium: An associated drug history, normal hair pull tests or the presence of dystrophic anagen hairs rather than telogen hairs points towards this diagnosis.

Loose anagen syndrome: In these cases, examination of shed hair reveals predominance of anagen hairs (≥70%) devoid of the outer (ORS) and inner root sheath (IRS) and with 'floppy sock appearance' on trichogram (a characteristic feature). On histopathology, the characteristic findings are clefting between IRS, IRS and ORS, ORS and fibrous sheath and lack of inflammation.

Structural hair disorders: These are associated with easy breakage of the hair. Thus, a history of breakage of hairs rather than intact shedding of hair with a bulbous end, is characteristic. Additionally, diagnostic findings of a particular structural hair disorder on trichoscopy (usually at a higher magnification) helps differentiate these from TE.

Psychogenic pseudoeffluvium: TE must be differentiated from psychogenic pseudoeffluvium in which the patient seeking advice for hair loss is not necessarily balding. Normal dense scalp hair and absence of any clinically convincing evidence of hair loss is regarded as the feature of imaginary hair loss or psychogenic pseudoeffluvium. In these cases, patients might need psychological counseling and consultation.

COURSE AND PROGRESSION

The progression of TE typically follows one of two courses (Headington JT).

- *Acute TE:* This is generally self-limiting, usually resolves once the triggering agent or the underlying cause is identified, removed or treated accordingly. Hair shedding takes about 3–6 months to cease, and simultaneously, hair regrowth can be noted. However, cosmetically significant regrowth may take up to 12–18 months.
- *Chronic TE:* Some of these patients develop a chronic-repetitive pattern of TE in which the chronic TE is punctuated by additional episodes of acute hair loss. With continued telogen hair loss, stimulated regrowth is also seen and overall a new balance is established between the two. There is overall reduction in hair density, reported as a thinning of ponytail or plait. However, there are no evident areas of balding or patterns.

MANAGEMENT

Most cases with ATE, particularly those associated with acute-onset events, like febrile illness, or parturition; or cases with mild seasonal TE; or the shedding upon initiation of topical minoxidil, are self-limiting and undergo normal reversal. Such patients can be counseled and reassured about the benign nature of hair loss after confirming the diagnosis.

For cases with chronic diffuse telogen hair loss, if the hair loss persists inspite of an extensive search for possible causes, a combination with female androgenetic alopecia should be considered. Ikeda and Yamada originally pointed out that the risk of developing TE increases in the presence of androgenetic alopecia.

A long list of possible causes for chronic diffuse telogen hair loss has been discussed above. Of these, **4 important ones** are: Systemic causes (e.g. iron deciency, thyroid dysfunction, systemic lupus erythematosus, or syphilis); intake of drugs; altered dietary habits; and seasonal variation. In our experience a profound hair loss is noticed in July to September in Delhi, which corresponds to the monsoon season. This probably could be the effect of sunlight and UV flux, that effects the biological clock to maintain hairgrowth during the summers. The medical measures given below may not be the "know it all" truth of TE, but in most cases, if the 4 factors above are excluded, most of the nutraceutical laced oral medicines may probably be working largely as a placebo.

Medical Line of Management

Evidence-based recommendations for treatment of primary CTE are scanty. Few reports exist about the usage of topical or systemic **corticosteroids,** topical **minoxidil,** and **dietary supplements** [including millet extracts, pantothenic acid, biotin, their combination, or combinations of L-cystine, medicinal yeast, and pantothenic acid (**CYP complex**)].

Topical Agents

Topical **minoxidil** can be used in CTE, as it promotes hair growth by prolonging anagen and shortening telogen, in an attempt to maintain hair density and stimulate regrowth of hair. Minoxidil 2% is applied twice daily to the entire scalp while 5% is usually used once per day. Minoxidil has to be used minimum of 1 year before concluding its infectiveness. Treatment must be continued indefinitely to maintain benefit (Sinclair R).

Hair growth **serums** containing biochanin, acetyl tetrapeptide-3 and other peptides can be of help during the acute shedding phase though sound scientific evidence is lacking. The diagram in Fig. 5.11 depicts the factors that "switch" telogen to anagen and unless hair serums demonstrate *in vitro* or preferably *in vivo* proof of their action via those factors, their use borders on a likely placebo effect.

Another useful agent is human placenta extract* which has a molecular basis for hair growth (*see* Chapter 14 page 315).

Oral Supplements

Iron: Dietary modification or oral iron supplementation for patients with TE can be considered, so as to obtain and maintain serum levels of ferritin well within the reference range (at least 70 µg/L); however, additional studies are necessary to clarify whether iron supplementation is of any benefit for non-anemic patients with TE. Olsen et al had compared the extent of iron deficiency in controls versus patients of TE and FPHL. They found that though iron deficiency is common in women in general, it is not much increased in patients with FPHL or CTE as compared to controls. Rushton has maintained that if a female patient of CTE has a level of ferritin lower than the low cut-off value for males, the patient should be treated with iron supplements. Based on available evidence if a female patient of TE has a serum ferritin

---

*Personal communication Dr PK Sharma.

<10 µg/L, oral iron supplements may help. However, in patients with no overt deficiency, the iron supplementation may also be beneficial, though no clear-cut evidence is available to support this. Finally, a caveat should be spoken against uncritical iron supplementation, since there is a possibility that increased iron storage could enhance DNA oxidative injury by inducing the Fenton reaction.

Other vitamins and sulfur containing AA

The impact of other supplements such as zinc (in the absence of symptomatic zinc deficiency), biotin, and vitamin D on TE is unclear (Feidler VC et al).

We have mentioned the role of CYP complex and there is a general belief that sulfur containing AA supplements has a beneficial effect in some cases of TE, but concrete data are lacking.

Psychological Support

The most important aspect in the management of TE is reassurance and counseling. The patient's concerns should be addressed by the clinician in a sensitive manner. The patient should be educated about the natural history of the condition explaining hair growth cycle and the expected course of TE (including an explanation that complete hair loss is not expected to occur). Follow-up evaluations can be helpful for reassuring the patient as well as for identifying patients who require further evaluation because of persistent TE.

Camouflage

Hair styling techniques, scalp coloring, and hair prostheses can be useful for camouflaging hair loss. Hair transplantation is not indicated for patients with TE (Sinclair R).

Treatment for inciting agent or disorder should be sought for in every case of TE.

Bibliography

1. Bregy A, Trueb RM. No association between serum ferritin levels >10 µg/L and hair loss activity in women. Dermatology 2008;217:1–6.
2. Camacho F, Moreno JC, Garcia-Hernández MJ. Telogen alopecia from UV rays. Arch Dermatol 1996;132:1398–99.
3. Cheung EJ, Sink JR, English Iii JC. Vitamin and Mineral Deficiencies in Patients with Telogen Effluvium: A Retrospective Cross-sectional Study. J Drugs Dermatol 2016 Oct 1;15(10):1235–37.
4. Dhurat R, Saraogi P. Hair Evaluation Methods: Merits and Demerits. International Journal of Trichology 2009;1(2):108–19.

5. Feidler VC, Hafeez A. Diffuse alopecia. Telogen hair loss. In: Olsen EA, editor. Disorders of hair growth, diagnosis and treatment. New York: McGraw-Hill 1994;p. 241–55.

6. Gilmore S, Sinclair R. Chronic telogen effluvium is due to a reduction in the variance of anagen duration. Australas J Dermatol 2010;51:163–7.

7. Gizlenti S, Ekmekci TR. The changes in the hair cycle during gestation and the post-partum period. J Eur Acad Dermatol Venereol Jul 2014;28(7):878–81.

8. Grover C, Khurana A. "Telogen Effluvium": Indian Journal of Dermatology, Venereology and Leprology 2013;79(5):591–603.

9. Hard S. Nonanemic iron deficiency as an etiologic factor in diffuse loss of hair of the scalp in women. Acta Derm Venereol 1963;43:562–9.

10. Headington JT. TE: New concepts and review. Arch Dermatol 1993; 129:356–63.

11. Ikeda T, Yamada M. Both telogen efuvium and traction alopecia mainly occur in patients with a condition of alopecia prematura. Acta Dermatol (Kyoto) 1967;62:47.

12. Kunz M, Seifert B, Trüeb RM. Seasonality of hair shedding in healthy women complaining of hair loss. Dermatology 2009;219:105–10.

13. Lynfield YL. Effect of pregnancy on the human hair cycle. J Invest Dermatol 1960;35:323–327.

14. Messenger AG, Sinclair RD, Farrant P, Berker DAR de. Acquired Disorders of Hair. Part 8, ch 89 http://www.rooksdermatology.com/: Accessed on 13/6/27.

15. Mirallas O, Grimalt R. The Postpartum Telogen Effluvium Fallacy. Skin Appendage Disord May 2016;1(4):198–201.

16. Mirmirani P. Hormones and clocks: Do they disrupt the locks? Fluctuating estrogen levels during menopausal transition may influence clock genes and trigger chronic telogen effluvium. Dermatol Online J. 2016 May 15;22(5).

17. Miteva M, Tosti A. Hair and scalp dermatoscopy. J Am Acad Dermatol 2012;67:1040.

18. Olsen EA. Disorders of Hair Growth—Diagnosis and Treatment. New York, NY: McGraw-Hill; 1997.

19. Olsen EA, Reed KB, Cacchio PB, Caudill L. Iron deficiency in female pattern hair loss, chronic telogen effluvium, and control groups. J Am Acad Dermatol Dec 2010;63(6):991–9.

20. Rebora A, Guarrera M, Drago F. Postpartum telogen effluvium. J Eur Acad Dermatol Venereol Mar 2016;30(3):518.

21. Rushton DH, Ramsay ID, James KC, Norris MJ, Gilkes JJ. Biochemical and trichological characterization of diffuse alopecia in women. Br J Dermatol 1990;123:187–97.

22. Rushton DH, Norris MJ, Dover R, Busuttil N. Causes of hair loss and the developments in hair rejuvenation. Int J Cosmet Sci 2002;24:17–23.

23. Rushton DH. Nutritional factors and hair loss. Clin Exp Dermatol 2002;27:396–404.

24. Rushton DH, Norris MJ, Dover R, Busuttil N. Causes of hair loss and the developments in hair rejuvenation. Int J Cosmet Sci. 2002 Feb;24(1):17–23.

25. Rushton DH, Ramsay ID. The importance of adequate serum ferritin levels during oral cyproterone acetate and ethinyl oestradiol treatment of diffuse androgen-dependent alopecia in women. Clin Endocrinol (Oxf) 1992 Apr;36(4):421–7.

26. SB Shrivastava. "Diffuse hair loss in an adult female: Approach to diagnosis and management." Indian Journal of Dermatology, Venereology and Leprology 2009;75(1):20–28.

27. Sinclair R. Chronic TE. A study of 5 patients over 7 years. J Am Acad Dermatol 2005;52:12.

28. Sinclair R. There is no clear association between low serum ferritin and chronic diffuse telogen hair loss. Br J Dermatol 2002;147:982–4.

29. Thai KE, Sinclair RD. Chronic telogen effluvium in a man. J Am Acad Dermatol 2002;47:605–7.

30. Whiting DA. Chronic telogen effluvium: increased scalp hair shedding in middle-aged women. J Am Acad Dermatol 1996;35:899–906.

31. Whiting DA. Update chronic telogen effluvium. Exp Dermatol 1999; 135(9):1123–24.

6

Pseudofolliculitis Barbae

Kabir Sardana, Ananta Khurana

Though pseudofolliculitis barbae (PFB) is a common follicular disorder and is most prevalent in men of African ancestry, it is also seen in Indian patients and is frequently misdiagnosed.

Pathogenesis

This condition is essentially a foreign-body reaction to the hair shaft. Individuals who have coarse, tightly curled hair and who shave are predisposed to this condition, owing to the tendency for the distal portion of tightly curled hair shafts to reenter the skin after shaving (Fig. 6.1).

The problem is shaving rather than infection. The shaved areas can become infected. Figure 6.1 shows how this condition arises. Hair grows from hair follicles. The hair grows outward and emerges from the surface of the skin hair follicle opening. When we shave, we try to get the closest possible shave. This is achieved by pulling on the skin and shaving against the grain. By pulling on the skin, the hair is made to stand farther out. After the razor passes over the hair and the skin

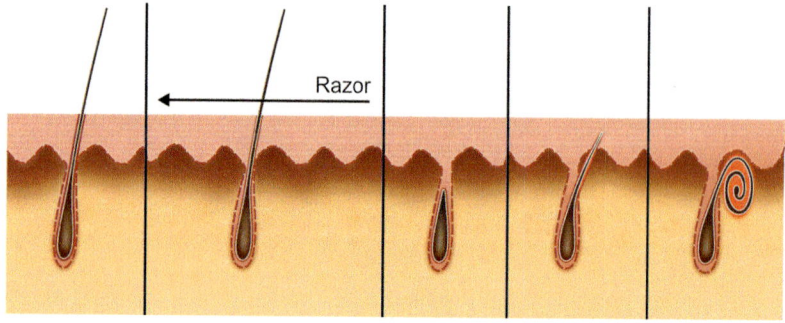

Fig. 6.1: A visualization of the mechanism of *PFB*, due to 'close' shaving

is released, the hair stubble retracts under the skin. Since you cannot feel it, it feels smooth. When the razor cuts across the hair, it frequently cuts it at an angle producing a sharp point similar to a hypodermic needle. As the hair grows out of the hair follicle again, the sharp point allows the hair to puncture the side of the hair follicle and move through the skin. In so doing, it carries bacteria and foreign material with it, which case an inflammation or infection in the hair follicle and surrounding skin (Fig. 6.2A). Sometimes in patients with curly hair, the hair grows into the skin (Fig. 6.2B) curling around to produce an ingrown hair.

Once the hair penetrates the dermis, an inflammatory reaction ensues. Hair growth usually continues into the dermis, reaching a depth of 2 to 3 mm. In the dermis, it produces an even greater inflammatory reaction, manifested by pustules and papules. The hair reaches the length of 10 mm after a growth period of up to 6 *weeks*. At this point, a spring action occurs that pulls out the embedded tip.

Thus, there are two mechanisms for causing PFB (Perry PK):

1. *Transfollicular penetration:* Here the sharp distal tip of a shaved hair shaft retracts beneath the skin surface, pierces the follicular wall, and enters the dermis. Stretching the skin during shaving or close shaving techniques can contribute to transfollicular penetration (Fig. 6.2A).

2. *Extrafollicular penetration:* Here the shaved hair shaft grows along its natural curvature and penetrates the epidermis 1 to 2 mm distal to the follicular opening (Fig. 6.2B).

A genetic risk factor has been identified that can affect a subset of men with PFB. A substitution mutation in the 1Aα-helical segment of the hair follicle specific keratin 75 (formerly K6hf) was found in 36% of PFB cases compared with 9% in controls. This single nucleotide polymorphism may be associated with a structurally weakened companion layer of the hair follicle which, along with curly hair shafts and close shaving, contributes to an increased risk for PFB (Winter H).

Clinical Features

The clinical hallmarks of PFB are follicular and/or perifollicular papules in an area where repetitive shaving has occurred (Fig. 6.3). In men, the most commonly affected area is the neck (Fig. 6.3) followed by the cheeks, whereas in women the chin (especially the submental region) is the most commonly affected area.

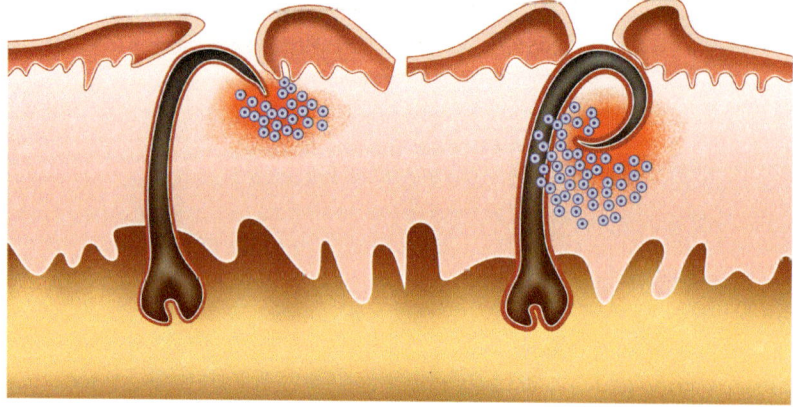

Fig. 6.2A: Pseudofolliculitis barbae: Mechanism of transfollicular penetration consequent to the fad "of stretching the skin to achieve a close shave"

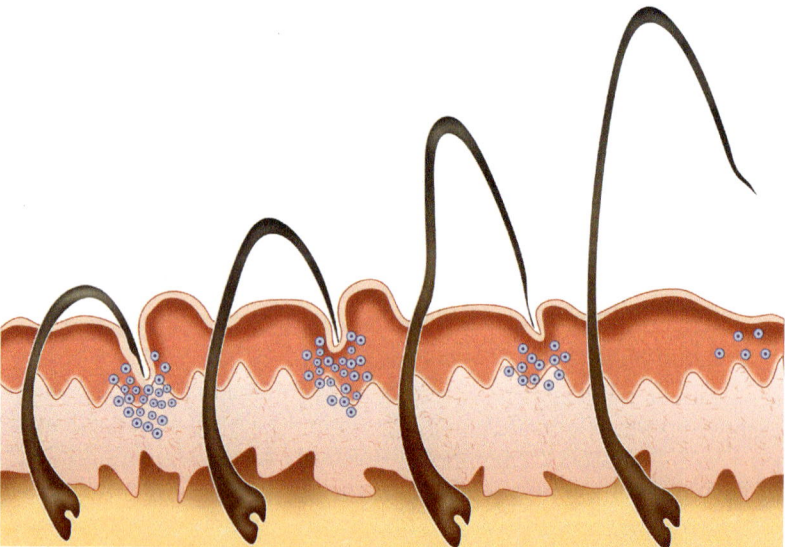

Fig. 6.2B: Mechanism of reentry of hair seen in curly hair

Of note, the moustache and nuchal areas are rarely affected. Hirsute women who shave or pluck unwanted hairs frequently develop PFB on the chin and neck area. Shaving the axillae and bikini region of the groin, a common practice among women of all races, can lead to pseudofolliculitis in these areas (Fig. 6.4).

The papules of PFB may be firm, skin colored, erythematous, or hyperpigmented. If secondary infection arises, pustules and papulopustules may be present. Some papules may contain visible

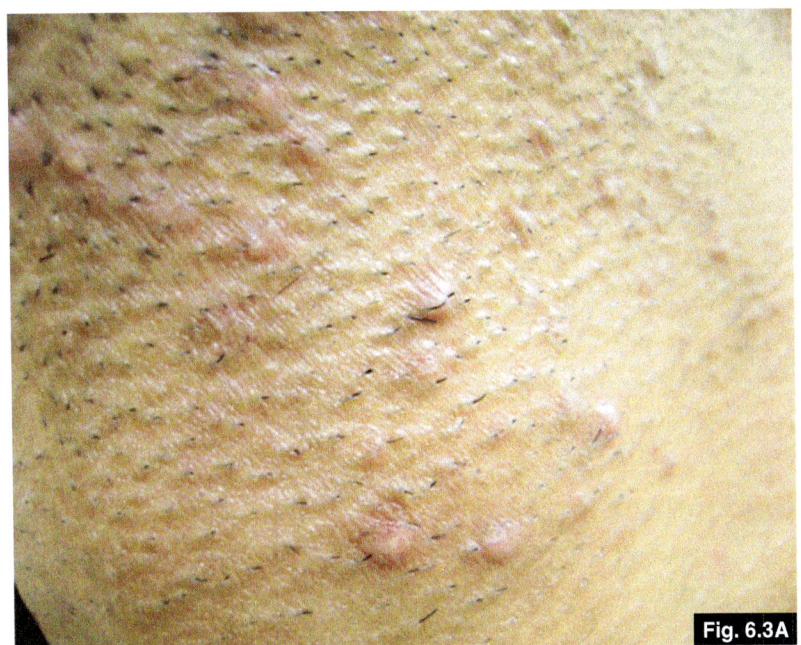

Fig. 6.3A

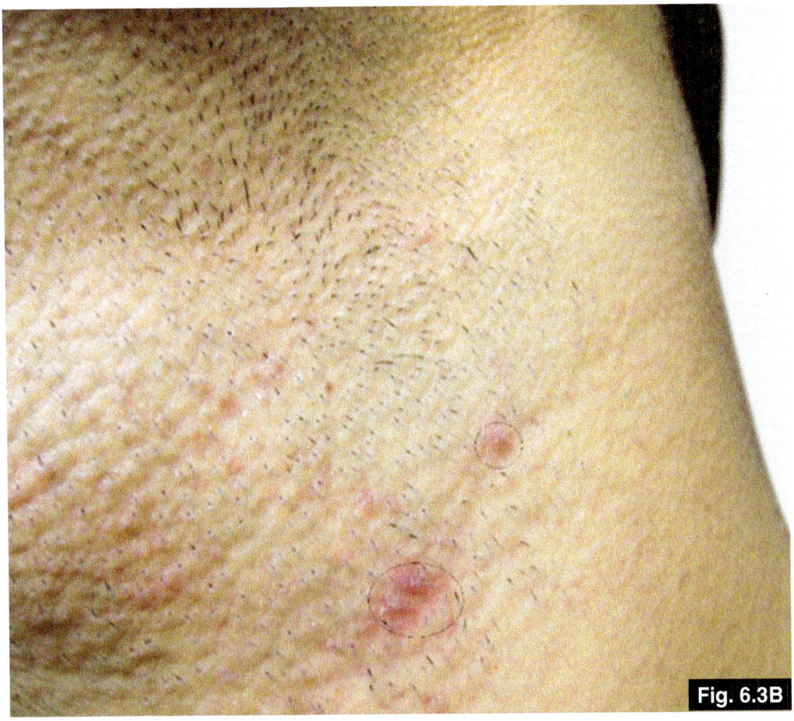

Fig. 6.3B

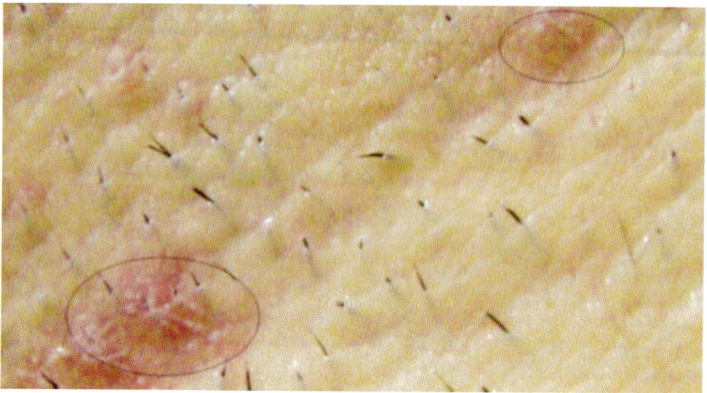

Fig. 6.3A to C: (A and B) A case of pseudofolliculitis, note the parallel orientation of hair which is embedded in the papule. This is a case of transfollicular penetration. (C) A case of recurrent pseudofolliculitis. A close up shows the embedded hair, the mechanical removal of which has miraculous results

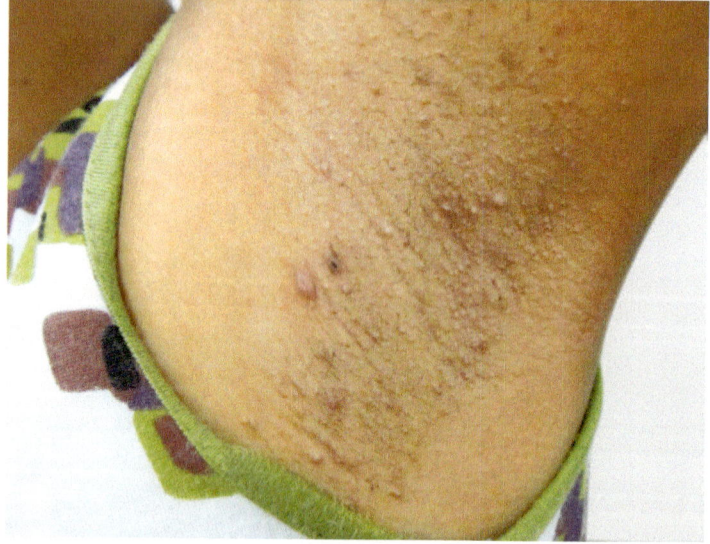

Fig. 6.4: A case of PFB in a female who gets waxed on a regular basis

hairs. Linear depressions in the affected areas likely represent hairs that are growing parallel to the surface of the skin (Fig. 6.3). Sequelae include post-inflammatory hyperpigmentation (PIH) and keloids.

Differential Diagnosis

Differential diagnosis of PFB includes acne vulgaris, sycosis barbae, and traumatic folliculitis.

Acne: No comedonal lesions are found in PFB, and acne vulgaris affects other areas of the face in addition to the beard area. Pustules are common in acne vulgaris, whereas they are rare in PFB.

Sycosis barbae: Perifollicular pustules are the primary and predominant lesions. Shaving improves sycosis barbae, whereas it makes PFB worse. Lesions in PFB are isolated, whereas in sycosis barbae they are confluent. Traumatic folliculitis, commonly known as razor burn, occurs when shaving is done too closely. Lesions are erythematous, painful, small follicular papules, which *disappear* within 24 to 48 hours after shaving.

Treatment

The only definitive cure is growing a beard or having the hairs permanently removed. A summary of options is listed in Table 6.1, but asking the patient to indefinitely avoid shaving maybe a excellent remedy, but is generally impractical to enforce.

General Shaving Advise

1. The first step is asking the patient to discontinue shaving for at least **1 month**, as this can be curative in some patients.
2. Modification of shaving practices, including the addition of pre-shave and post-shave regimens, is useful.
   a. Before shaving, the beard area should be prepped by washing with warm water and a mild soap-free cleanser.
   b. Using a wash cloth to apply gently rotating movement as this can gently release embedded hair shafts before shaving.
   c. Pre-shave washing regimens (using a scrub or brush) have been shown to reduce the percentage of trapped beard hairs (Cowley K).
   d. Shaving should be performed with a clean, sharp razor with the skin in its relaxed state (stretching of the skin should be avoided,

Table 6.1: Overview of measures for treating PFB	
General advise	Shaving techniques
Medical	Topical retinoids
	Low- to mid-potency topical corticosteroids
	Topical antibiotics
	Chemical depilatories
	Eflornithine hydrochloride
Cosmetic measures	Electrolysis/epilation
	Surgical depilation
	Lasers

as this may facilitate transfollicular penetration of hairs shaved slightly below the skin surface). This is converse to the media advertisements which emphasize the reverse.

e. Shaving in the direction of hair growth (i.e. with the grain) has been generally recommended; however, a recently published study found that men who reported shaving against the grain had lower papule counts (Daniel A).

f. Traditionally, single blade razors have been favored over multiple blade razors because of concerns about transfollicular penetration associated with the closer shave achieved with multiple blade razors. However, in a recent study, PFB was not exacerbated by the use of multiple blade razors (in conjunction with a pre-shavecleanser and post-shave lotion) (Daniel A).

g. Another option is to use a electric razor or clipper but leaving a stubble (approximately 1 mm in length). This can be easily accomplished with the use of electric clippers as they can be set to cut hair to a desired length (Halder RM). In my experience though a *single blade*, a *single pass* and *not stretching* the skin is always a more feasible option with consistently good results. Regardless ofchoice of a single blade or multiple blade razors, a clean, sharp razor blade should be used for each and every shave. Published comparative studies of single blade versus multiple blade razors or electric versus manual razors in patients with PFB are currently lacking, as are studies that prospectively investigate the effects of shaving direction on PFB severity.

The best method of effecting resolution is by removal of the embedded hair. I advise a judicious use of a hypodermic needle with excellent and consistent results (Figs 6.4 and 6.5). A list of measures has been detailed by Kelly AP et al and Sardana K is given in Table 6.2 as a ready reckoner.

Medical Therapy

The use of depilators and lasers to reduce hair maybe a option in females but in males neither of two are feasible and its not a advise that we render to our patients. Most of the medical therapies are directed at the end lesion and are akin to acne therapy.

Pharmacologic treatments for PFB include low-potency topical corticosteroids (e.g. desonide lotion), benzoyl peroxide formulations, topical antibiotics, and topical retinoids.

a. Topical **steroids** can be used (Flutibact ointment or Flutivate ointment) but should be limited to 2-week courses or used 1 to 3 times per week to minimize risk of atrophy and other side effects.

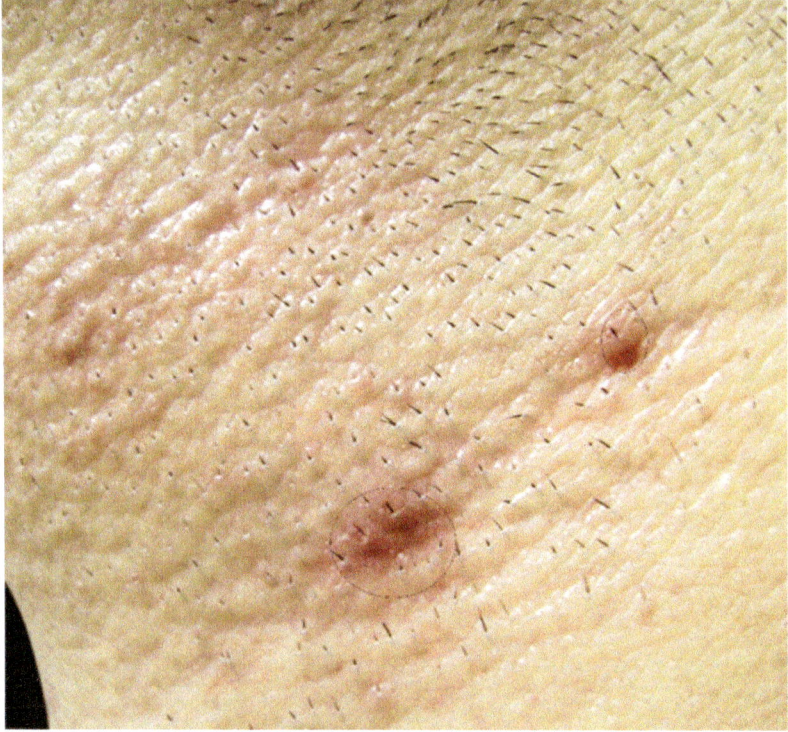

Fig. 6.5: Extraction of the hair with a hypodermic needle, note the minimal bleed. A complete resolution is seen after 10 days. The patient was asked to apply clindamycin gel (pseudofolliculitis: In Sardana K et al. Diagnosis and management of skin disorders: Wolter Kluwer, India, 2015)

b. **Benzoyl peroxide 5%/clindamycin** 1% gel has demonstrated significant reductions in combined papule and pustule counts (Cook-Bolden FE).

c. **Topical retinoids** (tretinoin, adapalene, or tazarotene) are recommended nightly, and are useful for improving both the clinical lesions of PFB (Kligman AM, Coley MK) and the associated post-inflammatory hyperpigmentation (Bulengo-Ransby SM). As there are various adapalene (ADP)—combinations with antibiotics notably clindamycin and nadifloxacin, these all commonly administered.

d. Chemical peels, containing glycolic acid and other β-hydroxy acids, can be used to reduce hyperkeratosis of the follicular infundibulum and thickening of the stratum corneum. This in turn allows the hair to grow out straighter and makes shaving easier.

Table 6.2: Overview of patient advise for prevention of PFB

Shaving should not be resumed until all the inflamed lesions have cleared and all the ingrown hairs have been released	1. Advise patients to discontinue shaving for **1 month** for mild cases, **2 to 3** months for moderate cases, and **3 to 6 months** for severe cases. During this shaving hiatus, beards can be trimmed with scissors or electric clippers to a minimum length of 1 cm
	2. Apply a warm water, saline, or Burow's solution compress for 10 to 15 minutes three times a day to soothe the lesions, remove the crust, stop drainage secondary to inflammation, and soften the epidermis, allowing for the easier and earlier release of ingrown hairs
	3. Apply a topical hydrocortisone cream or lotion (for 3 to 4 weeks only) to the shaved area
	4. An antibiotic or a short-course of oral steroid for 10 days may be needed
For those who need to shave	1. Ingrown hairs should *not* be plucked
	2. Use electric clippers to remove as much preexisting beard hair
	3. Apply warm water compresses for approximately 5 minutes
	4. Use any brand of shaving cream
	5. Choose a sharp razor that cuts best without irritation
	6. Shave *with* the grain of the hair, using short strokes while avoiding pulling the skin taut. Twice over one area is usually sufficient. Shave *gently*
	7. Use a magnifying mirror to search for any ingrown hairs. To release them gently, insert a toothpick under the loop or brush the beard area with a soft toothbrush
	8. In expert hands, a hypodermic needle can be used to release ingrowing hair (Figs 6.4 and 6.5)
	9. A steroid application can help in such inflamed areas post-release of the hair

Lasers

Lasers can be used. In Indian skin longer-wavelength lasers such as the diode (800–810 nm) and neodymium:yttrium-aluminum-garnet (Nd:YAG 1064 nm) lasers are preferred.

Combining topical eflornithine hydrochloride 13.9% cream (to slow down hair growth) along with long-pulsed 1064 nm Nd:YAG laser hair removal has been shown to be more effective than laser hair removal alone.

An algorithm is given below of the best available evidence for treating PFB and the crucial aspect, is modifying the ingrained shaving method of patients and learning the art of releasing the embedded hair (Fig. 6.6).

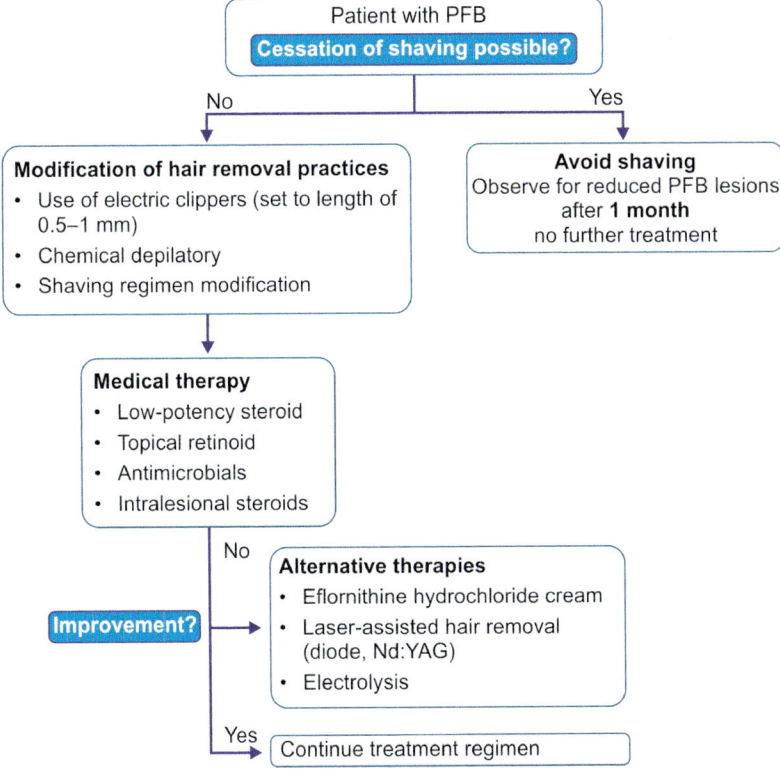

Fig. 6.6: Algorithm for management of PFB. (Adapted from: Coley MK, Kelly AP, Alexis AF. Pseudofolliculitis barbae and acne keloidalis nuchae. In: Alexis A, Barbosa VH, editors. Skin of color: A practical guide to dermatologic diagnosis and treatment, 1st edition. New York: Springer; 2013)

Bibliography

1. Bulengo-Ransby SM, Griffiths CE, Kimbrough-Green CK, et al. Topical tretinoin (retinoic acid) therapy for hyperpigmented lesions caused by inflammation of the skin in black patients. N Engl J Med 1993;328(20): 1438–43.

2. Cook-Bolden FE, Barba A, Halder R, et al. Twice-daily applications of benzoyl peroxide 5%/clindamycin 1% gel versus vehicle in the treatment of pseudofolliculitis barbae. Cutis 2004;73(Suppl 6):18–24. Coley MK, Alexis AF. Managing common dermatoses in skin of color. Semin Cutan Med Surg 2009; 28(2):63–70.

3. Cowley K, Vanoosthuyze K. Insights into shaving and its impact on skin. Br J Dermatol 2012;166(Suppl 1):6–12.

4. Daniel A, Gustafson CJ, Zupkosky PJ, et al. Shave frequency and regimen variation effects on the management of pseudofolliculitis barbae. J Drugs Dermatol 2013;12(4):410–8.

5. Halder RM, Robert CI, Nootheti PK, Kelly AP. Dermatologic disease in blacks. In: RM Halder, ed. Dermatology and Dermatological Therapy of Pigmented Skins. Taylor & Francis: Boca Raton, FL, 2006; pp. 331–55.

6. Kelly AP. Pseudofolliculitis barbae. In: Arndt KA, LeBoit P, LeBiot PR, et al, eds. Cutaneous Medicine and Surgery: An Integrated Program in Dermatology. Philadelphia, PA: WB Saunders; 1996:499–502.

7. Perry PK, Cook-Bolden FE, Rahman Z, et al. Defining pseudofolliculitis barbae in 2001: a review of the literature and current trends. J Am Acad Dermatol 2002;46(2 Suppl Under standing):S113–9.

8. Sardana K. Pseudofolliculitis barbae. In: Diagnosis and Management of Skin Disorders: Wolter Kluwer, India, 2015.CD.

9. Winter H, Schissel D, Parry DA, et al. An unusual Ala12Thr polymorphism in the 1A alpha-helical segment of the companion laser-specific keratin K6hf: evidence for a risk factor in the etiology of the common hair disorder pseudofolliculitis barbae. J Invest Dermatol 2004;122(3):652–7.

7

Alopecia Areata

Kabir Sardana, Khushbu Mahajan, Selma CH

Alopecia areata (AA) is a common form of nonscarring hair loss, which may involve any hair bearing region, but most commonly presents over the scalp, in a patchy distribution.

ETIOPATHOGENESIS

Current view purports that alopecia areata is a T-cell mediated autoimmune disease occurring in genetically predisposed individuals, with certain environmental factors acting as triggers.

Genetics: Studies focusing on genetic linkage have found that AA is localized to the HLA class II (HLA-D) region on human chromosome 6 but family-based linkage studies and GWAS analyses, enabled by the repository of the National Alopecia Areata Registry, identified linkage or association on many chromosomes, which suggests that alopecia areata is a very complex, *polygenic* disease.

Whereas most of the linked genes involve the immune system, a receptor for stress-induced proteins (NKG2D) is also strongly linked, which is of interest because a stressful event precedes the onset of AA in 9.5 to 58% of patients.

Hair dynamics: The hair dynamics in alopecia areata seemed to involve a rapid progression of hair follicles from the anagen phase to the catagen and telogen phases. Follicles that were less severely affected remained in the anagen phase but produced dystrophic hair shafts that eventually underwent progression to the telogen phase. The disorder affects anagen follicles and there is a little or no inflammatory infiltrate around the isthmus of the hair follicle, the site of hair follicle stem cells, which explains the non-scarring nature of the disorder.

Immune Response (Pratt CH et al)

An overview of the various aspects of the pathogenesis of AA is depicted in Fig. 7.1.

a. **Target:** The hair follicle matrix epithelium that is undergoing early cortical differentiation seems to be the primary target of an immune attack on the hair follicle based on several lines of evidence. *First,* the matrix cells exhibit vacuolar degeneration in affected anagen follicles (*see* below). These degenerative changes lead to a localized region of weakness in the hair shaft, which results in the hair shaft breaking when it emerges from the ostium at the skin surface, which explains the formation of the exclamation point hair shaft. *Second,* the affected hair follicles revert to the telogen phase, follicles re-enter the anagen phase normally but do not develop beyond the anagen III/IV phase, the point at which cortical differentiation commences. *Last,* aberrant MHC class I and class II expression occurs in the pre-cortical region where the inflammatory cell infiltrates are localized.

b. **Loss of immune privilege:** One of the reasons proposed to explain the pathogenesis of AA, is that there is a very low or absent expression of MHC class I proteins in the lower part of the follicular epithelium making the hair follicle an immunologically privileged site. This reduces the risk of attracting autoreactive cytotoxic CD8+ T cells that can recognize antigens in association with MHC class I. A loss of this immune privilege, leads to an attack by CD8+ cells (Fig. 7.1). A specific cytotoxic subset (CD8+ NKG2D+) is the main cell involved and this produces IFN-β that in turn activates interleukin-15 (IL-15) and IL-15Rα and sustains CD8+ T cell autoreactivity. There is involvement of the signaling pathway via the Janus kinase (JAK) receptors, which explains the potential use of JAK inhibitors in AA.

c. **Autoantigen epitopes:** The involvement of autoantigen epitopes in the initiation of alopecia areata has been hypothesized. An involvement of melanin, melanin-related proteins and keratinocyte-derived antigens has been suggested based on the observation that white hairs grow back after a period of alopecia areata and are often spared in further relapses.

Other implicated factors are listed in Table 7.1.

CLINICAL FEATURES

The onset may occur at any age with a peak incidence between 2nd and 4th decades of life. Most patients develop the condition before 40 years of age, with a mean age of onset between 25 and 36 years. Early-onset alopecia areata (a mean age of onset between 5 and 10 years)

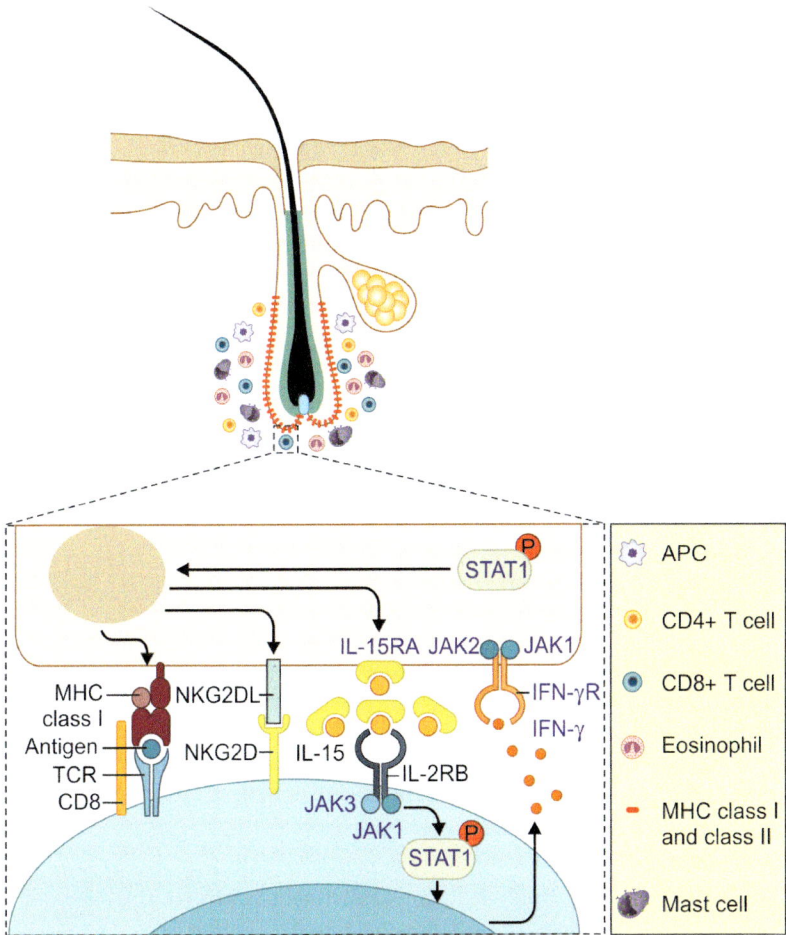

Fig. 7.1A: Late anagen hair follicles in patients with alopecia areata have perifollicular infiltrations of APCs, CD4+ and CD8+ T cells, and abnormal expression of MHC class I and class II molecules. CD8+ T cells also infiltrate into the hair follicle root sheaths. Molecules involved in the lymphocyte co-stimulatory cascade are involved in the pathogenesis of alopecia areata and provide targets for therapeutic intervention. No inflammatory cells are found in the surrounding of normal follicles in the late anagen phase

predominantly presents as a more severe subtype, such as alopecia universalis.

Patients usually complain of abrupt hair loss and marked hair shedding. The characteristic lesion of AA is a round or oval, bald, smooth patch involving the scalp or any hair-bearing area of the body (Fig. 7.1B). The patch has both intact and fractured hairs.

Table 7.1: Miscellaneous factors implicated in AA	
Oxidative stress	Oxidative stress and damage to SOD play a part in the induction of alopecia areata. High levels of malondialdehyde can be found in patients
Vasculature and lymphatic system	Lesions can have increased temperature, increased lympatics and increased inflammatory mediators
Environmental triggers	Emotional or physical stress, such as following bereavement or injury, vaccinations, febrile illness and drugs. Various infections that can trigger, include, Japanese encephalitis virus, hepatitis B virus, *Clostridium tetani*, herpes zoster virus, papillomavirus and swine flu virus infection

The fractured hairs develop owing to damage involving both the cortex and medulla, resulting in distal fractures. These are called *"exclamation mark"* hairs (Fig. 7.1B), because the distal segment is broader than the proximal end. These exclamation hairs are usually present at the margins and are not a very specific finding.

The disease is frequently asymptomatic, although a few patients may report paresthesias, mild to moderate pruritus, burning sensation or pain, before the appearance of hair loss.

The clinical presentation of AA can be classified on the basis of pattern or extent of the hair loss. According to **pattern**, the following forms are seen: *Patchy*, round or oval patches of hair loss (Fig. 7.1C); reticular variant (Fig. 7.2); *ophiasis* band-like hair loss in temporo-occipital scalp (Fig. 7.3); *ophiasis inversus* (sisapho) band-like pattern of hair loss in the frontoparieto-scalp; and **diffuse** AA, a diffuse decrease in hair density over the entire scalp. On the basis of **extent:** AA, partial loss of scalp hair; alopecia totalis (AT) (Fig. 7.4), total loss of scalp hair; and alopecia universalis (AU), total loss of hair on scalp and body have been described.

The initial regrowing hair in AA is often depigmented, followed later by repigmentation (Fig. 7.5). This loss of pigment may involve the whole scalp (thus the historical connotation of growing grey hair overnight). Sparing of white hair is a relative phenomenon and it is clear that the white hairs, although less susceptible to the disease, are *not* completely immune (Fig. 7.5B).

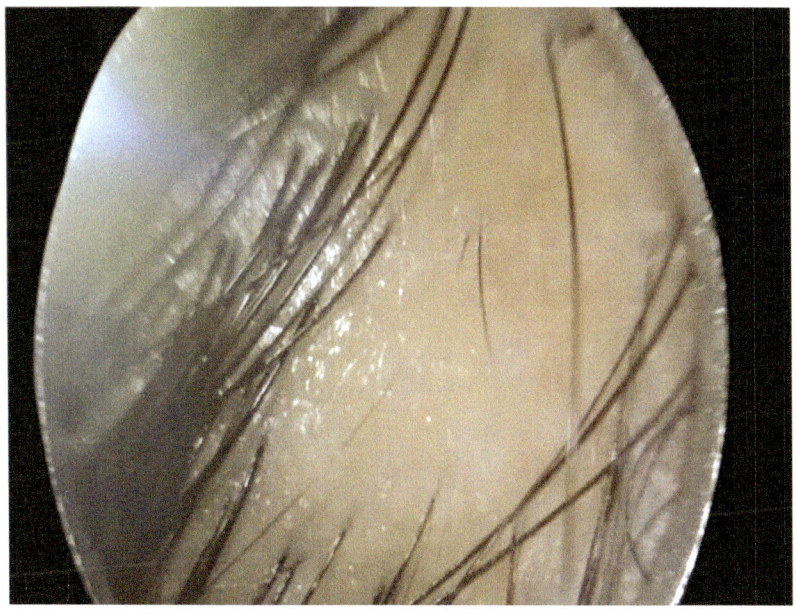

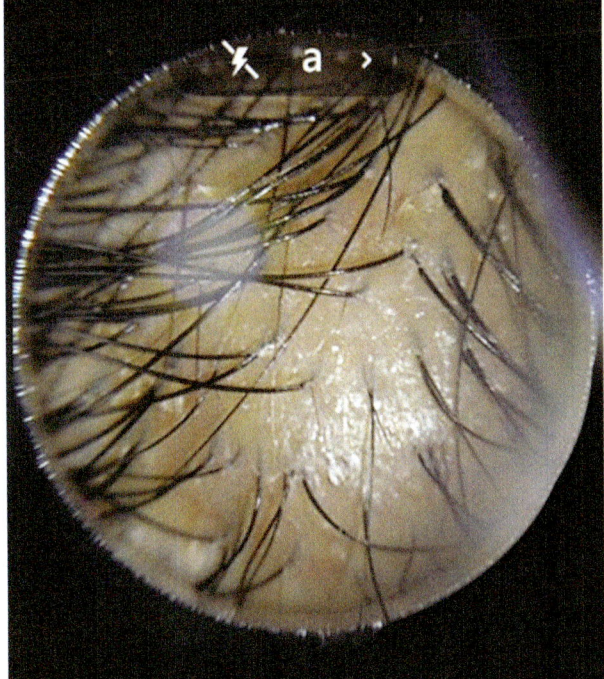

Fig. 7.1B: The top image shows a smooth scalp with loss of hair and multiple exclamation hairs, the second (bottom) image is 3 months after therapy with visible regrowth

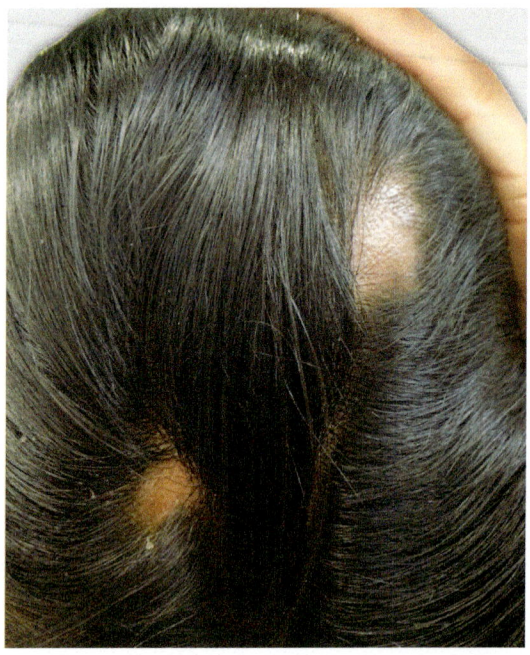

Fig. 7.1C: Localized patchy alopecia areata on the scalp. This responds readily to IL steroids

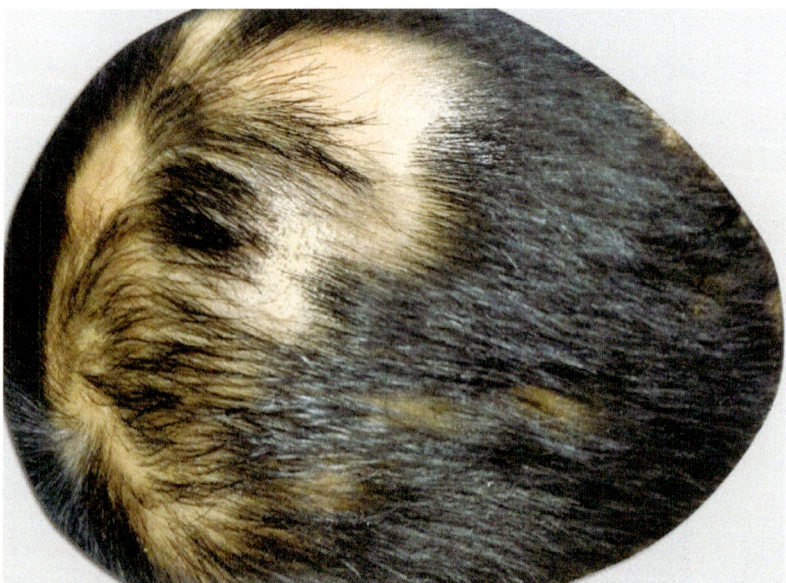

Fig. 7.2: Reticular variant of alopecia areata. This is an unstable variant and such patients often need systemic therapy

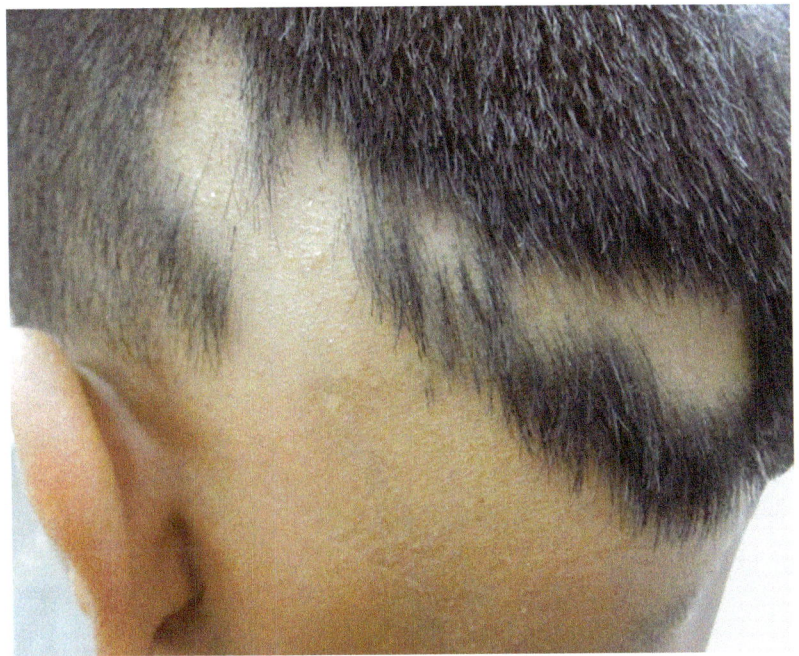

Fig. 7.3: Ophiasis in a child

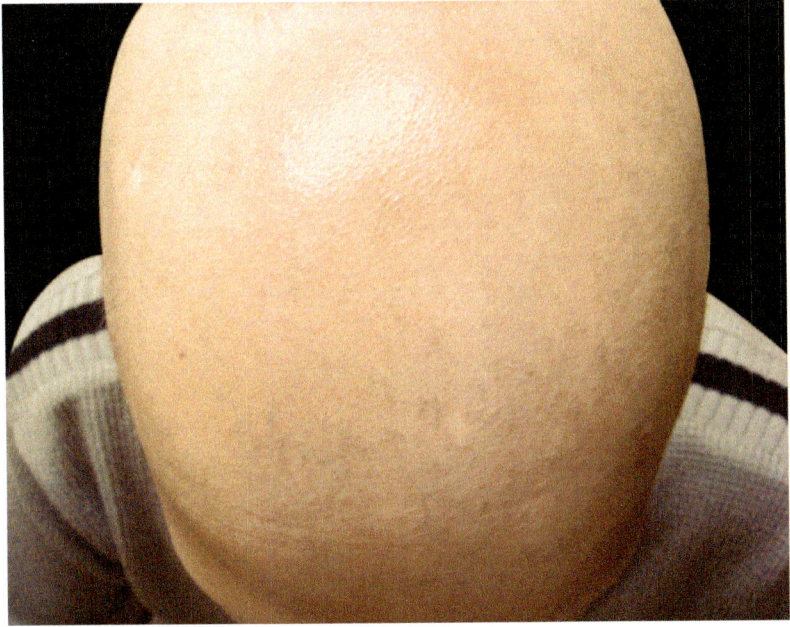

Fig. 7.4: Alopecia totalis in a child

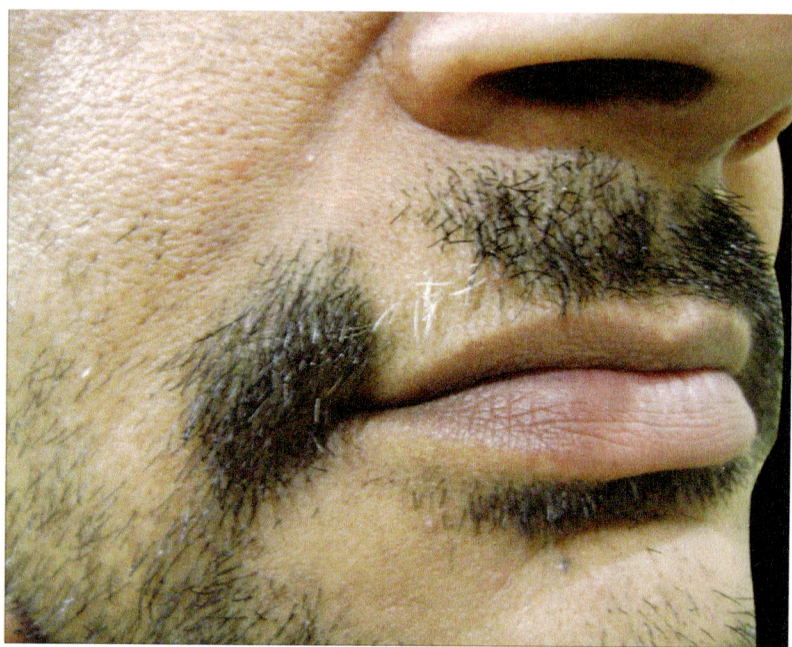

Fig. 7.5: Regrowth of hair, initially grey, in a case of alopecia areata of the moustache

Apart from the scalp, other commonly involved sites include the eyebrows (Fig. 7.6), eyelashes, beard (Fig. 7.7), limbs (Fig. 7.8) or thorax area and sometimes these may be the only site involved.

Patients may have associated nail changes and the incidence of nail changes in alopecia areata ranges from 10 to 66%. The most common nail change is fine nail pitting which occurs due to the presence of easily detachable parakeratotic cells in the superficial layers of the nail plate. Other reported changes include trachyonychia, onychorrhexis, spotting of the lunula, onycholysis and onychomadesis. Nail changes are more common in severe forms of AA.

Prognosis

It is said (Shapiro S and Otberg N) that "the only predictable thing about the progress of AA is that it is unpredictable". Patients usually present with several episodes of hair loss and hair regrowth during their lifetime. The recovery from hair loss may be complete, partial, or none. The majority of patients will regrow their hair entirely within 1 year without treatment. However, 7–10% can eventually end up with the severe chronic form of the condition. If hair loss progresses to

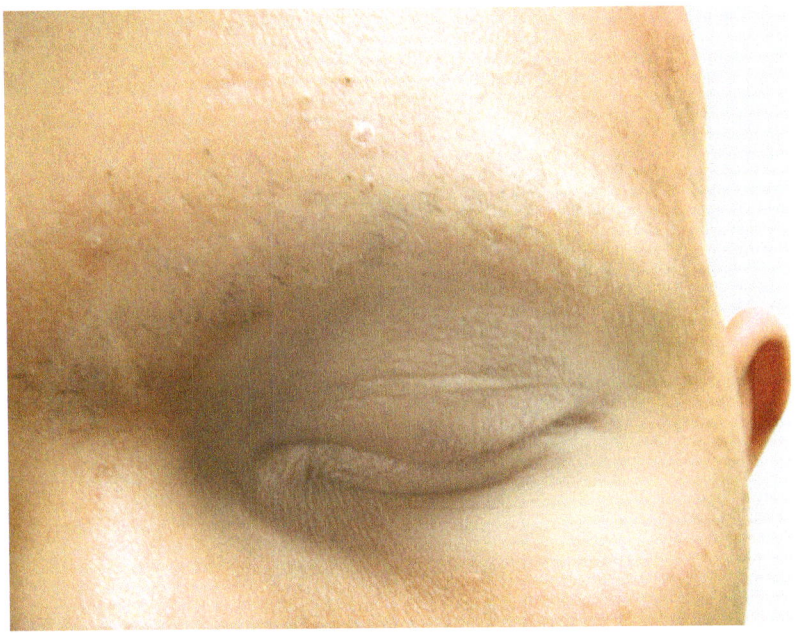

Fig. 7.6: Alopecia areata involving the eyebrows

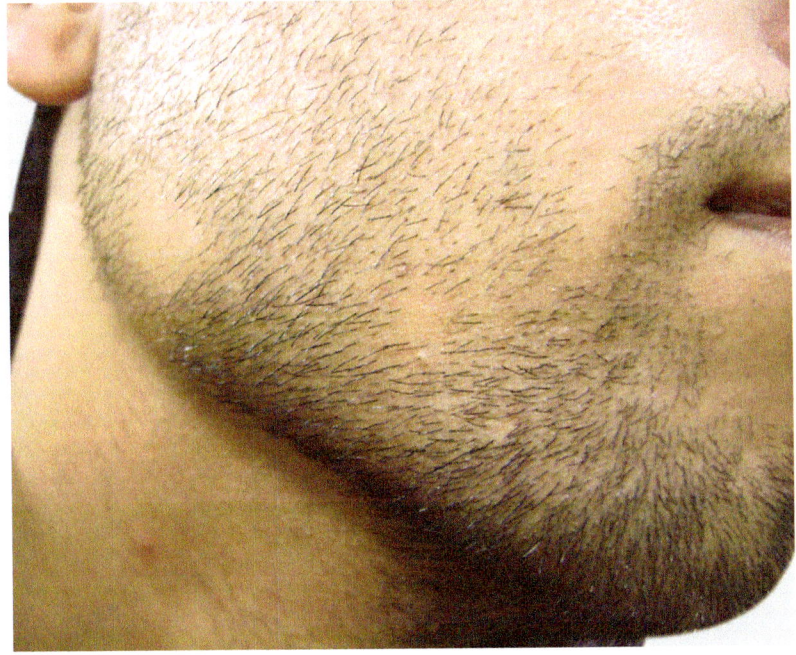

Fig. 7.7: Alopecia areata of the beard, a common cosmetic concern in males

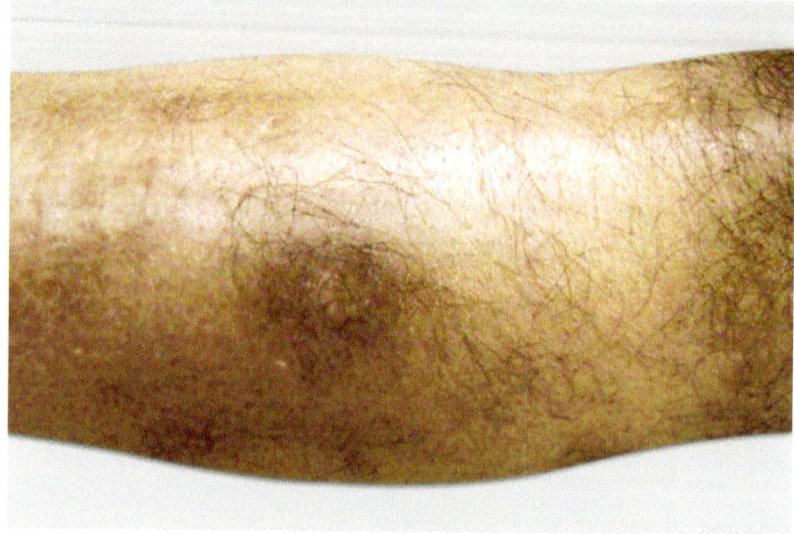

Fig. 7.8: Alopecia areata involving the limbs

involve all of the scalp (alopecia totalis) or the entire skin surface (alopecia universalis) spontaneous recovery is the exception rather than the rule (Messenger AG).

Poor prognostic indicators are listed in Box 7.1.

Associated diseases: Alopecia areata may be associated with several other autoimmune diseases including thyroiditis, lupus erythematosus, vitiligo and psoriasis. There may be an increased risk of type 1 diabetes in family members of AA patients; in contrast, the patients themselves may have a reduced incidence compared to the general population.

Box 7.1: Prognostic factors in AA

For the whole of the disease:
- Onset in childhood, especially where involvement is widespread
- Associated endocrine problems, atopy
- The presence of other autoimmune diseases
- A positive family history of AA

For the episode:
- How long the episode has been established
- The extent of the affected area
- Certain clinical forms: Ophiasis pattern, alopecia totalis, alopecia universalis, diffuse alopecia
- Hair loss and exclamation mark hairs at sites distant from the smooth patches
- Nail dystrophy

Atopic eczema, is also more common than expected in alopecia areata and is associated with an early onset and more severe forms of hair loss. Loss of function mutations in FLG (encoding filaggrin) have been associated with a more severe course.

DIFFERENTIAL DIAGNOSIS

In children, *tinea capitis* and *trichotillomania* are the most common diseases that are mistaken for alopecia areata. In addition, the early stages of scarring alopecia might be difficult to differentiate. The diffuse form of alopecia areata is perhaps the most difficult to identify and may require a detailed history to uncover previous episodes of hair loss, nail dystrophy and the usually rapid progression of the hair loss (Fig. 7.9).

The development of alopecia universalis in infancy should alert the clinician to the possibility of atrichia with papular lesions (also known as *papular atrichia*), which is due to rare, autosomal recessive mutations in the hairless (HR) or the vitamin D receptor (VDR) genes.

INVESTIGATIONS

The diagnosis of this disorder is purely clinical in majority of the cases.

1. Exclamation mark hairs as well as yellow and black dots can be identified with trichoscopy.
2. A hair pull test should be performed to estimate the disease activity on the margin of each lesion. The presence of exclamatory hairs at the border and a positive hair pull test with 6 or more hairs from the periphery suggests that the disease may be active and progressive.
3. In diffuse AA, a trichogram can be useful and will reveal an increased number of dystrophic anagen hairs.
4 In case of a diagnostic dilemma, a 4-mm punch biopsy is recommended from the margin of an active lesion which exhibits a perifollicular and intrafollicular inflammatory cell infiltrate composed of activated T cells (**'swarm of bees'** appearance) (Fig. 7.10). Early stages can show vacuolar changes in the hair shaft (Fig. 7.11). The infiltrate has a admixture of lymphocytes and eosinophils (Fig. 7.12).

   In the acute phase, when both CD8+ and CD4+ T lymphocytes infiltrate into the peribulbar area, the cell density is an indication of active disease progression. CD4+ T cells predominate in the infiltrate surrounding the hair follicle, while T cells within the follicular

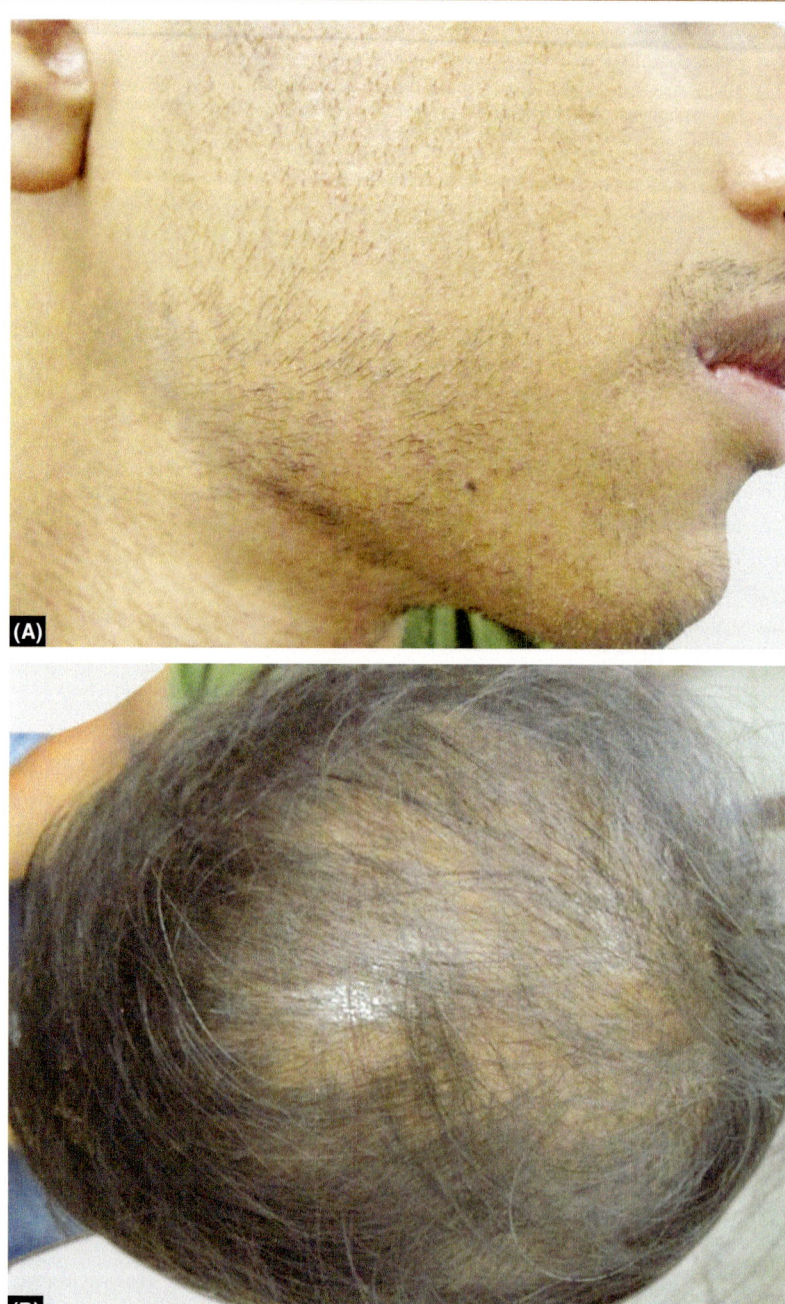

Fig. 7.9A and B: This case was being treated as a case of AA of the beard with MPHL, the latter diagnosis in a boy of 23 years old is an uncommon occurrence

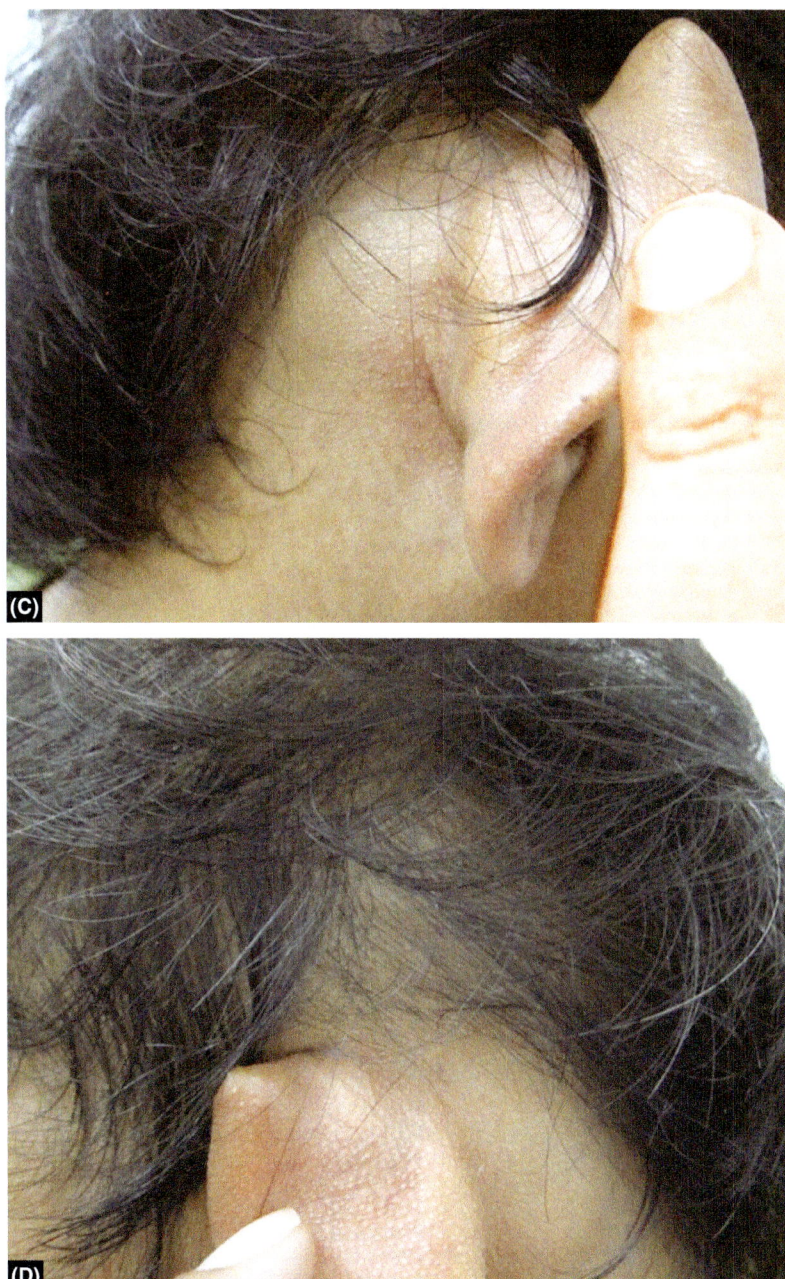

Fig. 7.9C and D: Close examination of the scalp found that there was a distinct ophiatic pattern. Also the rapid course of disease and past history of a few patches of AA confirmed the diagnosis of alopecia areata incognita aka diffuse AA

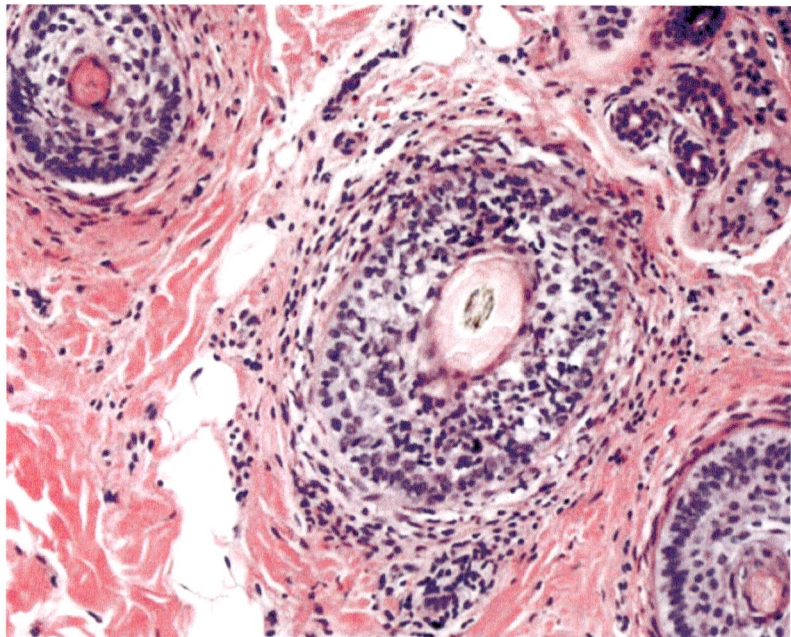

Fig. 7.10: In this patient with alopecia areata, the upper follicle is spared while the lower follicle is surrounded by lymphocytic inflammation as a result of which the outer root sheath, appears blurry (*Courtesy:* EA Knopp)

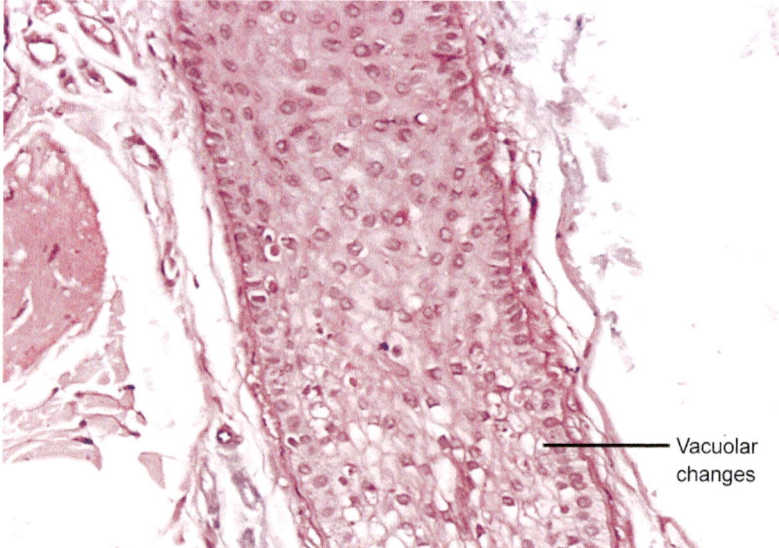

Vacuolar changes

Fig. 7.11: High power view: Intra- and intercellular edema and vacuolar changes in the hair shaft (Dr Purnima Malhotra)

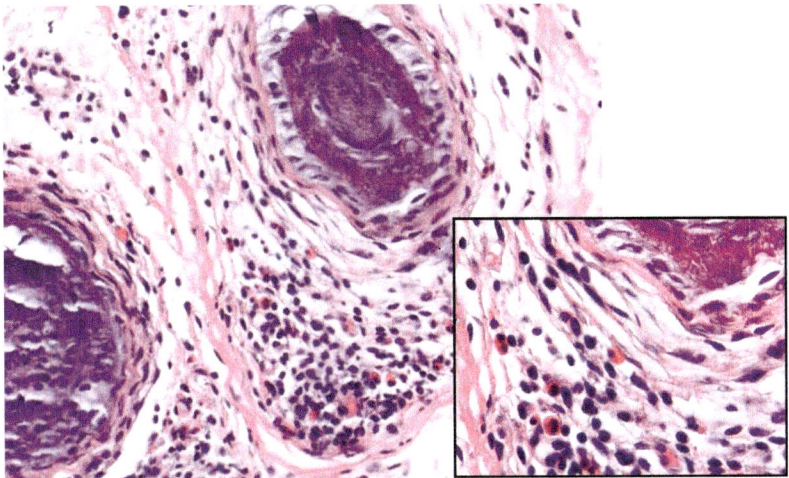

Fig. 7.12: Eosinophils are admixed with the peribulbar lymphocytic infiltrate. This explains the role on drugs like cetirizine and fexofenadine as an adjuvant in AA

epithelium are predominantly CD8+ (Fig. 7.1). This infiltrate is concentrated in and around the hair bulb and spares the isthmus of the hair follicle, the site of hair follicle stem cells.

5. In atypical cases dermoscopy may be of immense value (Fig. 7.13A to D)

6. Laboratory work up is done to rule out autoimmune thyroiditis (thyroid stimulating hormone—TSH, thyroid autoantibodies). Some clinicians test for ferritin, vitamin D, vitamin B$_{12}$, selenium, zinc, and copper to rule out other causes that might affect hair growth and regrowth, however such intensive work up is *not* needed in classical cases.

TREATMENT

There is no universally effective treatment for AA and the published data is difficult to interpret as the end point of successful therapy vary and studies do not stratify results according to the extent of AA. Another issue is that in localized AA there is a spontaneous remission in up to 80% of patients with a short duration hair loss (less than 1 year). Thus, an option of 'no treatment' can be given to patients presenting early in the course of disease though in India such an advise is a rarity.

All local treatments may help the treated areas, but do not prevent further spread of the condition. In addition, any mode of treatment may require long periods of usage, owing to the chronic nature of AA. At the present time, topical, intralesional, and systemic steroids,

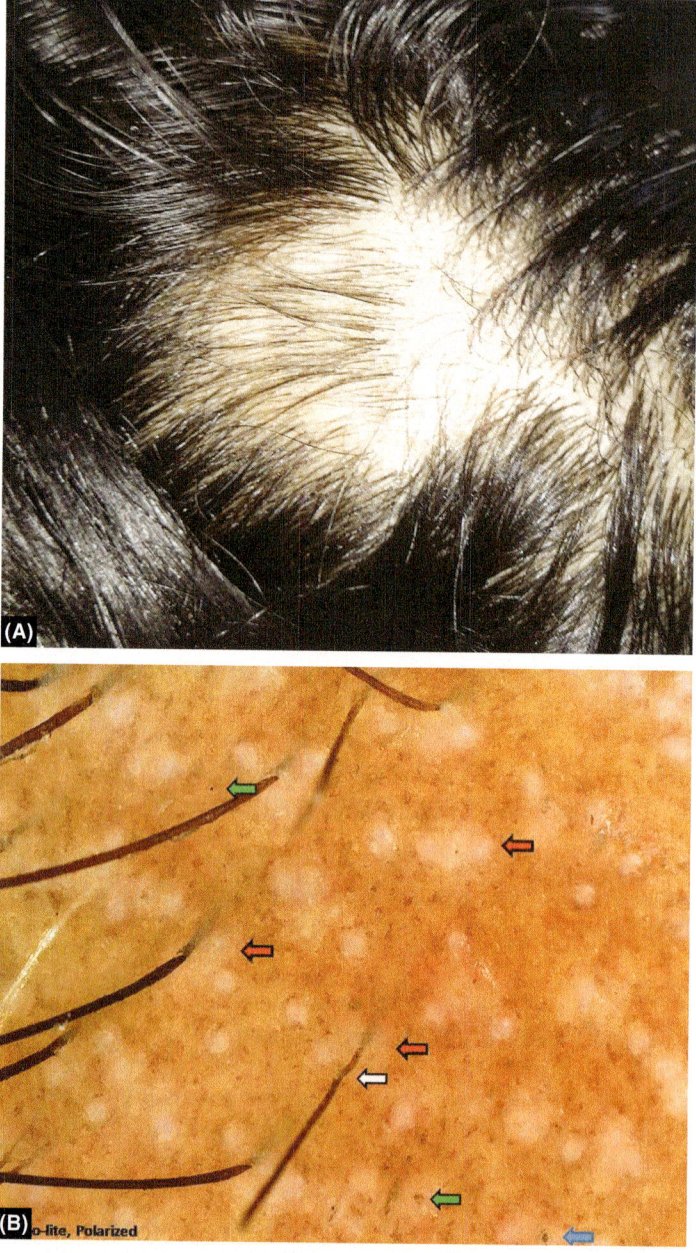

Fig. 7.13A and B: (A) A 22-year-old girl presented with 3 × 4 cm size patch of hair loss on vertex of scalp of 6 months duration. The patch showed partial regrowth in the central area. However, patient complained of increase in the size of the lesion; (B) Trichoscopic findings from the periphery of the lesion (follows)

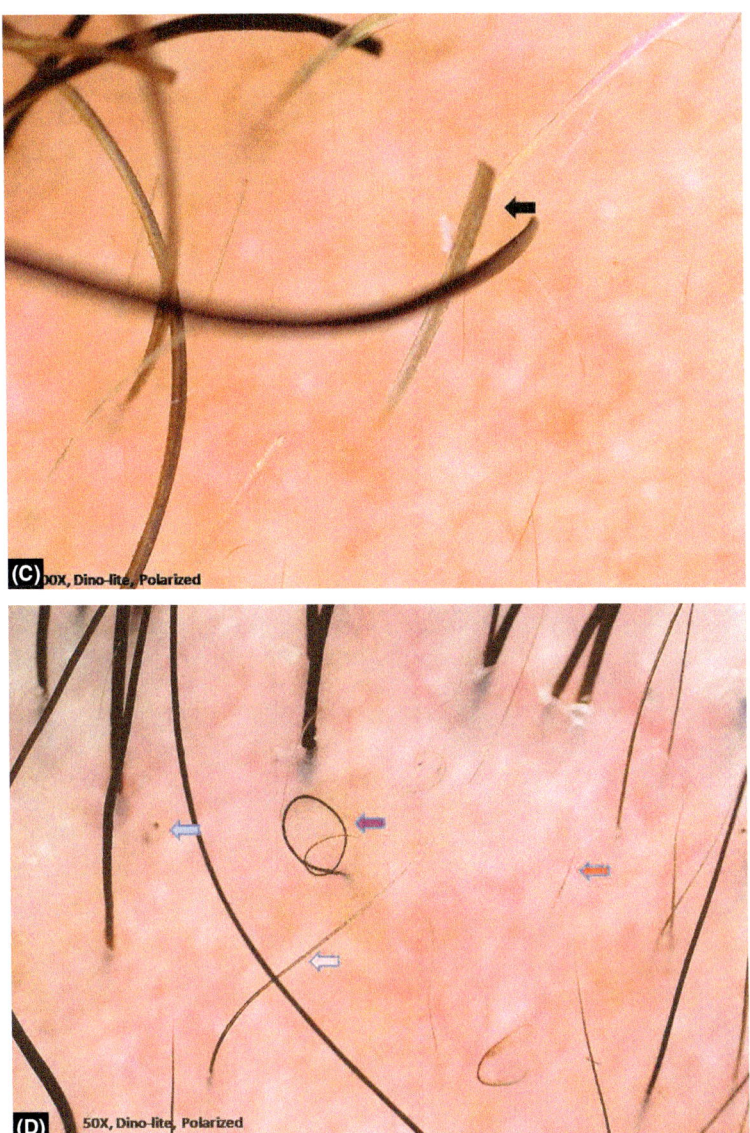

Fig. 7.13C and D: (B and C) Showed presence of yellow dots (red arrows), black dots (green arrows), cadaveric hair (blue arrow), caudability sign (white arrow) and exclamation mark hair (black arrow) consistent with alopecia areata in active phase whereas the trichoscopy of central area; (D) Showed pigtail hair (purple arrow), vellus hair (pink arrow) and tapering hair (brown arrow) consistent with alopecia areata in regrowing phase. Hence, patient was given injection triamcinolone acetonide 10 mg/ml only in the margins of the lesion for cessation of disease activity along with topical minoxidil

topical immunotherapy, anthralin, minoxidil, and photochemotherapy are available for the treatment of AA. The topical agents are to be used only for localized AA and are of no use for extensive AA.

Topical Agents

1. Corticosteroids

a. **IL steroids:** Intralesional corticosteroid injection is the first-line therapy for adult patients with less than 50% scalp involvement. Concentrations of triamcinolone acetonide vary from 2.5 to 10.0 mg/ml diluted either in xylocaine or sterile saline.

Scalp AA: 5 mg/ml with a maximum total volume of 3 ml.

Eyebrow/beard: 2.5 mg/ml

Method: 0.5 inch long 30-gauge needle is used to give multiple intradermal injections of 0.1 ml per site.

Results: Initial regrowth is often seen in 4–8 weeks. Treatments are repeated every 4 to 6 weeks. After **6 months** of treatment, if there is no response, treatment should be discontinued.

Side effects: Local atrophy is the most common side effect and an important reason for discontinuation of treatment (Fig. 7.14).

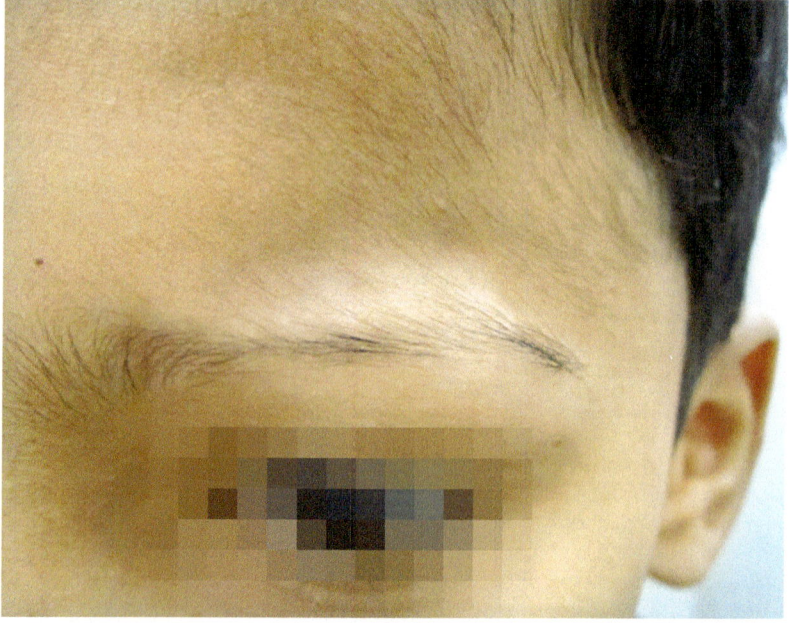

Fig. 7.14: Localized depigmentation and atrophy in a case following IL steroid injecton in the eyebrow

A recent study compared triamcinolone acetonide (TA) and betamethasone dipropionate (BD) injections and found the latter to be better in a ¼ dilution (Ustuner P et al).

b. **Topical corticosteroids:** Various steroids are used including, clobetasol propionate, betamethasone valerate, fluocinolone acetonide and halcinonide. Fiedler et al used a combination of 0.05% betamethasone dipropionate cream and minoxidil and found it to be more beneficial than either alone. The crucial aspect while using steroids on the scalp is using them in the correct base, that is a lotion, foam or shampoo formulation may be better than an ointment or cream base. Treatment should be continued for at least **3 months**.

However, topical treatment has been found to be less effective than IL route, and thus this should be used mainly in children or patients not willing for IL injections.

2. Minoxidil

Topical minoxidil solution is also used with 5% being the most effective concentration.

Indications: Patchy AA.

Application: It must be applied twice daily.

Results: Usually seen after 12 weeks.

Combination: Although combination therapy has been found to be more effective than monotherapy, this therapy is not effective in patients with AT/AU.

a. Anthralin is applied 2 hours *after* the minoxidil application.

b. Betamethasone dipropionate cream is applied twice daily, 30 minutes *after* each use of minoxidil.

3. Anthralin

Anthralin may have a nonspecific immunomodulating effect (anti-Langerhans' cell), as it does in psoriasis. Its mode of action is via its inhibition of the JAK pathway. Clinical irritation is not necessary for efficacy. As is the case with most topical agents, it is to be used for localized AA. Experiments showed that expression of tumor necrosis factor-α and interferon-γ was inhibited by anthralin, whereas expression of interleukin-1 αβ and their receptor antagonist, interleukin-1RA, and interleukin-10 was stimulated by anthralin.

Use: Anthralin 0.5–1.0% cream is applied once daily. Short contact therapy is preferred. It is applied daily for 15 to 20 minutes initially then washed. The contact time is increased by 5 minutes weekly up to 1 hour or until low-grade dermatitis develops. The contact time is then fixed and continued daily for at least 3 months before judging the response to treatment. It is mistakenly believed that anthralin should produce a mild irritant reaction to be effective. Use of topical CS at the same time is not advisable.

Avoid: Eyebrows or the beard area.

Results: New hair growth is usually seen within 3 months.

A recent study has examined its use in extensive AA in children (Özdemir M). Using a 1% anthralin, the mean time to first response in terms of new hair growth was 3 months and the mean time to maximal response was 9 months. Those that responded can continue the therapy for 12 months. About 33% achieved complete response. In the first 12-month period, 10 patients (33.4%) achieved complete response and of the 36% with partial response, 6 patients achieved a complete response before the end of the study.

If used properly the results of this can compare with most other topical therapies.

4. Topical Immunotherapy

Contact immunotherapy is an effective treatment for some patients with patchy alopecia areata. The application of a potent allergen to a small area on the scalp sensitizes the patient. The same allergen, in a concentration that is sufficient to induce a mild contact dermatitis, is then applied weekly. Contact allergens used in this treatment include dinitrochlorobenzene, squaric acid dibutylester and diphenylcyclopropenone, with diphenylcyclopropenone being most commonly used.

MOA: Though the mode of action of contact immunotherapy is unknown, antigens might induce 'antigenic competition' and attract CD4+ T cells away from the perifollicular region (Happle R). Other proposed mechanisms include the nonspecific stimulation of suppressor T cells in the skin (Bröcker EB), increased local expression of transforming growth factor-β and the activation of myeloid suppressor cells.

Results: Although the published response rates vary widely (9–87%), in general, 20–30% of patients achieve a response that is considered to be worthwhile to enable the patient to manage without a wig (Rokhsar CK). Longer treatments have a better response. Less favourable responses were reported in patients with extensive hair loss and the response in patients with alopecia totalis and alopecia universalis was only 17%, which did not improve upon prolonged treatment beyond 9 months.

Relapse: Unfortunately, 62% of successfully treated patients showed relapse.

Side effects: The side effects can be a big drawback to its use, including dermatitis, cervical lymphadenopathy, hyperpigmentation and hypopigmentation (including vitiligo) and most importantly health professional developing sensitization.

Photochemotherapy

The mechanism of action of PUVA on AA is believed to be a photoimmunologic and it acts by affecting the T cell function and antigen presentation, and possibly inhibits the local immunologic attack against the hair follicle by depleting Langerhans' cells.

It can be administered topically (0.1% 8-methoxypsoralen) followed by UVA with excellent regrowth in 8/22 (36.3%) and good regrowth in 2/22 (9%). The mean total UVA exposure is 171.1 joules/cm², with a mean 47 treatments. Whole body PUVA can also be used with variable results. A cheaper option is PUVASOL, wherein almost (71.42%) of patients showed complete hair regrowth in 14 weeks. In this 8 methoxy - psoralen (0.75% solution) was applied half an hour prior to the exposure to sunlight, for 30 seconds which was gradually increased to 2 minutes (Sharma PK).

Efficacy: Photochemotherapy with all types of PUVA (oral or topical psoralen, local or whole body UVA irradiation) claims success rates of up to 60–65% for alopecia areata in uncontrolled studies, with inconsistent results.

The major problem with PUVA therapy is the high relapse rate that frequently sets in after tapering the treatment.

308 nm Excimer Laser Therapy

Excimer laser therapy is believed to employ a 308-nm wavelength ultraviolet (UV) B light to induce T cell apoptosis and has been previously used in the treatment of psoriasis, vitiligo, mycosis fungoides, atopic dermatitis, lichen planus, and prurigo nodularis. There is evidence that laser therapy may also be beneficial for AA; however, additional long-term data are required (McMichael AJ, Byun JW).

Systemic Agents

1. Corticosteroids

Systemic corticosteroids have been used for many years in patients with rapidly progressive and extensive AA. They are the most frequently prescribed therapy in AA with myriad regimens including single dose administration, alternate day doses of prednisone, short-term high dose intravenous methylprednisolone, tapered doses and interval therapy with tapered doses over 1 week every month for

3–6 months. In general, success rate is found to be much better in multifocal AA compared to ophiasic, totalis, and universalis AA.

The common oral regimens practiced include:

i. Prednisolone 40 mg daily tapered over 6 weeks
ii. Dexamethasone 5 mg on 2 consecutive days weekly
iii. Dexamethasone 0.5 mg daily for 6 months.

A study by Kurosawa et al compared different treatment modalities. They used either (a) dexamethasone 0.5 mg/day for 6 months or (b) intramuscular triamcinolone acetonide 40 mg once a month for 6 months followed by 40 mg once every 1.5 months for 1 year or (c) pulse therapy with oral prednisolone at 80 mg for 3 consecutive days once every 3 months. Response rates were found to be better with intramuscular triamcinolone acetonide as compared to the dexamethasone group in patients with multifocal AA. Relapse rates in patients with AT/AU were found to be the lowest in the patients who received pulse therapy with oral prednisolone. Thus, this could be a simple intervention method for the practitioner without resorting to IV pulses of steroids.

The use of steroids till Cushing threshold might possibly result in long-term suppression of disease activity without incurring the dreaded side-effects of systemic corticosteroid therapy. It should be noted that the **Cushing threshold dose** is the lowest dose that causes iatrogenic Cushing's syndrome with typical symptoms of abdominal obesity, buffalo hump, moon face, red striae, virilization as well as osteoporosis, amenorrhea, adynamia, parchment skin, and diabetes—varies between different corticosteroids. While betamethasone and dexamethasone have a Cushing threshold of only 1.5 mg/day, it is 40 mg/day for 'conventional' cortisone and 7.5 mg/day for prednisolone. In children, the threshold dose for the most commonly used corticosteroid–prednisolone has been calculated at 6 mg/day/m^2 body surface (BSA) (Mosteller formula).

Other regimens are given in Box 7.2, but in essence, one should desist from using intermediate and long-acting steroids as their

---

Box 7.2: Overview of steroid regimens

Systemic corticosteroid regimens include:

1. Prednisolone 40 mg daily tapered over 6 weeks
2. Dexamethasone 5 mg on 2 consecutive days weekly
3. Intravenous methylprednisolone 250 mg twice daily on 3 consecutive days monthly
4. Dexamethasone 0.5 mg daily for 6 months
5. Intramuscular triamcinolone acetonide 40 mg monthly
6. Prednisolone 80 mg daily on 3 consecutive days every 3 months

potential for suppression of the HPA axis is more. Thus the oft used pulse therapy of such steroids (betamethasone or dexamethasone) in India, is converse to pharmacological principles where such pulsed regimens are more suited for short and intermediate acting steroids.

2. Cyclosporine

Due to the cost of the drug, its side-effect profile, the high recurrence rate following discontinuation of the treatment, the long treatment periods, and the inability to change the ultimate prognosis of the disease, this treatment should be reserved for exceptionally recalcitrant AA cases.

3. Sulfasalazine

This treatment has been used from time to time by some researchers and has results that require confirmation.

MOA: Sulfasalazine has both immunomodulatory and immuno-suppressive actions, including inhibition of T cell proliferation, natural killer cell activity, and antibody production. Sulfasalazine also inhibits the T cell cytokines IL-2 and IFN-γ and the monocyte/macrophage cytokines IL-1, TNF-α, and IL-6.

Results: In an open-label study done on patients with severe AA, complete hair regrowth was achieved in 27.3% of patients (Aghaei S).

Dose: Sulfasalazine was started at 0.5 g twice daily for 1 month, 1 g twice daily for 1 month, and then 1.5 g twice daily for 4 months. The relapse rate was 45.5%. Thirty-two percent of patients suffered from adverse effects, which included gastrointestinal distress, rash, headache, and laboratory abnormalities. A similar response rate (25.6%) was shown in another uncontrolled trial of 39 patients with AA.

4. Methotrexate

Methotrexate (MTX) is often combined with steroids. A study by Chartaux E and Joly P showed a success rates of 63–64% using a combination of MTX 15 mg weekly and prednisone at 10 mg or 20 mg daily. Hair regrowth in 57% of patients with AT and AU was achieved using MTX alone. The onset of hair regrowth was noted after a median delay of 3 months. Interestingly this drug has been used in *children* also and Royer et al treated 14 children aged 8–18 years with MTX at doses between 15 and 25 mg/week and found that 5/14 children showed more than 50% regrowth.

A recent study has again examined its role but without steroids and has found that in a dose of 10–15 mg/week it is efficacious, more so in patients with a disease duration <24 months (Lim SK et al).

Importantly the use of methotrexate alone makes more sense as the results of the combination with steroids is only marginally better, but the relapse rates are higher in the steroid group.

5. Azathioprine

It is a cytotoxic and immunosuppressive drug that has been used in the treatment of autoimmune diseases for more than 50 years. It seems to impair T cell function and IL-2; it seems to be more *selective* for T lymphocyte than for B lymphocyte.

Some authors are inclined towards using azathioprine in a dose of 50 mg twice a day for 2–3 months for extensive alopecia areata (Vañó-Galván S). It is a reasonably effective drug for use in AA, but has a slow onset of action.

6. Biologicals

The response of alopecia areata to biologic drugs has so far proven to be disappointing and several reports exist of alopecia areata occurring in patients receiving anti-TNF biologic drugs for other conditions (Ferran M et al). In an open-label study in 17 patients with moderate to severe alopecia areata there was no response to treatment with etanercept. In a randomized controlle trial in 45 patients with severe alopecia areata, there was no significant response to alefacept, compared with placebo (Galán-Gutiérrez M).

1. **Janus kinase inhibitors:** Tofacitinib citrate (Xeljanz®) abrogates IL-15 signaling and the IL-15 activation of lymphocytes. Ruxolitinib and baricitinib are JAK1/2 inhibitors while tofacitinib, is a pan-JAK inhibitor. Both tofacitinib and ruxolitinib have shown promising efficacy in preventing the development of AA in mouse models when administered systematically. Clinical case studies have shown similarly promising results. Although the number of reports is small, and no randomized, placebo-controlled studies have yet been performed, the response in patients with severe alopecia areata (in which spontaneous remission is rare) strongly suggests a therapeutic effect.

   Three patients with moderate to severe AA demonstrated hair regrowth when administered systemic ruxolitinib and on histopathology, a decrease in perifollicular T cell infiltration and dermal inflammation was observed (Xing L). Hair regrowth was also observed in a patient, diagnosed with AU, who was given ruxolitinib for thrombocythemia. Similarly, three patients with AU treated with systemic tofacitinib in two different studies experienced significant hair regrowth. Thus, there is potential for efficacy with JAK inhibitors. Although no serious adverse effects were observed, previously noted concerns include an increase in infection, anemia, neutropenia, headache, and mild nausea with tofacitinib and moderate to severe thrombocytopenia, anemia, and 'ruxolitinib withdrawal syndrome' with ruxolitinib (Gupta AK).

Of these the drug tofacitinib citrate (Xeljanz®) is available in India and is used for RA. A recent 3 months open-label trial of 66 patients with AA, was conducted by Liu et al with AA (14.4%), AU (83.3%), or AT (2.2%). Tofacitinib 5 mg twice daily was given for the first 2–3 months of treatment. After this induction phase, 29% of patients received a higher tofacitinib dose (up to 10 mg orally twice daily), and 28% of patients started adjuvant therapy with pulsed prednisone. 77% of cases achieved a clinical response after 4–18 months of therapy and 20% showed a complete response (full hair regrowth) after a median of 15 months of treatment.

Importantly, like other systemic agents, patients with AA were better responders than those with AT or AU. Also the trial did not include long-standing cases of AA (>10-year duration).

An informative case depicts the lack of efficacy in treatment resistant case of AT (Fig. 7.15). It seems the suppression of AA by tofacitinib is an active process that, if too weak, may not tip the balance towards stable hair regrowth but instead allow a reversion to a completely alopecic state. In essence the exact duration of therapy is not yet decided hence, the relapses and lack of consistent response should not be ignored.

Thus, we should be cautious and read the fine print, as was the case with the initial use of anti-TNF-α biologicals like etanercept in psoriasis. A few points to ponder and practice include:

a. Do the costs justify the therapy as in AT/AU the results are not encouraging?

b. What are the relapse rates of this drug therapy?

c. Oral JAK inhibitors used to treat rheumatoid arthritis have been associated with significant adverse events, including rare cancers (soft tissue and lymphoma) and serious infections. Whether these risks are unique to patients with rheumatoid arthritis because of comorbidities and concurrent medications, remains to be determined in AA.

Hopefully more trials will be able to shed light on these issues.

2. **IL12/23:** Suárez-Fariñas M et al found that in AA signatures with Th2, Th1, IL-23, and IL-9/TH9 cytokine activation, were seen in scalp biopsies, suggesting consideration of anti-Th2, anti-Th1, and

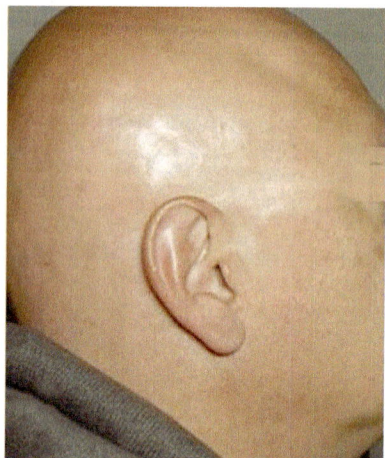

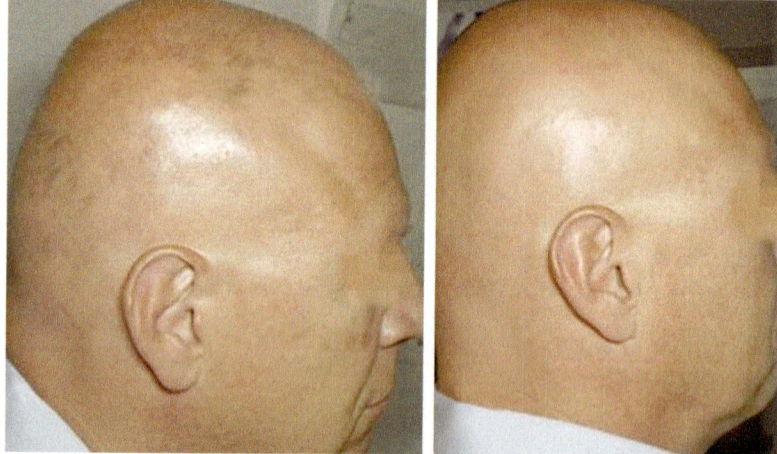

Fig. 7.15: An illustrative case of a failure of JAK inhibitors in a case of AT (figure used with the Permission of Dr. Alexander A. Navarini)

anti-IL-23 targeting strategies. As patients with alopecia areata had a significant increase in the levels of IL-12 and IL-23 in their skin compared with normal patients **ustekinumab**, a human monoclonal antibody that is targeted against these cytokines can be used. A small series of patients had a gradual improvement at 20 and 28 weeks of treatment and full hair regrowth by week 49 (Guttman-Yassky E). Clinical trials are in progress for using this drug to treat patients with alopecia areata.

3. **Apremilast:** Apremilast is an oral agent that blocks the action of phosphodiesterase (PDE)-4, preventing the production of IFN-γ and leading to a decrease in MHC class II expression (Schafer PH). Given

these anti-inflammatory properties and FDA approval for use in the treatment of additional autoimmune diseases, including psoriasis, apremilast was further investigated for the treatment of AA in murine models. Study results showed that apremilast treatment prevented collapse of immune privilege and the onset of AA. The ability of apremilast to induce hair growth in established AA is yet to be determined (Keren A).

4. **Low-dose interleukin-2:** A deficiency in T-regulatory cells is believed to contribute to AA (Shin BS). There is evidence that low-dose IL-2 promotes recruitment of these immune suppressing regulatory cells and is thus this a potential future option for disease that has not responded to previous therapies. In a clinical trial, four of five patients with AU displayed partial regrowth after 6 months of subcutaneous low-dose IL-2. Adverse events were considered mild to moderate, as there were reports of asthenia, arthralgia, urticaria, and local injection-site reactions (Castela E).

5. **Stem cell approaches:** Stem cell educator therapy (Li, Y) has shown some initial success with a "closed-loop" system to isolate mononuclear cells derived from patients with alopecia areata, allowing them to interact with human cord blood-derived multipotent stem cells and then return the 'educated' cells into the patient's circulation. Using this treatment, patients with severe alopecia areata had improvement in both hair regrowth and QOL. The underlying mechanism seemed to be the upregulation of T helper 2 (Th2) cytokines and the restoration of balancing Th1, Th2 and Th3 cytokine production.

7. Statins

Simvastatin/Ezetimibe: A combination of simvastatin and ezetimibe was effective in the treatment of a case of AT and AU. Furthermore, a prospective pilot study (N = 19) reported 20% hair regrowth after 24 weeks of treatment in 70% of participants.

Simvastatin is believed to inhibit the loss of immune privilege in the hair follicle through downregulation of adhesion molecules on leukocytes and endothelial cells. Simvastatin also blocks major histocompatibility complex (MHC) class II expression whereas ezetimibe is believed to contribute additional immunomodulatory and anti-inflammatory effects (Gupta AK).

Platelet-rich Plasma

Platelet-rich plasma (PRP) is an autologous plasma preparation of concentrated platelets. Growth factors within the platelets are released when PRP is activated and have been shown to stimulate angiogenesis, proliferation, and differentiation in hair follicles, leading to an increase in duration of anagen phase and promotion of hair growth.

In particular, the transforming growth factor (TGF)-β is a known immunosuppressant, and may have a role in restoring follicular immune privilege. In a randomized trial in 45 participants 1–3 years into relapse, PRP treatment increased hair growth and cell proliferation compared with triamcinolone acetonide or placebo. At 12 months after the first treatment, 60% of patients had achieved complete remission.

It has been suggested that PRP be reserved for mild cases. PRP treatments were administered over 6 months and assessed at 1 year. Only one relapse was reported, suggesting a benefit. Thus far, side effects are mild to non-existent, and no adverse effects have been reported (Gupta AK).

COSMETIC STRATEGIES

Women with extensive alopecia might decide to wear a wig, hairpiece or bandana. Men tend to shave their heads, although some opt for a wig. The former is the technique adopted by a famous actor now director, who in his acting career was always seen in a wig. His son another famous actor, luckily, has his hair intact. The use of semi-permanent tattooing can be helpful to disguise loss of eyebrows.

Patients can be asked to refer to patient support organizations, for example, the National Alopecia Areata Foundation (https://www.naaf.org) and Alopecia UK (http:// www.alopeciaonline.org.uk).

APPROACH TO TREATMENT

The therapy in AA depends on patient's age, extent of alopecia, and motivation for treatment. In India, there is an issue with patients who either want a guaranteed cure or those who have a steroid phobia and are unwilling to even use these as topical agents. It is thus a good advice to tell the patient about the course of the disease and the possibility of relapse and also reiterate the safety of topical steroids on the scalp.

Another method of examining the therapy options is to understand the pathogenesis and place, the various options on the pathways depicted in Flowchart 7.1. Of course, the issue always lies in understanding which of the pathways is important, though for now agents that target the CD8+ cells or the JAK pathways seems to be the "flavor of the year".

In children (<10 years), topical therapies with minoxidil, corticosteroids, and anthralin can be considered, whereas in adults other options to be considered include intralesional corticosteroids or

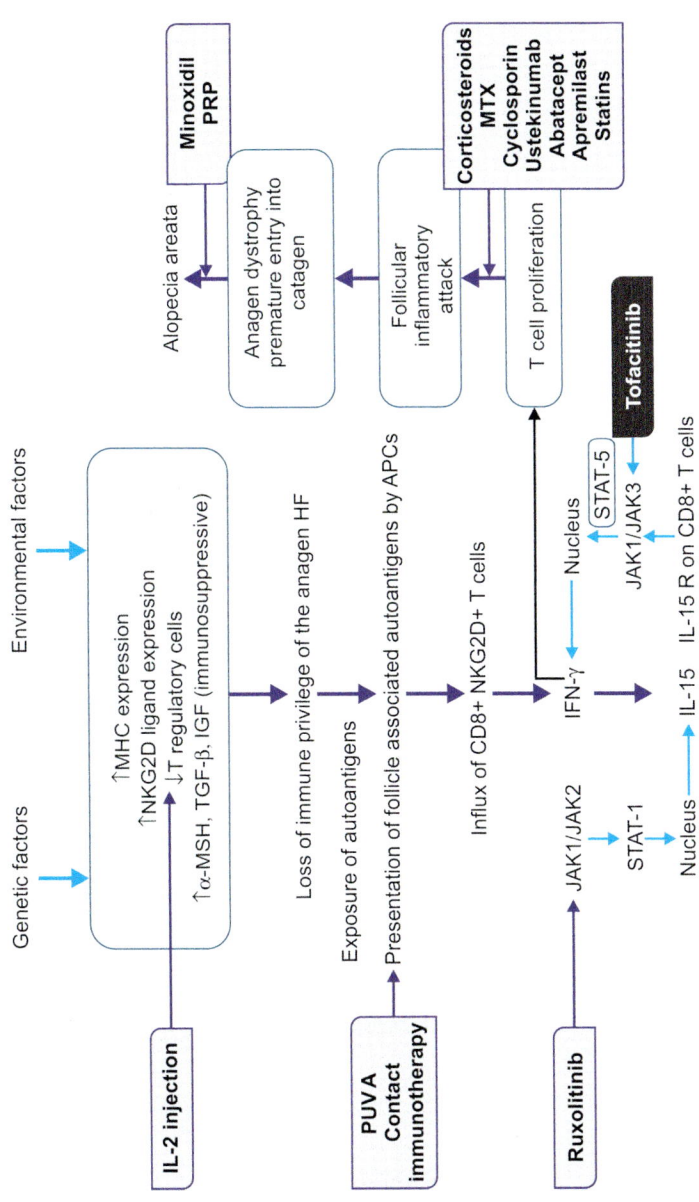

Flowchart 7.1: Practical treatment algorithm for treatment of alopecia areata, based on the salient pathogenetic steps

immunotherapy. Flowchart 7.2 systemic therapy should only be carefully considered in adults with rapid progressive AA or therapy refractory AA.

For adult patients with less than 50% scalp hair loss intralesional corticosteroid injection is a valid intervention (Flowchart 7.2). In case of no response after 3–4 months, minoxidil 5% solution twice daily followed by a superpotent corticosteroid cream such as clobetasol propionate applied 30 minutes after the minoxidil is a useful regimen. Another option is to add short-contact anthralin therapy combined with topical minoxidil 5% solution applied twice daily.

For those patients with more than 50% scalp involvement, a good first-line option, if the clinician is adequately trained in it, is topical immunotherapy with DPCP. If there is no response by 52 weeks, topical immunotherapy should be discontinued. This is apart from the other options discussed above including systemic PUVA. A scalp prosthesis/wig should be advised to all patients with more than 50% scalp involvement.

Children, older than 10 years are treated with the same protocols as in adults. In those younger than 10 years, minoxidil alone or in combination with a midpotency topical corticosteroid or anthralin is a valid option.

Flowchart 7.2: Treatment of AA based on age and area of involvement

SPECIAL SCENARIOS

A summary of various scenarios that the clinician may encounter is detailed below as a guide, though most clinicians use a combination of regimens.

1. **Alopecia areata that is minimal** (affects <25% of the scalp surface or moderate (<50%), that is spreading slowly and/or spread some time ago):
   - IL steroids
   - Topical CS
   - Minoxidil
   - Anthralin
   - Combinations of the above
2. **Major alopecia areata in adults** (affects >50% of the scalp, widespread ophiasis pattern, alopecia totalis, alopecia universalis):
   - PUVA
   - Contact immunotherapy
   - Methotrexate
3. **Rapidly spreading alopecia** (non-ophiasis pattern)
   - Methylprednisolone pulses
   - Oral: Prednisolone pulse
4. **Children with AA**

   Localised AA/multifocal AA

   1. The most commonly used therapy for more limited AA in children is topical corticosteroids, with or without occlusion class I steroid used as an intermittent pulse therapy.
      - Clobetasone for 3 months
      - Intradermal corticosteroid injections: Uncomfortable
      - Triamcinolone acetonide: 2.5 mg/ml (eyebrow area) to 10 mg/ml (scalp). 0.1 ml interval of 4 to 6 weeks.
   2. Minoxidil: 2 to 5%: Regrowth is seen in 20 to 45% of patients in a BD dose combination with corticosteroids or anthralin (Price VH).

      SE: Local irritation, allergic contact dermatitis, and hypertrichosis, tachycardia, palpitations, and dizziness (Georgala S).
   3. Prostaglandin F2α analogues (e.g. latanoprost, bimatoprost, travoprost): Not useful, can cause periorbital hyperpigmentation.
   4. Anthralin cream (1%): SCT (30 min–2 hr). No concomitant corticosteroids. Growth is seen in 3–6 months.
   5. Topical calcipotriol: Not very effective

6. Excimer laser therapy, 2/weekly: 60% regrowth of recalcitrant patches of AA × 3 months

Extensive AA

1. Immunotherapy: Difficult to perform in children
2. PUVA: Erratic results
3. Oral CS

    Most responders are patients with duration of less than 6 months and an onset at younger than 10 years of age and multifocal *vs* diffuse disease respond better. Most relapse back. Continuing application of topical minoxidil after a steroid taper has been shown to decrease hair loss.

    a. Prednisone: 0.5 to 1 mg/kg per day × 4 weeks until hair loss ceases. Tapered to alternate-day therapy for a few months.

    b. Sequential high and low dose steroid: 2 mg/kg × 9 weeks: Tapered to below the individual Cushing threshold (6 mg/m^2/day). Maintenance therapy consist of doses between 75% and 25% of the Cushing threshold dose. Response: 66% in 6 weeks (Jahn-Bassler K).

    c. Pulse therapy with intravenous methylprednisolone 250 mg BD for 3 days.

    d. Intravenous methylprednisolone 8 mg/kg for 3 days × 5 to 6 months. Complete response in 38% and no response in 33%, but 81% relapsed within 9.5 months after therapy (Friedland R).

4. Methotrexate (0.3 to 0.6 mg/kg per week): >50% hair regrowth in 5 of 12 children (>40%) with recalcitrant AA × 2 months. Mean time to regrowth was 4.4 months, and all responders experienced improvement within 6 months (Royer M).

5. Sulfasalazine 1.5 g twice daily (starting with 0.5 g/dose and then 1 g/dose for the first and second month, respectively).

6. AA: Topical pJAK3 and pJAK1 inhibitors.

CONCLUSION

There are still no FDA approved treatments for alopecia areata. For AA, most therapies revolve around the clinical types, which may be an outdated concept, specially when molecular level targets have been identified. The need of the hour is to re-look at treatment based on their effect on the molecular targets (Fig. 7.1). Hopefully such studies will change the way we treat alopecia areata in the future and the Flowchart 7.2 that details therapies based on area of involvement becomes redundant.

Bibliography

1. Aghaei S. An uncontrolled, open-label study of sulfasalazine in severe alopecia areata. Indian J Dermatol Venereol Leprol 2008;74(6):611–3.

2. Bröcker EB, Echternacht-Happle K, Hamm H Happle R. Abnormal expression of class I and class II major histocompatibility antigens in alopecia areata: modulation by topical immunotherapy. J Invest Dermatol 1987; 88:564–68.

3. Byun JW, Moon JH, Bang CY, Shin J, Choi GS. Effectiveness of 308 nm excimer laser therapy in treating alopecia areata, determined by examining the treated sides of selected alopecic patches. Dermatol Basel Switz 2015;231:70–6.

4. Castela E, Le Duff F, Butori C, Ticchioni M, Hofman P, Bahadoran P, et al. Effects of low-dose recombinant interleukin-2 to promote T-regulatory cells in alopecia areata. JAMA Dermatol 2014;150(7):748–51.

5. Chartaux E, Joly P. Long-term follow-up of the efficacy of methotrexate alone or in combination with low doses of oral corticosteroids in the treatment of alopecia areata totalis or universalis Article in French. Ann Dermatol Venereol 2010;137(8–9): 507–13.96(5):69S–70S.

6. Fiedler VC. Alopecia areata: Current therapy. J Invest Dermatol 1991;.

7. Ferran M, Calvet J, Almirall M, et al. Alopecia areata as another immune-mediated disease developed in patients treated with tumour necrosis factor-α blocker agents: report of five cases and review of the literature. J Eur Acad Dermatol Venereol 2011;25:479–84.

8. Friedland R, Tal R, Lapidoth M, et al. Pulse corticosteroid therapy for alopecia areata in children: a retrospective study. Dermatology 2013;227(1):37–44.

9. Galán-Gutiérrez M, Rodríguez-Bujaldón, Moreno-Giménez JC. Update on the Treatment of Alopecia Areata. Actas Dermosifiliogr 2009;100:266–76.

10. Georgala S, Befon A, Maniatopoulou E, et al. Topical use of minoxidil in children and systemic side effects. Dermatology 2007;214:101–2.

11. Gupta AK, Carviel J, Abramovits W. Treating Alopecia Areata: Current Practices Versus New Directions. Am J Clin Dermatol 2017;18(1):67–75.

12. Guttman-Yassky E. et al. Extensive alopecia areata is reversed by IL-12/IL-23 p40 cytokine antagonism. J Allergy Clin Immunol 2016;137:301–4.

13. Happle R. Antigenic competition as a therapeutic concept for alopecia areata. Arch Dermatol Res 1980;267:109–14.

14. Jahn-Bassler K, Bauer WM, Karlhofer F, Vossen MG, Stingl G. Sequential high- and low-dose systemic corticosteroid therapy for severe childhood alopecia areata. J Dtsch Dermatol Ges 2017 Jan;15(1):42–47.

15. Joly P. The use of methotrexate alone or in combination with low doses of oral corticosteroids in the treatment of alopecia totalis or universalis. J Am Acad Dermatol 2006;55(4): 632–6.

16. Keren A, Shemer A, Ullmann Y, Paus R, Gilhar A. The PDE4 inhibitor, apremilast, suppresses experimentally induced alopecia areata in human skin *in vivo*. J Dermatol Sci 2015;77(1):74–6.

17. Kurosawa M, et al. A comparison of the efficacy, relapse rate and side effects among three modalities of systemic corticosteroid therapy for alopecia areata. Dermatology 2006; 212(4): 361–5.

18. Liu LY, Craiglow BG, Dai F, King BA. Tofacitinib for the Treatment of Severe Alopecia Areata and Variants: A Study of 90 Patients . J Am Acad Dermatol 2017;76:22–28.

19. Lim SK, Lim CA, Kwon IS, Im M, Seo YJ, Kim CD, Lee JH, Lee Y. Low-dose Systemic Methotrexate Therapy for Recalcitrant Alopecia Areata. Ann Dermatol 2017 Jun;29(3):263–67.

20. Li Y, et al. Hair regrowth in alopecia areata patients following stem cell educator therapy. BMC Med 2015;13:87.

21. Messenger AG, McKillop J, Farran P, McDonagh AJ, Sladden M. British Association of Dermatologists' guidelines for the management of alopecia areata. Br J Dermatol 2012;166:916–26.

22. McMichael AJ. Excimer laser: a module of the alopecia areata common protocol. J Investig Dermatol Symp Proc 2013;16(1):S77–9.

23. Özdemir M, Balevi A. Bilateral Half-head Comparison of 1% Anthralin Ointment in Children with Alopecia Areata. Pediatr Dermatol 2017 Mar;34(2):128–32.

24. Pratt CH, King LE Jr, Messenger AG, Christiano AM, Sundberg JP. Alopecia areata. Nat Rev Dis Primers 2017 Mar 16;3:17011.

25. Price VH. Topical minoxidil in extensive alopecia areata, including 3-year follow-up. Dermatologica 1987;175(Suppl. 2):36–41.

26. Rashidi T, Mahd AA. Treatment of persistent alopecia areata with sulfasalazine. Int J Dermatol 2008 Aug;47(8):850–2.

27. Rokhsar CK, Shupack JL, Vafai JJ, Washenik K Efficacy of topical sensitizers in the treatment of alopecia areata. J Am Acad Dermatol 1998;37:751–61.

28. Royer M, Bodemer C, Vabres P, et al. Efficacy and tolerability of methotrexate in severe childhood alopecia areata. Br J Dermatol 2011;165(2):407–10.

29. Schafer PH, Day RM. Novel systemic drugs for psoriasis: mechanism of action for apremilast, a specific inhibitor of PDE4. J Am Acad Dermatol 2013;68(6):1041–2.

30. Shapiro S ,Otberg N. Hair Loss and Restoration, second edition, English 2015. CRC Press, Taylor and Francis Group. © 2015 by Taylor & Francis Group, LLC.

31. Sharma PK, RK Jain, AK Sharma. PUVASOL therapy in alopecia areata. Ind J of DermatolVenereolLeprol. 1990; 56(4):301–303.

32. Shin BS, Furuhashi T, Nakamura M, Torii K, Morita A. Impaired inhibitory function of circulating CD4+, CD25+ regulatory T cells in alopecia areata. J Dermatol Sci 2013;70(2):141–3.

33. Ustuner P, Balevi A, Özdemir M. Best dilution of the best corticosteroid for intralesional injection in the treatment of localized alopecia areata in adults. J Dermatolog Treat 2017 May 30:1–9.

34. US National Library of Medicine. ClinicalTrials.gov https://clinicaltrials.gov/ ct2/show/NCT02599129(2017).

35. Vañó-Galván S, Hermosa-Gelbard Á, Sánchez-Neila N, Miguel-Gómez L, Saceda-Corralo D, Rodrigues-Barata R, Jaén P. Treatment of recalcitrant adult alopecia areata universalis with oral azathioprine. J Am Acad Dermatol 2016 May;74(5):1007–8.

36. Xing L, Dai Z, Jabbari A, Cerise JE, Higgins CA , Gong W, et al. Alopecia areata is driven by cytotoxic T lymphocytes and is reversed by JAK inhibition. Nat Med 2014;20:1043–9.

8

Cicatricial (Scarring) Alopecias

*Kabir Sardana, Masarat Jabeen,
Ananta Khurana, Selma CH*

INTRODUCTION

Cicatricial (scarring) alopecias comprise a diverse group of scalp disorders that probably represent the only so-called **"hair emergency"**; as, if untreated they invariably result in irreversible hair loss, which is not always amenable to even surgical therapy.

All scarring alopecias are characterized clinically by a loss of follicular ostia and pathologically by a replacement of hair follicles with fibrous tissue. They are divided into two types: *Primary* (PCA) and *secondary* cicatricial alopecias.

The location of the destructive process is crucial in determining the irreversibility of alopecia. Follicular stem cells are located in the bulge area, where the arrector pili muscle inserts into the follicles. As the hair cycles through the various stages anagen, catagen, and telogen, the upper portion is permanent while the lower portion is non-permanent. Pluripotent hair follicle stem cells are responsible for the renewal of the upper part of the hair follicle and sebaceous glands, and for the restoration of the lower cyclical component of the follicles at the onset of a new anagen period. Thus, when the inflammation is located deep, around the non-permanent portion, scarring alopecia is unlikely to develop. If the inflammation is located within the upper permanent portion, affecting the *bulge area* and the *sebaceous* gland within the isthmus then a cicatrizing alopecia is likely to occur (Cotsarelis G).

In primary scarring alopecias, the pathology primarily affects the hair follicles as opposed to secondary scarring alopecias, which affect the dermis and secondarily cause follicular destruction (Fig. 8.1).

For a proper diagnosis of these disorders, appropriate investigations and their interpretation is crucial. Various types of cicatricial alopecia have been classified based on the infiltrate seen on histology (Table 8.1 and Fig. 8.2A).

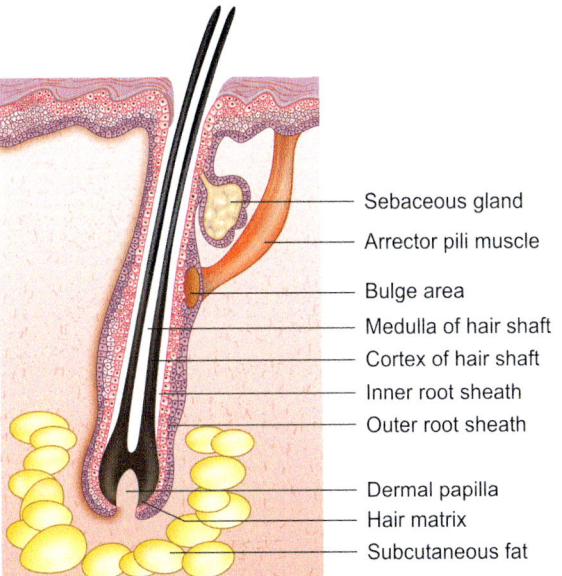

Sebaceous gland
Arrector pili muscle

Bulge area
Medulla of hair shaft
Cortex of hair shaft
Inner root sheath
Outer root sheath

Dermal papilla
Hair matrix
Subcutaneous fat

Fig. 8.1: A depiction of the hair follicle: The portion above the bulge area is permanent, i.e. it does not change through the phases of hair growth. Hence, any affliction in that area, specially the bulge area, leads to scarring alopecia

Table 8.1: Classification of primary scarring (permanent) alopecias (North American Hair Research Society, 2001)	
Lymphocyte-associated	Chronic cutaneous lupus erythematosus
	Lichen planopilaris
	Classic lichen planopilaris
	Frontal fibrosing alopecia
	Graham Little syndrome
	Classic pseudopelade (Brocq)
	Central centrifugal cicatricial alopecia
	Alopecia mucinosa
	Keratosis follicularis spinulosa decalvans
Neutrophil-associated	Folliculitis decalvans
	Dissecting cellulitis/folliculitis
Mixed inflammatory	Folliculitis (acne) keloidalis
	Folliculitis (acne) necrotica
	Erosive pustular dermatoses
Nonspecific primary scarring alopecia*	

*Nonspecific scarring primary alopecia, is defined as an idiopathic scarring alopecia with inconclusive clinical and histopathological findings, which is usually the end stage of a variety of inflammatory primary scarring alopecias, such as lichen planopilaris and folliculitis decalvans. But, this should not be labeled as pseudopelade which is a distinct entity.

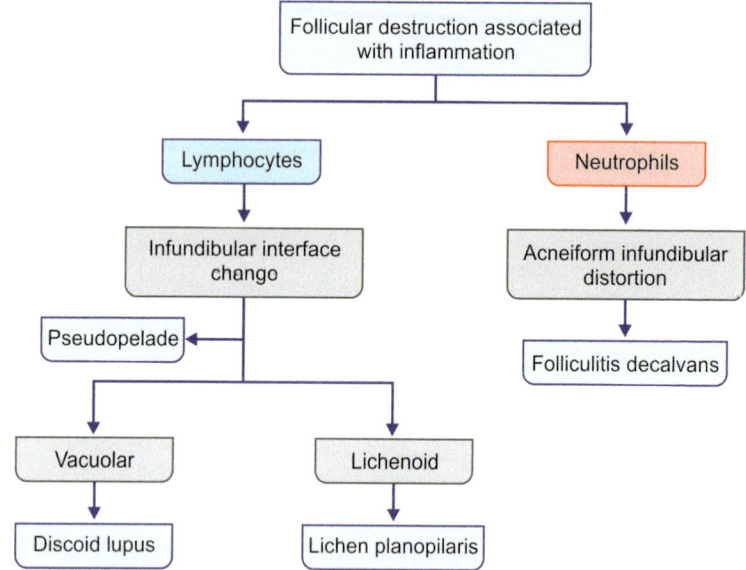

Fig. 8.2A: An overview of histological diagnosis of common cicatricial alopecias (Kossard S)

Investigations commonly employed to aid diagnosis are:
- Dermoscopy
- Biopsy (histopathology and direct immunofluorescence)

1. Dermoscopy/Trichoscopy

Trichoscopy is an excellent first-line, noninvasive method for assessing scalp and hair characteristics in clinics, giving important clues to diagnosis. It can be done by both hand-held dermatoscope using polarized light as well as with video dermatoscopy, which ensures up to 1000 times magnification (Inuis S).

Dermoscopy of PCA reveals absence of follicular ostia in 100% cases even if it is not evident clinically. Other findings suggestive of PCAs are tufted hairs, follicular hyperkeratosis, pili torti, and pink-white appearance. Trichoscopy also helps clinicians assess PCA disease activity, e.g. "follicular red dots", erythematous polycyclic, concentric structures regularly distributed in and around the follicular ostia, are suggestive of active lupus erythematosus of the scalp.

2. Biopsy for Scarring Alopecias

As evidenced by the classification above, scalp biopsies are crucial to confirm the diagnosis of scarring alopecia and to identify the type and localization of the inflammatory infiltrate. The following recommendations were developed at the consensus meeting on cicatricial alopecia (Olsen EA) in 2001.

1. A 4 mm punch biopsy should be taken from a clinically active area, following local anesthesias with 1/2% of xylocaine with epinephrine. At least 1 ml of the solution must be injected and it is ideal to wait for 15 minutes for epinephrine to be effective in reducing bleeding. The punch is placed parallel to the direction of the hairs (which is mostly not perpendicular to scalp) and inserted to the depth of the bevel. The biopsy should include the subcutaneous fat, because this is the location of terminal anagen hair bulbs.

2. The biopsy site is then closed with a blue 3–0 or 4–0 nylon suture. The blue suture allows for easier recognition and differentiation from hair during suture removal (done 7–10 days later).

The tissue is then processed for horizontal sections and stained with hematoxylin and eosin, elastin (acid alcoholic orcein), mucin, and periodic acid–Schiff (PAS) stains. Compared with vertical sectioning where 3 to 4 follicles may be acquired from one biopsy sample, horizontal sectioning allows up to 30 follicles to be examined from one sample.

A second 4 mm punch biopsy from a clinically active disease-affected area should be cut vertically into two equal pieces. One half provides tissue for transverse cut routine histological sections, and the other half can be used for direct immunofluorescence (DIF) studies. Recently, the "HoVert" (Horizontal and vertical) technique, a novel processing technique that produces transverse (horizontal) and vertical sections from a single biopsy has been described (Fig. 8.2B). This overcomes the limitation of multiple scalp biopsies (Ngyen et al).

TREATMENT PRINCIPLES

The treatment principles vary but some of these disorders can be treated using a common therapeutic protocol (Fig. 8.3). The evidence for most PCAs is generally poor, based on case series and reports. The aims of treatment are:

1. Disease arrest and symptom control. Some hair regrowth may occur, but this is uncommon.

2. Treatment is directed to areas demonstrating disease activity, rather than the irreversibly scarred areas.

3. Potent topical and intralesional steroids into the area of active inflammation are the mainstays in most PCAs. Tacrolimus can be used over long-term.

4. Minoxidil stimulates hair growth and is generally co-prescribed.

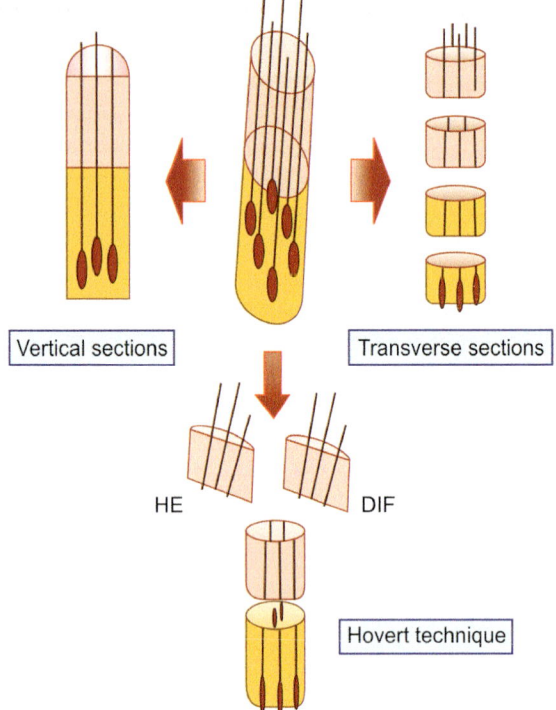

Fig. 8.2B: A diagrammatic description of Hovert technique

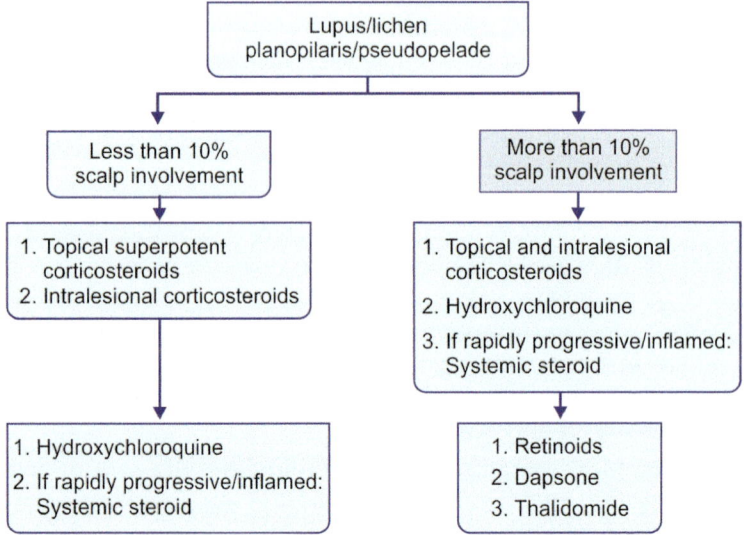

Fig. 8.3: Treatment protocol for common cicatricial alopecias

5. It must be remembered that even if PCA is controlled for a prolonged period, it may recur at any time.
6. Topical drugs may be continued as maintenance 2–3 times per week following clinical remission to prevent relapses.

A treatment overview is given in Table 8.2.

Prior to counseling the patient on treatment options, it is essential to explain that the goal of treatment is to (a) alleviate the symptoms and clinical signs and (b) retard or slow the progression of the disease. The patient should also understand that regrowth of hair is not possible and activity may recur after months or years. With this understanding, the clinician and the patient can work together to evaluate the efficacy of treatments. The therapeutic plan is generally based on the extent of the inflammatory infiltrate on biopsy (sparse, moderate, dense) and on clinical assessment of the disease.

Components of the clinical assessment include:

1. Symptoms (itching, pain, burning)
2. Clinical signs (perifollicular erythema, perifollicular scale, erythema, pustules, crusting, pull test: Anagen/total)
3. Spreading of hair loss (determined by patient self-report, review of photographs, clinical exam, and measurements if practical)

Table 8.2: Treatment overview of cicatricial alopecias		
1st line	*2nd line*	*3rd line*
Lymphocytic cicatricial alopecia		
Hydroxychloroquine 200 mg twice daily for 6–12 months or Doxycycline 100 mg twice daily for 6–12 months	MMF 0.5 gm BD × 1 month; then 1 gm BD for 5 months Cyclosporine 3–5 mg/kg per day or 300 mg/ day for 3–5 months	Pioglitazone 15 mg daily or Rosiglitazone 4 mg daily for 3–6 months
Neutrophilic/plasmacytic cicatricial alopecia		
Folliculitis decalvans	Clindamycin 300 mg BD, ciprofloxacin 750 mg BD, doxycycline 100 mg BD	Rifampicin 600 mg × 10 days
Dissecting cellulitis	Isotretinoin 10–20 mg per day for 6–12 months	Infliximab, adalimumab, etanercept

This can be evaluated once in 3 months. If there is no improvement after 3 months, then an alternative systemic drug is considered. With improvement in the outcome measures, this drug is continued for 6 to 12 months.

LYMPHOCYTIC CICATRICIAL ALOPECIAS

1. Chronic Cutaneous Lupus Erythematosus (CCLE)
(Discoid Lupus Erythematosus—DLE)

DLE and lichen planopilaris (LPP) constitute the most common causes of inflammatory cicatricial alopecias. Women are more often affected than men and the disease is more common in adults (with first onset typically at the age of 20–40 years).

Clinical Features

DLE usually presents as erythematous (Fig. 8.4), atrophic, and alopecic patches. Follicular hyperkeratosis (Fig. 8.5), hyperpigmentation, hypopigmentation (Fig. 8.6), and telangiectasia can be seen. Hyperpigmentation is frequently found in the lesion. Changes described are seen in the *centre* of the patch rather than the *edges* c.f. LPP where the activity is at the edges only. Plaques most commonly

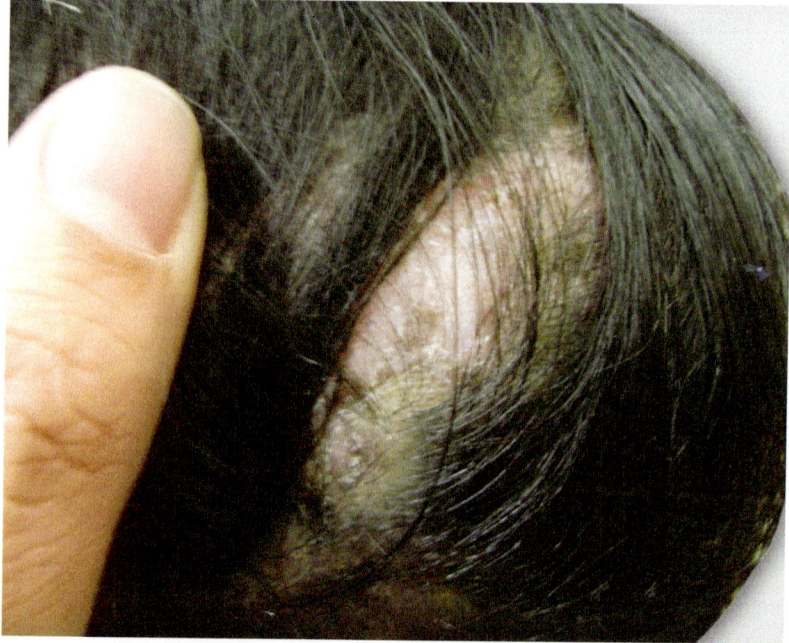

Fig. 8.4: A patient of DLE on the scalp; early stage with erythematosus plaques

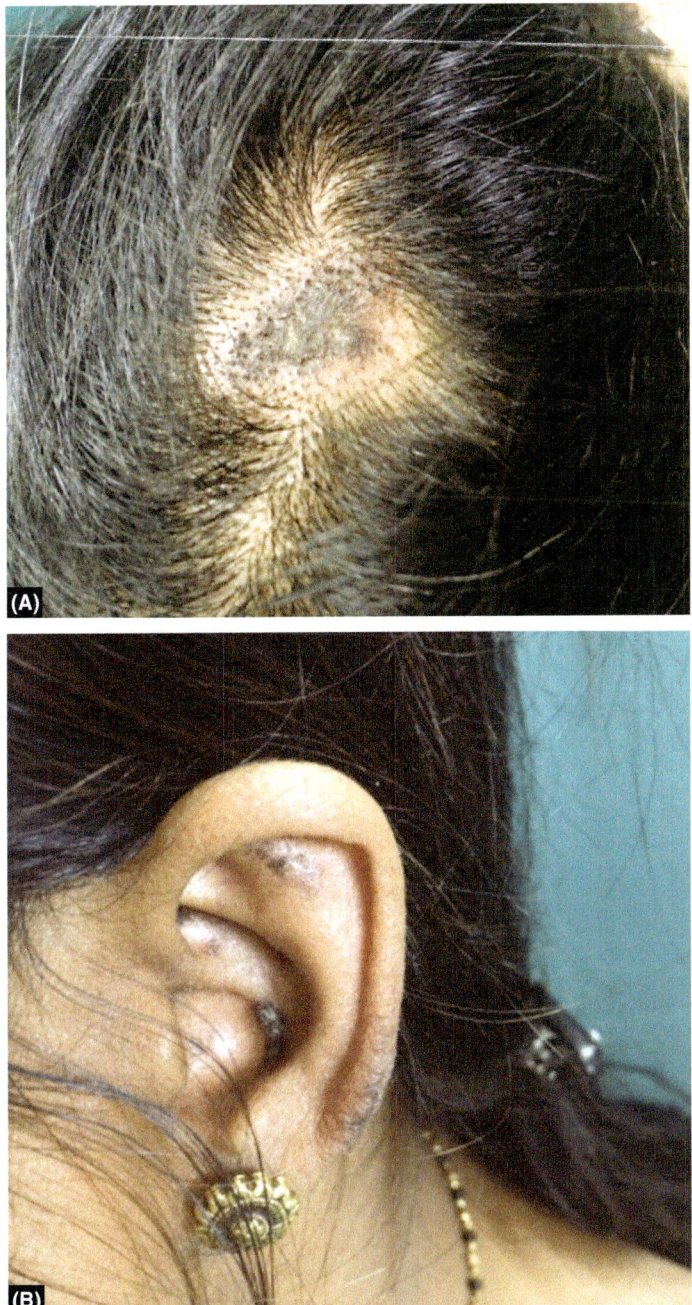

Fig. 8.5A and B: (A) A patch of discoid lupus erythematosus with hyper-pigmentation and hyperkeratosis; (B) Same patient with lesions of DLE in the ear

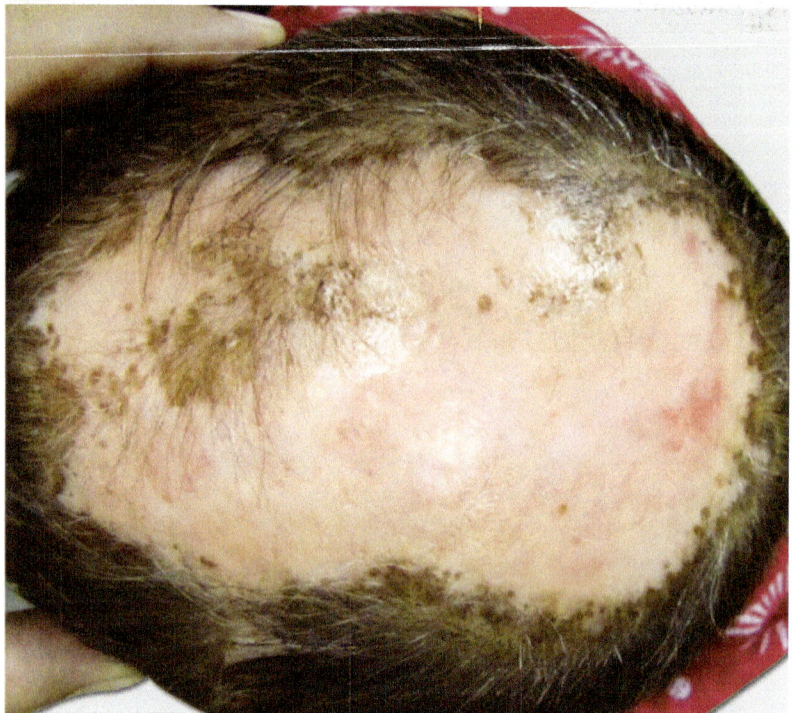

Fig. 8.6: A late stage of DLE with depigmentation of the scalp with scarring

develop over the vertex area. Active lesions can be sensitive or pruritic, and the patient might report a worsening after UV exposure. Thirty percent of these patients will also have lesions of DLE elsewhere on the body. Signs and symptoms of systemic LE must be looked for in all patients, although the incidence is low if the lesions are confined to head and neck only (1–2%). Antinuclear antibody titers are positive in 15 to 45% of cases and lupus band test positive in 60 to 80% of cases.

Investigation

Biopsy

a. Dense lymphocytic infiltrate is seen predominantly in the upper part of the follicle (at the infundibulum more than the isthmus). It may also involve the interfollicular epidermis.

b. Lymphocyte-mediated interface dermatitis with vacuolar degeneration of the follicular basal cell layer and apoptotic keratinocytes, a thickened basement membrane, and destruction of sebaceous glands is seen. Deep dermal mucin is variably present.

c. Follicular infundibula is filled with laminated keratin.

d. DIF typically shows a linear granular deposition of IgG and C3 at the dermoepidermal junction in both cutaneous and follicular epidermis. IgM, C1q, and rarely IgA can also be found.

Dermoscopy: It reveals mottled dyschromia, follicular plugs, telangiectasias, and white central plaques. In addition, blue-gray dots irregularly distributed in a speckled pattern between the hair follicles may be seen. **Red dots** can help to distinguish DLE of the scalp from lichen planopilaris (LPP) (Fig. 8.7A to C).

Treatment

DLE of scalp usually responds well to treatment. As the disorder can progress to scarring, aggressive management is required and thus steroids are invariably the first-line of therapy. They can be used topically or intralesionally in localized disease. Multimodal aggressive therapy in rapidly progressive DLE might reverse early alopecic patches and save hair follicles from the destructive process.

Patients should wear a hat and avoid sun exposure, the last of which is an issue in India in patients with outdoor jobs. Some compact fluorescent bulbs that provide indoor lighting emit more UV B than incandescent bulbs; thus their shielding is a useful measure.

1. **Oral corticosteroids** (1 mg/kg/day prednisolone) are useful in active and rapidly progressive disease and can be tapered over 2–4 months. High-potency topical steroids have been used with variable success, including 0.025–0.05% fluocinonide, clobetasol lotion or cream and intralesional triamcinolone acetonide (10 mg/ml). In some cases, oral steroids can be used as a **"bridge"** therapy while antimalarials are initiated.

2. **Antimalarials,** including 200–400 mg/day hydroxychloroquine (preferred) or 250 mg/day chloroquine, are usually initiated as the first-line treatments, but they might take 3 months for maximum efficacy. If hydroxychloroquine fails to take effect in this much time, switching to chloroquine is another option. The duration of treatment ranges from 9 to 24 months, depending on the response. The risk of ophthalmological side effects is less if a dose of 400 mg hydroxychloroquine or less per day is taken. The risk is higher when a person takes the medication over 5 years or has a cumulative dose of >1000 g. A yearly ocular evaluation is sufficient. A point in favor of anti-malarials is the observation that early hydroxychloroquine treatment is associated with a delayed systemic LE onset and with a delay in integument damage development in patients with systemic LE.

3. Other systemic agents include thalidomide, retinoids and dapsone. Oral retinoids such as acitretin have been investigated

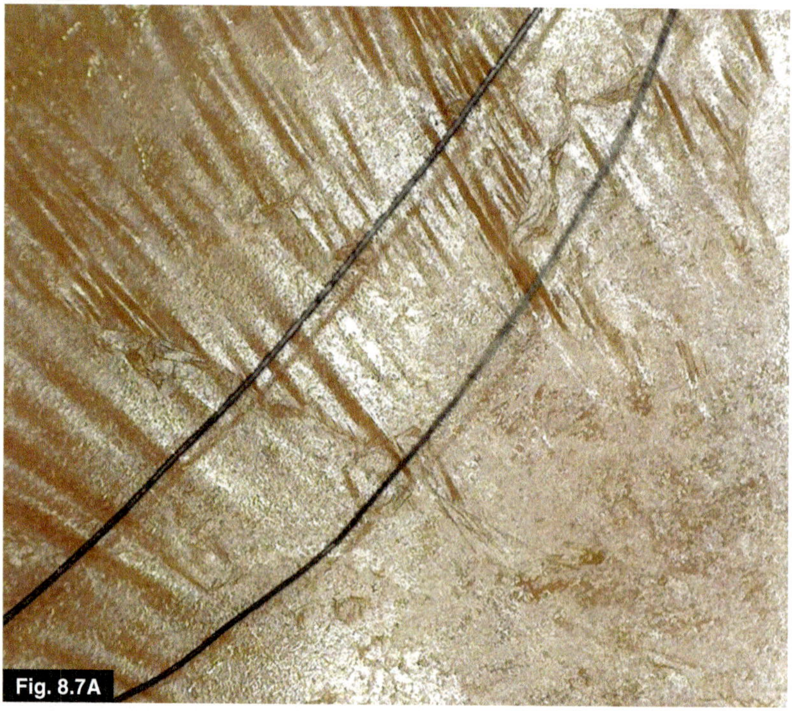

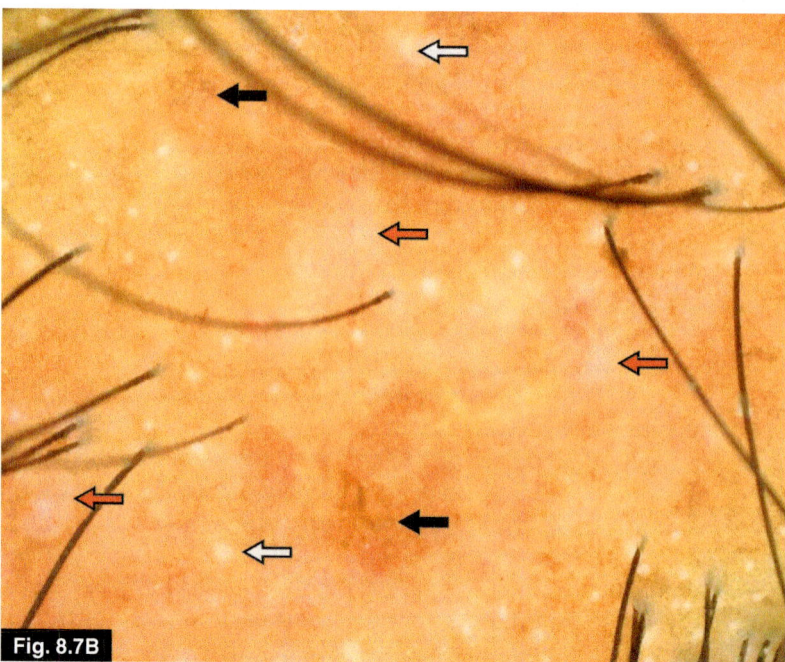

Fig. 8.7A

Fig. 8.7B

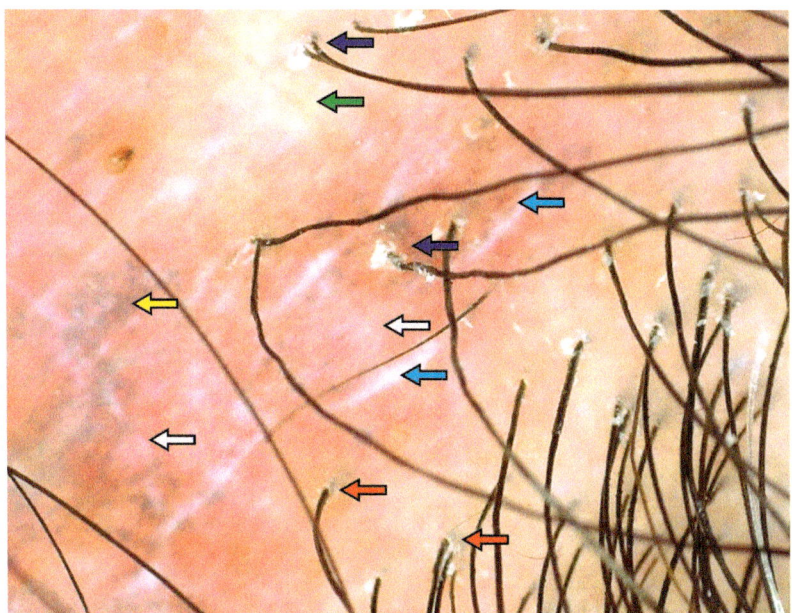

Fig. 8.7A to C: A 30-year-old male presented with multiple patches of scarring alopecia in frontal as well as vertex region of scalp. Trichoscopy of the patch present on the vertex region (A and B) showed marked atrophy, marked loss of follicular openings, pink-white areas (red arrows), white dots (white arrows), exaggeration of normal pigment network (black dots) absence of blue-grey dots, white dots, and perifollicular casts suggestive of an inactive disease. Whereas trichoscopy of a single 2–3 cm size lesion present on anterior scalp (C) showed presence of blue-gray dots (yellow arrow), perifollicular casts (blue arrows), yellow-white areas (green arrow), pink-white areas (white arrows), follicular sinking (red arrows) and Wickham's striae (light blue arrows), which were suggestive of active lichen planopilaris. The findings were further confirmed by biopsy. Patient was started on oral steroid in combination with methotrexate to control the disease activity

in randomized controlled trials and found to have similar efficacy to antimalarial treatment.

4. Unresponsive patients can be given methotrexate (7.5–25 mg/week), cyclophosphamide, mycophenolate mofetil and azathioprine. Ustekinumab has shown efficacy in case reports. Anti-TNF drugs are **not** effective and may even induce or exacerbate LE.

5. In cases of extensive cutaneous disease, rituximab, which is a chimeric monoclonal antibody that targets CD20, has been tried.

6. Vitamin E, oral gold, clofazimine have also been tried.

An overview of DLE is given in Box 8.1.

Box 8.1: DLE in nutshell

Clinical features
- Erythematosus atrophic scaly plaques
- Hyperkeratotic adherent follicular plugs
- Pigmentary disturbances

Histopathology
- Vacuolar interface alteration of follicular epithelium
- Perivascular and interstitial lymphocytic infiltrate with dermal mucin
- Atrophy of sebaceous glands and follicular plugging

DIF: Deposits of immunoglobulin IgG or IgM and C3 in a granular or homogeneous band like pattern at the dermal interface within the follicular epithelium and interfollicular epidermis.

Treatment

First line: Class 1 or 2 topical corticosteroid, IL triamcinolone acetonide injections

Second line: Antimalarials, oral corticosteroids, retinoids (acitretin 50 mg/day)

Third line: Thalidomide, methotrexate, topical immunomodulators, dapsone, azathioprine, cyclosporine.

2. Lichen Planopilaris (syn Follicular Lichen Planus)

The term "lichen planopilaris" is lichen planus with follicular keratotic lesions. Clinical *variants* include classic LPP, frontal fibrosing alopecia (FFA), and Graham Little syndrome.

Clinical Features

During the early phases, patients may not show patches of hair loss, only exhibiting small atrophic areas and pin-sized follicular papules around the hairs at the periphery. During the late stages, inflammatory signs may be completely absent. If the patch is extending, horny plugs may still be present in follicles around its margins.

In classic LPP, the affected areas are mostly located at the crown and vertex area and usually show scaling, perifollicular erythema and follicular hyperkeratosis (Fig. 8.8) in the initial stages. Typical papules of lichen planus are generally not seen. The alopecic areas of LPP are often *smaller*, *irregularly shaped*, and interconnected which can lead to a *reticulate* (Fig. 8.9A) clinical pattern which *differentiates* it from DLE. In late stages, the characteristic pigmentation is diagnostic (Fig 8.9B). However, overlapping clinical features with those of DLE are frequently seen. Patient's symptoms include itching, burning sensations, and sensitivity of the scalp. In late stages, smooth, atrophic plaques may be seen, sometimes with pseudopelade like features.

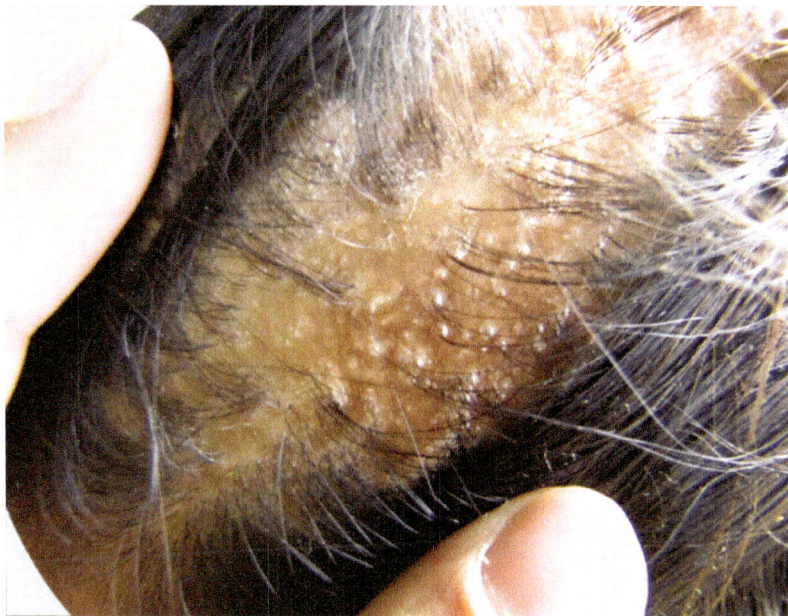

Fig. 8.8: Lichen planopilaris on the scalp; note the lack of follicular ostia and multiple follicular hyperkeratotic lesions

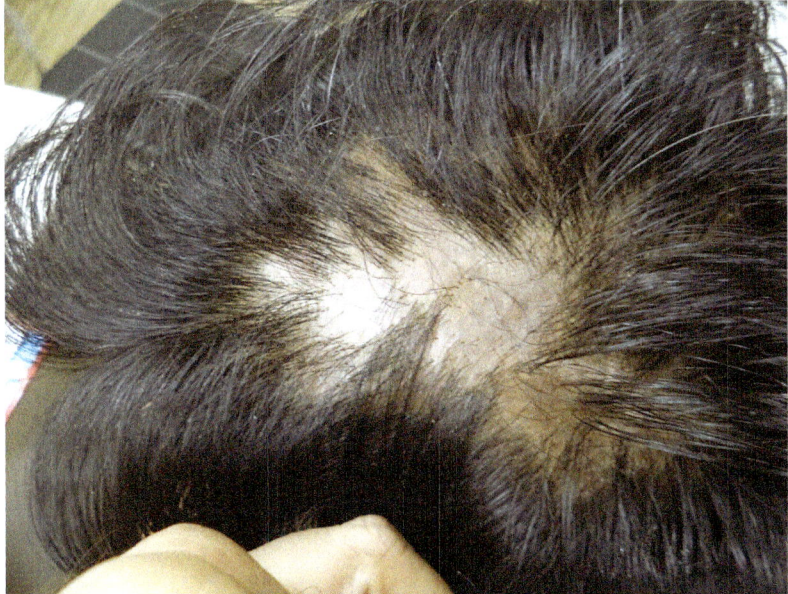

Fig. 8.9A: A case of lichen planus with cicatricial alopecia. Note the irregular, reticular pattern of alopecia with the violaceous hue

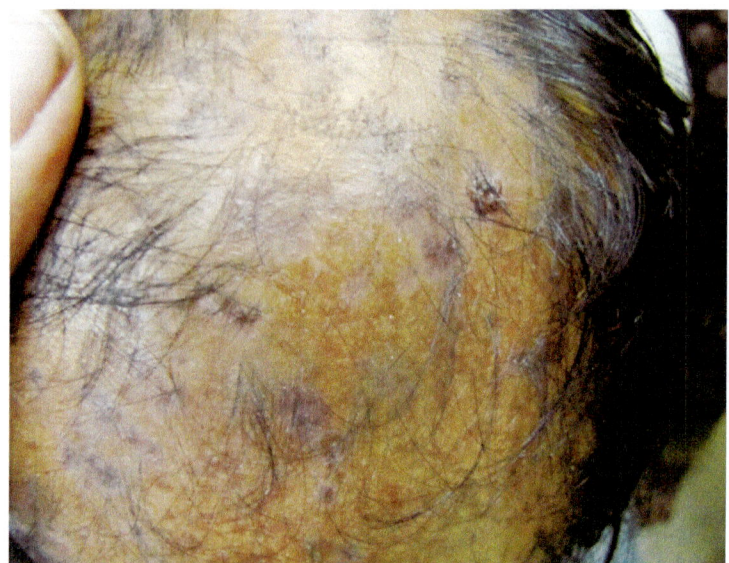

Fig. 8.9B: A case of cicatricial alopecia with characteristic violaceous pigmentation

Lesions of LP may be present elsewhere (Fig. 8.10A to C). An incidence of up to 50% for associated cutaneous lesions and <10% for nail and mucosal involvement is reported in literature.

Frontal fibrosing alopecia (FFA) was first described by Kossard S as a scarring alopecia predominantly affecting women after menopause.

Skin along the hairline is pale and contrasts with the photo-damaged skin of the lower forehead, with the line of demarcation indicating the location of the original hairline (Fig. 8.10D). In some patients, the pale skin of the receded hairline appears atrophic. The band-like frontal recession may progress laterally to above and behind the ears and less often to the occipital hairline (Fig. 8.10D and E).

Perifollicular erythema at the receding hairline is a helpful sign and indicates active follicular inflammation. Perifollicular scale is usually slight or absent in FFA. Prominence of veins on the forehead may be seen in patients with FFA, including those who have never received intralesional corticosteroids (loss of eyebrows may be complete or partial and is supportive of the diagnosis of FFA).

Recession of frontal hairline is the cardinal feature of FFA in contrast to AGA, frontal hairline recedes in a straight line rather than bitemporally and side burns are commonly lost.

Lichen planopilaris may develop in some patients with FFA. Cutaneous or mucous membrane lichen planus may also occur but is less common in patients with FFA than in patients with LPP.

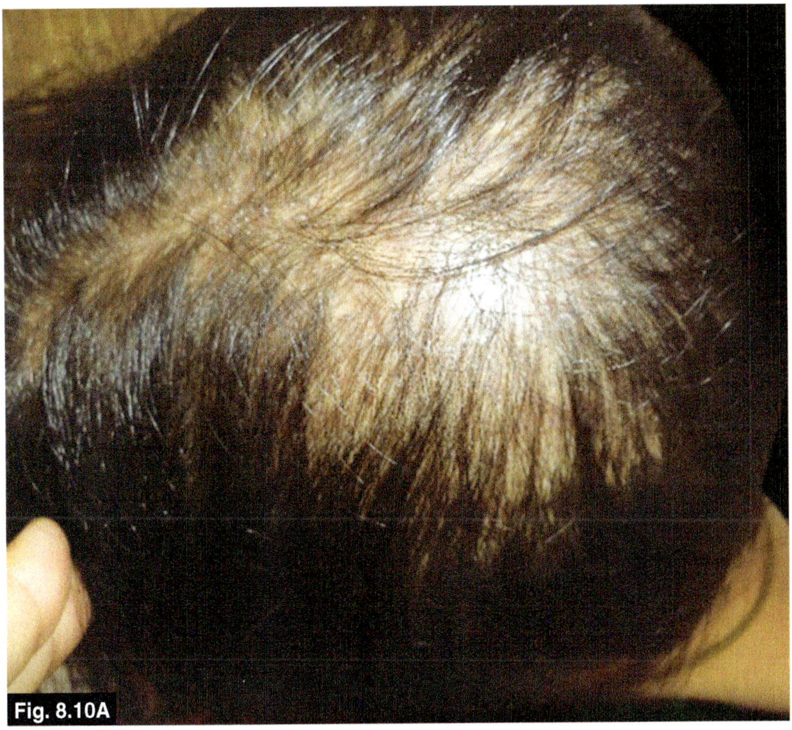

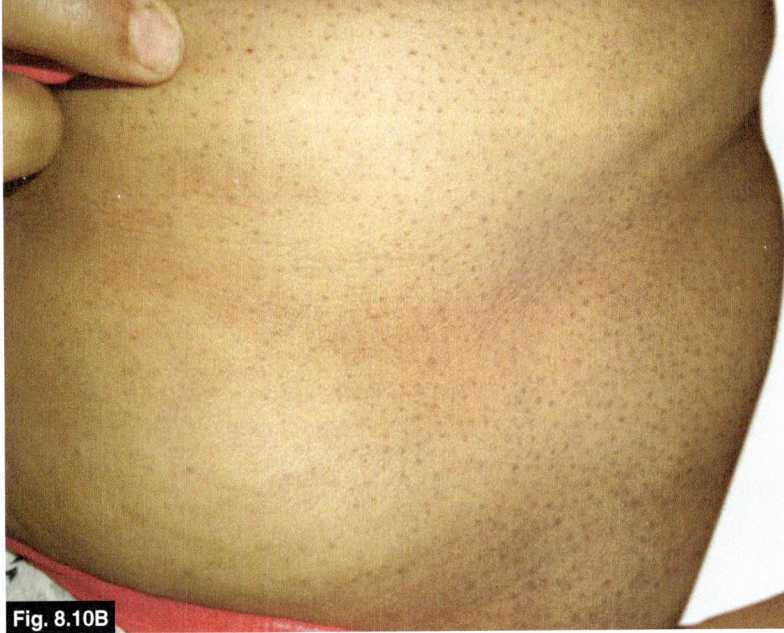

Fig. 8.10A

Fig. 8.10B

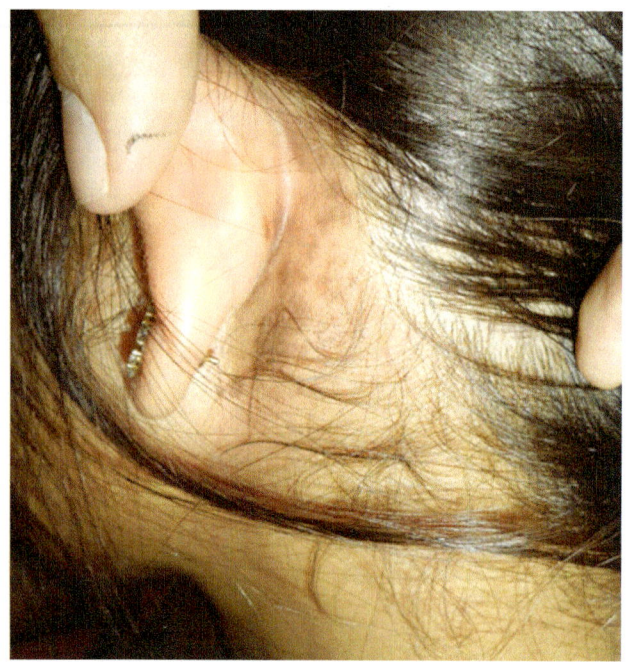

Fig. 8.10A to C: A case of early LPP with persistent itching of scalp, close examination revealed papules on the scalp, follicular papules on the trunk and pigmentation in the postauricular area

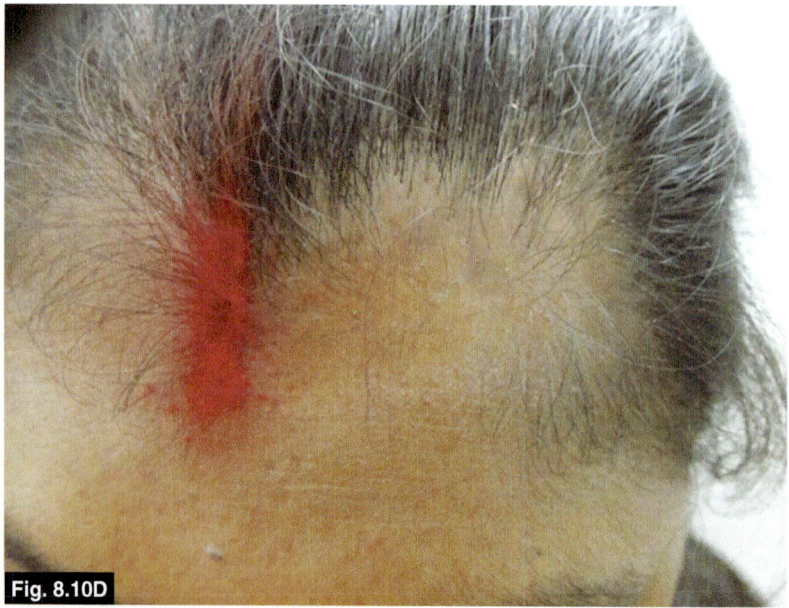

Fig. 8.10D

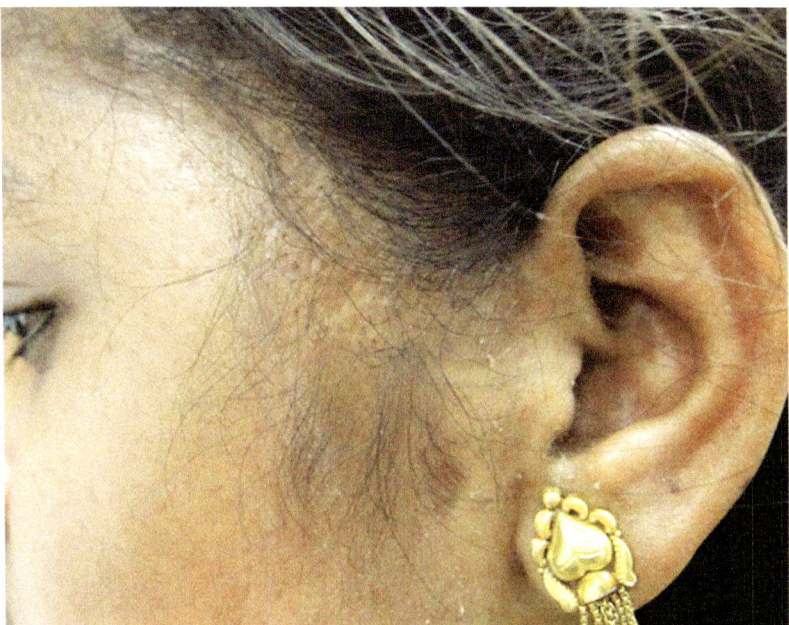

Fig. 8.10D and E: Fibrosis with alopecia in the frontal and preauricular area (FFA). The patient had concomitant lichen planus pigmentosus (*Courtesy:* Dr Niharika Dixit)

Graham Little-Piccardi-Lassueur syndrome is a very rare condition that predominantly affects female adults. It is characterized by LPP of the scalp; non-cicatricial alopecia of the eyebrows, axilla, and groin; and follicular papules on the trunk and extremities.

Differentials

In LPP, hair follicles around the margins of the bare areas show perifollicular erythema and perifollicular scale, whereas the center of the bare patches is smooth and devoid of inflammation. This is in contrast to discoid lupus erythematosus (DLE) where the center of the bare patches shows inflammation with follicular plugging, erythema, telangiectasia, and varying degrees of hypo- and hyperpigmentation. In alopecia areata, the patches may be distinguished by their peach color and the presence of normal follicular ostia.

Histology

a. A lymphocytic infiltrate and interface dermatitis are predominantly found in and around the upper permanent part of the hair follicle, mainly the infundibulum, with isthmus being involved in about one-third of cases (Fig. 8.11). Colloid bodies are seen in upper part of dermis (more frequent than in DLE, but less frequent than epidermal lichen planus). Follicular hypergranulosis is generally present (c.f. DLE). The interfollicular epidermis is rarely involved.

b. Perifollicular fibrosis and chronic inflammation without interface changes may be seen in later stages, and the infiltrate seems to "back away" from the zone of fibrosis.

c. Eventually, the follicles are replaced by columns of sclerotic collagen (follicular scars). LPP typically presents with a loss of elastic fibers only in the area of the follicular infundibulum.

d. Unlike DLE, the vascular plexus is not affected by inflammation and mucin deposits are absent.

e. DIF typically shows globular cytoid depositions of IgM, and rarely IgA, IgG, or C3 in the dermis around the infundibulum.

Treatment

The course of LP pilaris is quite *unpredictable*. In some, it may rapidly result in extensive and permanent alopecia, while in others the progression may be slow. Unfortunately, an absence of visible signs of inflammation and symptoms does not imply disease arrest, as the disease may progress insidiously for years.

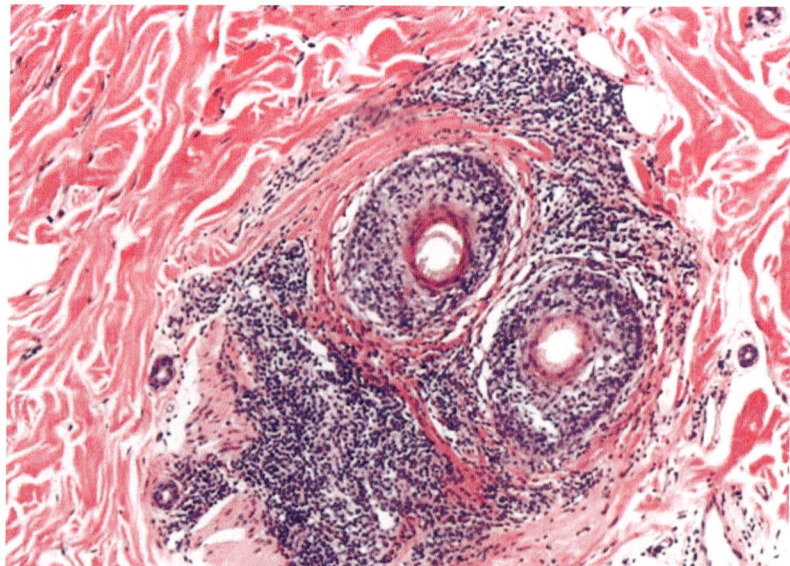

Fig. 8.11: Two adjacent follicles demonstrating brisk lymphocytic inflammation in the vicinity of the insertion point of the arrector pili muscle. Inner root sheaths are intact (*Courtesy:* Dr EA Knopp)

It is the view of some clinicians that, even a solitary active area is an indication for therapy to try to prevent progression.

Response to therapy is typically partial and often unsatisfactory. Steroids are useful to prevent progression and scarring and are often used as a bridge therapy. Treatment is only given in **active stage** of disease, evident clinically as violaceous papules or expanding patches and histopathologically by presence of significant inflammatory infiltrate.

Potent and very potent topical and systemic steroids (IM triamcinolone acetonide 0.5 mg/ kg/month or 25–50 mg/day of oral prednisone) are considered the mainstays of therapy for this disease. Oral corticosteroids (1 mg/kg/day of prednisolone) can be particularly helpful in cases of rapidly progressive disease and can be tapered over 1–2 months. Intralesional triamcinolone injections into the hair bearing regions can help arrest the inflammatory process. There is no evidence that intradermal injection (targeting the zone of inflammation) is superior to subcutaneous injections (which are less painful and reduce the risk of atrophy). The injections are initially repeated 4–6 weekly. The interval can later be increased to up to 12 weeks depending on the response.

A recent case series (Dhonncha et al, 2017) reported full clinical response with HCQS in 61% of patients and partial response in another 9%. Other agents that have been used with variable success include doxycycline 200 mg/day, 2.5–5 mg/kg/day cyclosporine, 2 gm/day mycophenolate mofetil, 100 mg/day oral thalidomide, 100 mg/day azathioprine, 2% topical minoxidil and 0.1% topical tacrolimus. Specific PPAR-γ-targeted therapy with agents such as pioglitazone is not consistently effective.

In FFA, topical therapy alone has shown limited effectiveness. Intralesional triamcinolone acetonide at a dose of 2.5–5 mg/ml can be combined with topical corticosteroids, tacrolimus, or pimecrolimus. A concomitant therapy with topical minoxidil, systemic dutasteride, or finesteride has shown some beneficial effects.

Camouflage

Patients should be advised about camouflage techniques, hairpieces, and wigs. Women with extensive LPP lesions on the crown and vertex can benefit from a hairpiece, particularly if the *frontal hairline* is *preserved*, and this is usually more comfortable to wear compared to a full wig.

Surgery

Hair restoration surgery is an option if no disease activity occurs on the scalp for at least **1 year** without therapy. The patient has to be warned about a possible disease recurrence and limited graft survival.

But most patients are very grateful for the cosmetic improvement and might accept lower hair density and even the mild flare of their LPP after surgery.

An overview of LPP is given in Box 8.2.

3. Classic Pseudopelade of Brocq

"Pelade" is the French term for alopecia areata, and the name "pseudo-pelade" emphasizes the resemblance to alopecia areata. Pseudopelade of Brocq (PPB) is classified as an idiopathic lymphocytic primary cicatricial alopecia that predominantly affects the scalp and is seen in women between 30 and 50 years of age. This is considered a primary disorder to be differentiated from the pseudopelade that results from various inflammatory processes. Recent microarray analysis (Yu M) compared the gene expression profiles of LPP and PPB and clearly indicated that PPB is a distinct active disease and not a late- or end-stage phase of LPP. However, there is no consensus on this point yet. Some authors believe it to be a distinct entity while others consider it as a common final stage of a different primary cicatricial alopecia.

The lack of consensus emanates from the fact that it is not easy for some to distinguish PPB from LPP histologically which is true to some extent.

Thus, the preferred terminology is pseudopelade (Brocq) (PPB) to describe the primary lymphocytic cicatricial alopecia, as detailed in this chapter, and the term "end-stage nonspecific cicatricial alopecia" to describe end stage of any primary cicatricial alopecia when the clinical features are no longer distinguishable and histology shows sparse hair follicles, many scarred fibrous tracts, and absent sebaceous glands.

Clinical Features

It usually affects the vertex and occipital areas of the scalp and presents with small flesh-colored smooth atrophic alopecic patches with irregular margins, the pattern being referred to as "footprints in the snow pattern" (Fig. 8.12). The hair in the uninvolved scalp is normal, but if the process is active the hairs at the edges of each patch are very easily extracted. The course is of a slow development of small, round patches of alopecia over many years that ultimately converge to produce larger irregular areas of hair loss.

This can also present as a noninflammatory centrifugally spreading patch of alopecia, which might be seen as a variant of central centrifugal cicatricial alopecia (CCCA) in Caucasians.

This condition should meet the diagnostic criterion as laid down in Table 8.3.

Box 8.2: Lichen planopilaris at a glance

Classical LPP
- Multifocal alopecic patches
- Perifollicular, erythematous or violaceous papules
- Spinous follicular hyperkeratosis at hair bearing margin

Frontal fibrosing alopecia (FFA)
- Postmenopausal women
- Progressive symmetrical cicatricial alopecia usually in frontotemporal area

Graham Little-Piccardi (GLP) syndrome

Triad of:
- Progressive scarring scalp alopecia (patchy)
- Non-scarring loss of pubic and axillary hair
- Widespread keratosis pilaris like horny follicular papules

Histopathological clues
- Follicular lymphocytic interface dermatitis
- Dense band-like lymphocytes around the upper follicle and infundibulum obscuring DEJ.
- Infundibular hyperkeratosis and hypergranulosis.
- Cytoid bodies scattered along the BMZ.

Treatment

1. LPP

First-line: Potent topical corticosteroid, IL triamcinolone acetonide, minoxidil, tacrolimus

Second-line
- Oral corticosteroids
- Oral cyclosporine

Third-line

Oral retinoid, antimalarial, mycophenolate mofetil, azathioprine, thalidomide

Newer therapies

PPAR-γ agonist

2. FFA

Intralesional and topical corticosteroid, oral steroids, oral retinoid

3. GLP
- Topical and oral steroids
- Oral retinoid

Histology

a. Early PPB lesions typically show a sparse to moderate lymphocytic infiltrate around the follicular infundibulum with a complete destruction of the sebaceous glands.

b. In later disease, hair follicles are completely replaced by fibrous tracts.

c. This is differentiated from DLE and LPP, as the interface dermatitis is usually absent and the elastic fibers are preserved and thickened in PPB.

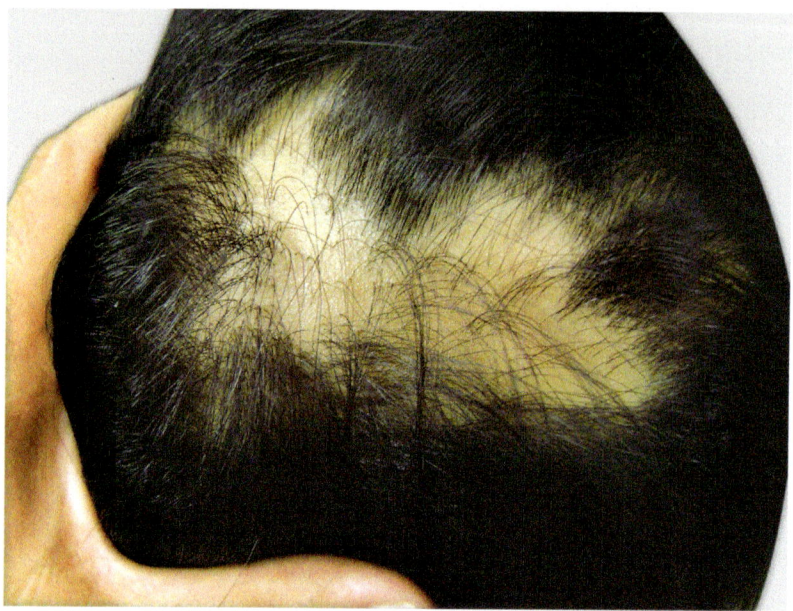

Fig. 8.12: A case of pseudopelade of Brocq with scarring alopecia demonstrating the reticular elongation also known as "footprints in the snow pattern""

Table 8.3: Diagnostic criteria for pseudopelade of Brocq	
Clinical criteria	Irregularly defined and confluent patches of alopecia
	Moderate atrophy (late stage); mild perifollicular erythema (early stage)
	Female–male ratio 3:1
	Long course (more than 2 years)
	Slow progression with spontaneous termination possible
Histological criteria	Absence of marked *inflammation*
	Absence of widespread *scarring* (best seen with elastin stain)
	Absence of significant *follicular plugging*
	Absence, or at least a decrease of *sebaceous glands*
	Presence of normal epidermis (only occasional atrophy)
	Fibrotic streams into the dermis
Direct immunofluorescence	Negative (or only weak IgM on sun-exposed skin)

Management

There are two schools of thought on its management, one believes that medical intervention in the early stages may be of help. But a contrarian view is that, it is irreversible and does not respond to medical therapy and thus no treatment can arrest its progression (Messenger AG, et al).

Intralesional triamcinolone acetonide at a concentration of 10 mg/ml × 2 ml every 4–6 weeks in combination with topical corticosteroids is the treatment of first choice. Topical tacrolimus 0.1% has been used as well.

Hydroxychloroquine (200 mg BD), oral prednisone (0.5 mg/kg), isotretinoin (1 mg/kg/day) and mycophenolate mofetil (starting from 1 g/day) have shown some effectiveness in treating PPB.

Hair restoration surgery is an option for PPB if the condition is stable without treatment and the patient has a suitable donor supply. A small test area with a limited number of grafts (20–30 grafts/cm^2 with a maximum total of 100 grafts) 6 months to 1 year before a larger session, is helpful to minimize the risk of disease progression and assure the success of a hair transplant procedure.

4. Central Centrifugal Cicatricial Alopecia

CCCA is a primary lymphocytic cicatricial alopecia of the central scalp which is not seen commonly in India and is restricted largely to Afro-Americans.

It has multiple causes including: Chemical processing, heat, traction, or traumatic hair practices. Premature desquamation of the inner root sheath (below the level of the isthmus where it keratinizes) is a pathological feature of CCCA and affects not only the follicles showing inflammation and fibrosis but also the unaffected follicles.

Clinical Features

There is a skin-colored patch of scarring alopecia on the crown, which progresses centrifugally to the parietal areas. The symptoms reported include itching, tenderness, and "pins and needle" sensations.

Management

Minimal hair grooming is recommended, topical and intralesional corticosteroids are usually the first-line. Intra-lesional triamcinolone (5–10 mg/ml) is injected into the periphery of the patch monthly. Doxycycline, minocycline and tetracycline have been used to reduce inflammatory symptoms initially (for 2–6 months). Anecdotal evidence favors the use of antimalarials, minoxidil, thalidomide, cyclosporine and mycophenolate mofetil. Short courses of oral steroids can be used in cases of active inflammation. But the main intervention is to switch to more natural, less traumatizing, hair care practices. Wigs and transplant are valid interventions in severe cases.

An overview of CCCA is given in Box 8.3.

Differentiating the Various Lymphocytic Cicatricial Alopecia

Over time, or with treatment, the clinically distinct features of the primary cicatricial alopecias become less distinct. Thus, in untreated or end stage disease, the characteristic features of these diseases are no longer present. What is seen is the bana morphology of bare patches coalescing into large bare areas devoid of follicular ostia and devoid of inflammation.

The singular enception being that of DLE, which in the late or end stage can be distinguished by the hypo- and hyperpigmentation of the scalp and ears and follicular plugging in the ears.

The one important point is that in acute stage PPB or CCCA there is very little clinical signs or symptoms and this may be misdiagnosed as end-stage disease. In PPB and CCCA, clinical spreading and extent of inflammatory infiltrate (in a scalp biopsy) may be the only two indicators of ongoing activity and signal the need for treatment.

Table 8.4 enumerates the differences between the salient lymphocytic cicatricial alopecias and alopecia areata.

Box 8.3: CCCA in a nutshell

Clinical features
- Slowly progressive scarring of vertex
- Spreads symmetrically and centrifugally
- Islands of unaffected hairs within scar area

Histopathology
- Premature disintegration of inner root sheath resulting in outward migration of the hair shaft through the ORS at the level of the isthmus
- Lamellar fibroplasias and variably dense lymphocytic inflammation surround the follicle at this level
- Follicular destruction and fibrous tract formation

Treatment options
- Potent topical and intralesional corticosteroid
- Minoxidil
- Hydroxychloroquine, isotretinoin
- Thalidomide, cyclosporine, mycofenolate mofetil

Table 8.4: Differentiating features between lymphocytic cicatricial alopecias and alopecia areata

	PPB	LPP	CCCA	AA
Symptomatic	No	No	Yes	No
Perifollicular erythema/scaling	No	Yes	No	No
Loss of follicular ostia	Yes	Yes	Yes	No
Color of affected patches	White	White	White	Peach coloured

PPB: Primary pseudopelade of Brocq; LPP: Lichen planopilaris; CCA: Central centrifugal cicatricial alopecias

NEUTROPHILIC CICATRICIAL ALOPECIAS

1. Folliculitis Decalvans

Folliculitis decalvans, along with tufted folliculitis, represents the primary cicatricial alopecias with a suppurative phase. Decalvans is a term derived from Latin meaning "making bald".

Folliculitis decalvans (FD) is a disorder that affects young- and middle-aged adults. It is believed to be consequent to a bacterial infection involving *Staphylococcus aureus* in combination with hypersensitivity reaction to "superantigens" and a defect in host cell-mediated immunity. Sometimes, scalp trauma and surgery can be an inciting factor.

Clinical Features

The condition starts in the vertex area of the scalp. The areas of alopecia have follicular pustules and follicular hyperkeratosis (Fig. 8.13A). The symptoms include pain, itching, dysaesthesia, and/or burning. Importantly *trichodynia* and *pruritus* predict a relapse. The inflammatory process is followed by the formation of one or more areas of scarring alopecia. In advanced cases there are patches of alopecia over the vertex of the scalp surrounded by crusting and a few follicular pustules. Unlike CCLE and LPP, the *scar* is *indurated* and *boggy* rather than atrophic, at least in the early stages.

Although the inflammatory severity fluctuates, the disease course is prolonged and progressive. Tufted folliculitis (Fig 8.13B) is typically found in FD but can also occur in other cicatricial inflammatory alopecias. Tufted folliculitis is characterized by multiple hairs (5–30) emerging from one single dilated follicular orifice (Box 8.4).

Histology

Early lesions: Keratin aggregation in the infundibulum with numerous neutrophils, as well as an intrafollicular and perifollicular neutrophilic infiltrate. Sebaceous glands are destroyed.

Advanced lesions: Follicular abscesses with infiltrate consisting of neutrophils, lymphocytes, and plasma cells.

End stage: Follicular and interstitial dermal fibrosis as well as hypertrophic scarring can be observed.

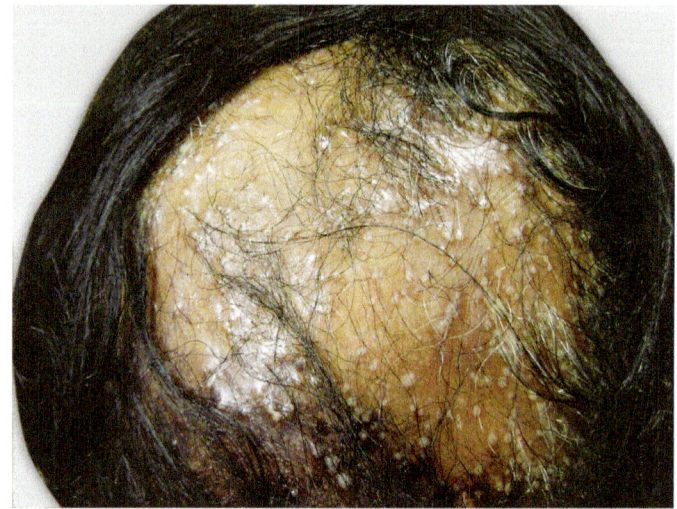

Fig. 8.13A: Multiple pustules with associated cicatricial alopecia in a case of folliculitis decalvans

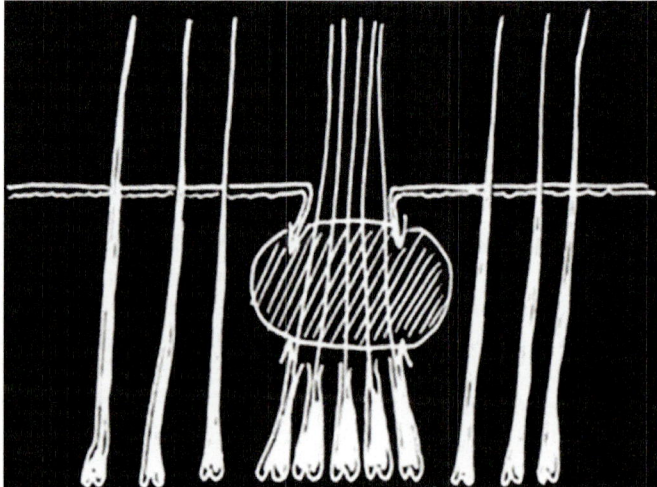

Fig. 8.13B: Tufted folliculitis: Multiple hair shafts emerge from a single dilated follicular opening (tuft consists of a central anagen hair surrounded by telogen hairs, each arising from independent follicles, converging towards common dilated follicular infundibulum)

Box 8.4: Tufted folliculitis at a glance

Clinical features
- Destructive, suppurative folliculitis
- Caused by *Staphylococcus aureus*
- Painful/pruritic erythematous pinpoint follicular pustules, papules with boggy swelling
- Crusting and scarring in the centre
- Tufts of hair appear from dilated follicular opening giving 'Dolls hair' appearance

Histopathology
- Perifollicular neutrophilic inflammation around the upper follicle
- Later develops into a more mixed inflammatory infiltrate of neutrophils, lymphocytes and plasma cells
- In burnt out stage, follicular and adventitial fibrosis is seen

First line
Oral plus topical antibiotics (oral clindamycin, doxycycline, minocycline ciprofloxacin, clarithromycin)

Second line
Oral rifampicin, oral fusidic acid, oral zinc, dapsone, oral cyclosporine, excision, laser

Management

Treatment is difficult and disease activity can persist over many years. The basic principle is to initiate an effective agent that targets *Staphylococcus aureus*, with long-term remission. Thus, a combination of antibacterial shampoo, topical antibiotic cream and systemic antibiotic is ideal. If severe itching suddenly becomes a predominant symptom, a fungal infection may be superimposed on the underlying scarring alopecia.

Though other agents have been tried including zinc, dapsone and isotretinoin, the main therapy revolves around the use of antibiotics. The duration of treatment with antibiotics may range from few weeks to a year. Isotretinoin has been used to alter the follicular environment to make it less suitable for *S. aureus* colonization, but it may increase cutaneous carriage of this organism and make the condition worse.

There are **two** different approaches to therapy, one involves the use of antibiotics and the other of retinoids. Two studies published have reported divergent views with regard to the remissions achieved. Vañó-Galván S et al found that oral antibiotics (tetracyclines and the combination of clindamycin and rifampicin) improved 90% and 100% of the patients, with a mean duration of response of 4.6 and 7.2 months respectively. Another study by Tietze JK et al found that the combination of clindamycin and rifampicin showed the lowest success rate in achieving long-term remission, since 80% of the patients relapsed shortly after the end of treatment. Clarithromycin and dapsone were more successful with long-term and stable remission rates of 33% and 43%, respectively. Treatment with isotretinoin was the most successful oral treatment with 90% of the patients experiencing stable remission during and up to two years after cessation of the treatment.

We feel that to minimize long-term use of antibiotics, a short-term use for 6 weeks can be followed by dapsone or isotretinoin to maintain remission.

1. Eradication of *S. aureus* with doxycyline, minocycline, erythromycin, cephalosporines, and sulfamethoxazole–trimethoprim has shown some effectiveness. Relapse can often be observed after the antibiotics are discontinued. If 2–3 courses are given the relapses are less.

   Rifampicin forms the main therapy. It must not be used alone in order to avoid resistant forms of Staphylococcus emerging and to prevent resistant tuberculosis in India. Hence, it is often combined with **doxycycline**, **ciprofloxacin**, or **clarithromycin**.

   One regimen involves the use of rifampicin 600 mg/day combined with clindamycin at a dose of 600 mg/day for ten weeks. Other adjuvants that can be used include **doxycycline** 100 mg, minocycline 100 mg and **azithromycin** 250 mg thrice a week all for 3 months.

2. **Isotretinoin** has also been found to be useful in a dose of 0.2–0.5 mg/kg/d × 5–7 months tapered down to 10 mg thrice a week for 2 months.

3. Oral therapy should be combined with topical antibiotics such as mupirocin, 1.5% fusidic acid, 2% erythromycin and antibacterial cleansers. Topical tacrolimus has also shown some effectiveness.

4. Intralesional triamcinolone acetonide at a concentration of 10 mg/ml every 4–6 weeks might help to reduce the inflammation and reduces symptoms such as itching, burning, and pain. Intranasal eradication of *S. aureus* with topical antibacterial agents has also been found to be useful.

Hair transplant surgery should only be considered for exceptional cases in which the patient did not show any signs of inflammation for several years without any treatment. The risk of reactivation after surgery is much higher in FD compared to other inflammatory cicatricial alopecias. Laser hair removal is another option in recalcitrant cases, if acceptable to the patient.

2. Perifolliculitis Capitis Abscedens et Suffodiens
(Dissecting Cellulitis)

It occurs predominantly in males during their second to fourth decades of life.

Clinical Presentation

It begins as simple folliculitis of the vertex and/or occiput with clusters of perifollicular pustules that are rapidly followed by formation of an abscess and sinus (Fig. 8.14). Nodules may be firm or fluctuant. Seropurulent fluid may be expressed from fluctuant nodules. Lesions may persist for years and frequently heal with scarring alopecia.

This disorder has been suggested to result from occlusion of the pilosebaceous unit. Acne conglobata and hidradenitis suppurativa may be associated. With follicular occlusion, the retention of material dilates

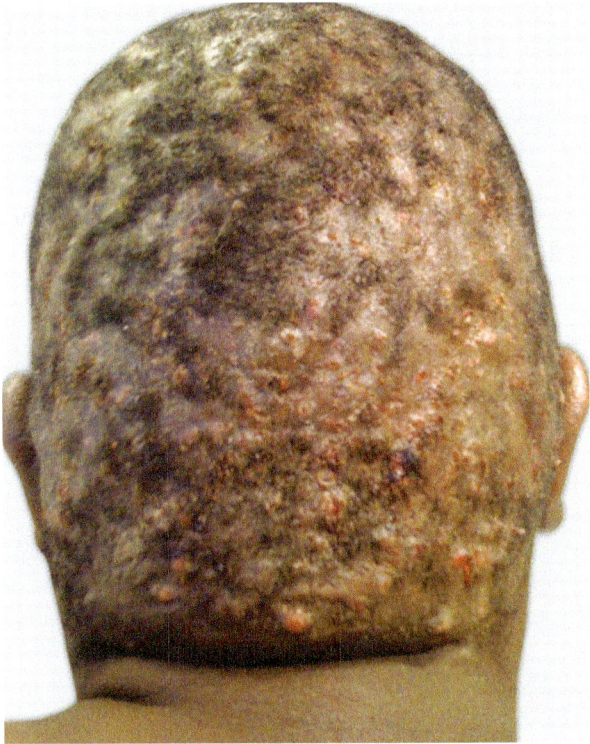

Fig. 8.14: Boggy, fluctuant, draining tracts, multiple erosions, and patches of alopecia were present on the scalp, most prominently in the occipital area (*Courtesy:* Dr Jyoti P Mundi, MD, New York)

the follicle, leading to its rupture, resulting in the exposure of keratin to the skin and organisms. This in turn causes inflammation with neutrophilic and granulomatous responses. A bacterial infection likely develops secondarily because most bacteriological cultures are negative. The most frequently isolated pathogens include *S. aureus*, *S. epidermidis*, and *S. albus*.

Management

Medical therapy

Topical isotretinoin 0.05% and clindamycin 1% have been used in early cases. Isotretinoin in a dose of 0.5–1 mg/kg/day has achieved prolonged remission and should be considered as a first-line treatment. Prolonged remissions following discontinuation have been reported. In general, higher doses and longer periods of treatment are required compared to acne. Some suggest starting with the dose of 1 mg/kg/day. Isotretinoin is resumed in case of relapse. Usually a combination of systemic antibiotics (minocycline, tetracycline, cloxacillin, erythromycin, cephalosporin, or clindamycin), intralesional corticosteroids, and oral prednisolone is administered. The benefits of systemic antibiotics are most likely due to their anti-inflammatory effects rather than to their antibacterial action. A good response has been reported with infliximab and adalimumab. Etanercept, however, was ineffective.

Surgery

Incision and drainage of therapy resistant, painful nodules and marsupialization with curettage of the cyst wall have been tried.

Laser depilation, external beam radiation and complete scalp excision up to the galea followed by split thickness skin grafting has been effective in severe recalcitrant cases.

Scalp reduction can be considered for smaller burnt-out areas. Hair restoration surgery is difficult because of the hypertrophic or keloidal scar tissue. An overview is given in Box 8.5.

MIXED PRIMARY CICATRICIAL ALOPECIAS

1. Acne Keloidalis Nuchae (AKN)/Folliculitis Keloidalis Nuchae

This disorder is primarily seen in young men aged from 14 to 25 years. It is believed to be triggered by trauma (shirt collars, helmets, wooden combs) or infection (demodex or bacteria). Hormonal factors possibly

Box 8.5: Dissecting cellulitis at a glance

Clinical features
- Suppurative painful fluctuant nodules and abscesses
- Interconnecting sinuses
- Multifocal lesions
- Ultimately depressed, hypertrophic or keloidal scars

Histopathology
- Infundibular acneiform distension with intrafollicular and perifollicular neutrophilic infiltration
- The inflammation is much deeper than in folliculitis decalvans, being concentrated around lower half of follicles and superficial fat
- Abscess formation on follicular rupture is composed of neutrophils, lymphocytes and plasma cells
- Abscess becomes partially lined by squamous epithelium forming sinus tracts

Treatment
First line: Oral isotretinoin, intralesional triamcinolone acetonide
Second line:
- Oral antibiotics plus topical antibiotics/topical retinoids
- Aspiration and intralesional triamcinolone acetonide

Third line
- Low dose corticosteroids
- Dapsone
- Excision and skin grafting
- Lasers

play a role as AKN is rarely reported in females. Ingrowing hair is unlikely to be an inciting factor and this has now been well demonstrated by trichoscopy and histopathology of AKN lesions.

The term AKN is commonly used although it is generally agreed that the condition is not a keloid, and affected individuals do not have a tendency to develop keloids in other areas of the body. Also, the histological features are not those seen in keloids.

Clinically, skin-colored follicular papules, pustules, and plaques as well as keloid-like scarred lesions are seen classically in the occipital scalp (Fig. 8.15). The onset is usually preceded by pruritus a few hours to days after a haircut or some form of mild irritation from use of a headwear such as a sports helmet.

Treatment is usually difficult and protracted. Monthly intralesional triamcinolone acetonide (10–40 mg/ml) alone or combined with topical 2% clindamycin or oral (tetracyclines) antibiotics is the treatment of

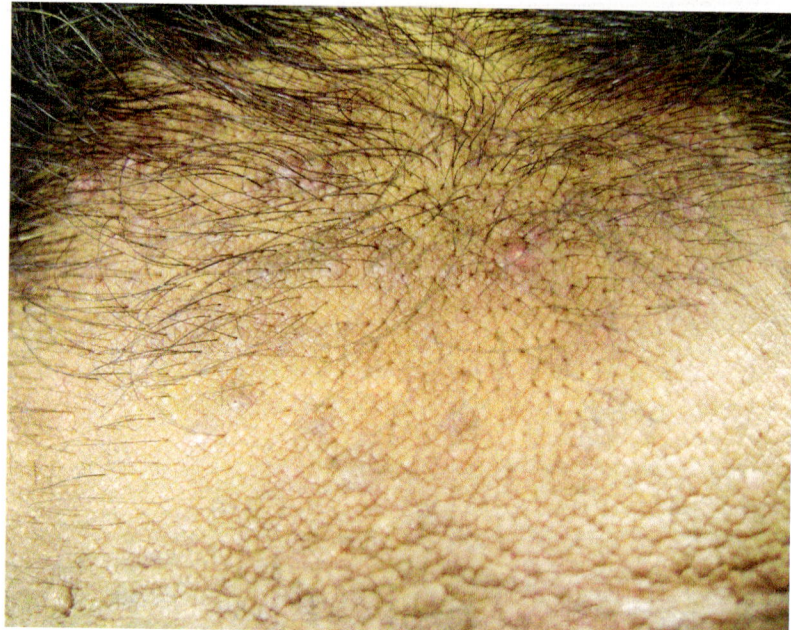

Fig. 8.15: Multiple skin-colored and pigmented follicular papules in the occipital scalp

first choice. Topical potent steroids alone or in combination with topical antibiotics or topical retinoids for mild cases of AKN. Cryotherapy has been found useful in both early and keloidal lesions. It has been known to cause softening of keloidal lesions making intralesional injections easier. Treatment with 1064 nm Nd:YAG and the 810 nm diode lasers has been found useful. Excision by carbon dioxide laser has also been reported to improve lesions of AKN.

Targeted ultraviolet B radiation for 16 weeks was also found to be useful in improving the appearance of fibrotic papules.

Surgical excision of extensive keloidal lesions may be considered but should be reserved for therapy refractory, extensive, and symptomatic cases.

Hair transplantation is not recommended as any surgical procedure on the scalp may aggravate the disease and low graft survival can be expected when transplanting into hypertrophic scars.

2. Acne Necrotica (Varioliformis)

This is a rare, chronic condition that predominantly occurs in adults.

Frontal and parietal scalp, as well as seborrheic areas of the face, are most commonly affected. It presents with umbilicated, pruritic, or painful papules that undergo central necrosis. The condition leaves varioliform or smallpox-like scars. Oral antibiotics, isotretinoin, intralesional, or topical corticosteroids have been tried.

SECONDARY SCARRING ALOPECIAS

This entity has numerous disorders which are beyond the scope of this book. They include diverse entities, including infections, trauma (Fig. 8.16), sclerosing disorders, granulomatous disorders, neoplasias and congenital disorders. A few common disorders are detailed below.

1. **Traction alopecia:** Prolonged traction may lead to transient alopecia or sometimes, with prolonged traction, follicular atrophy and permanent alopecia. Chronic traction can be caused by tight ponytails, braids, heavy dreadlocks, or extensive use of rollers. In India, it is seen in women who tightly braid their hair and causes alopecia in the frontal hairline or temples. This is also seen in Sikh boys, whose hair is usually tied up in a bind.

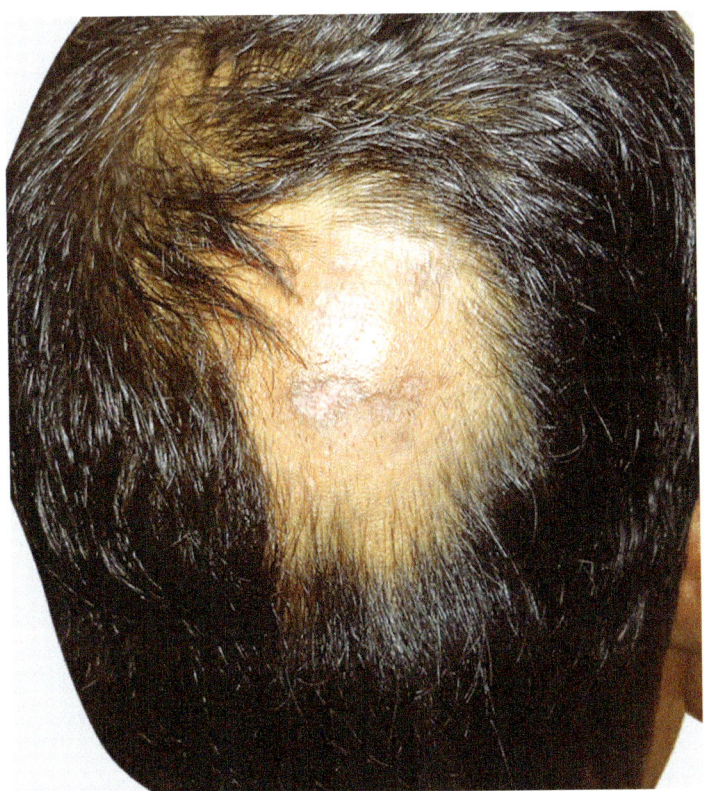

Fig. 8.16: Scarring alopecia due to trauma, note the central scar

2. **Trichotillomania** (Greek: Tricho = hair, tillo = pull, mania = excessive excitement) is a form of traumatic alopecia caused by an irresistible compulsion to pull out, twist, or break off one's own hair.

In the infantile or early onset trichotillomania there is a short duration of history and it may resolve spontaneously or with simple interventions. Trichotillomania that starts around or after puberty shows a more chronic course and is usually a sign of a more severe underlying psychopathology (Fig. 8.17). Women are far more often affected than men (up to 7:1).

There are single or multiple asymmetrical, occasionally geometrically shaped areas of hair loss on the scalp or other areas of the body. The areas of hair loss display short or bristly anagen hair with classical presence of hair of unequal length. Dermoscopy is useful in diagnosing difficult cases (Fig. 8.18A to C).

Counselling is advised but a better method could be to ask the patient to wear a loose fitting cap or head dress, which reminds the patient of the habit and can help break the cycle of pulling out the hair (further details in the chapter 'Hair Loss in Women').

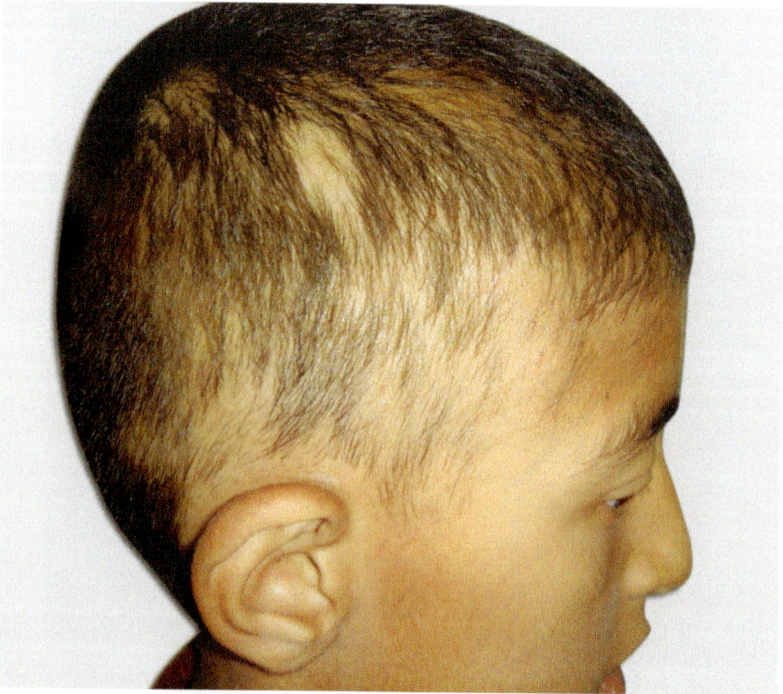

Fig. 8.17: A boy with multiple asymmetrical areas of hair loss which show short hair with unequal length

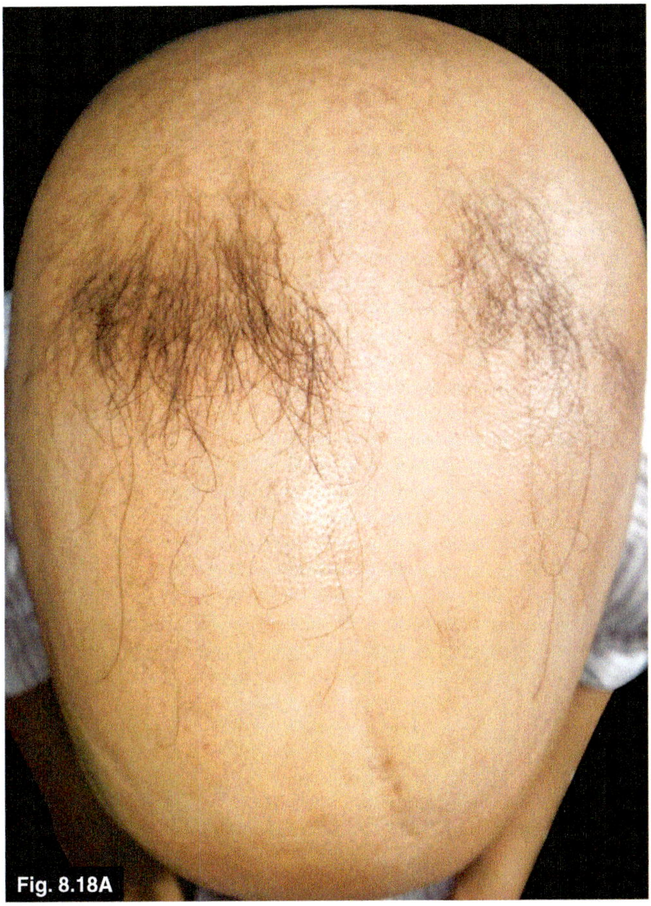

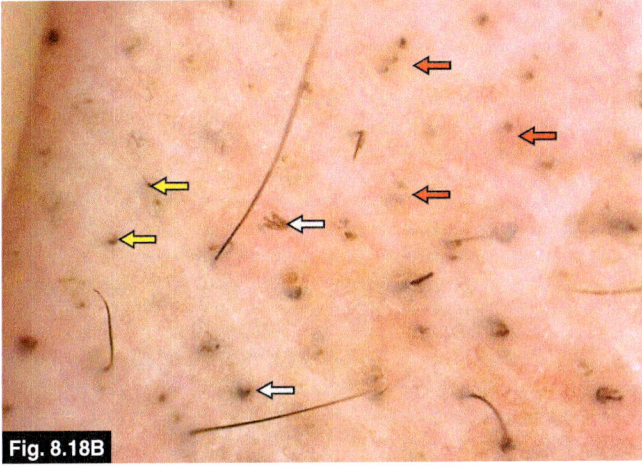

Fig. 8.18A

Fig. 8.18B

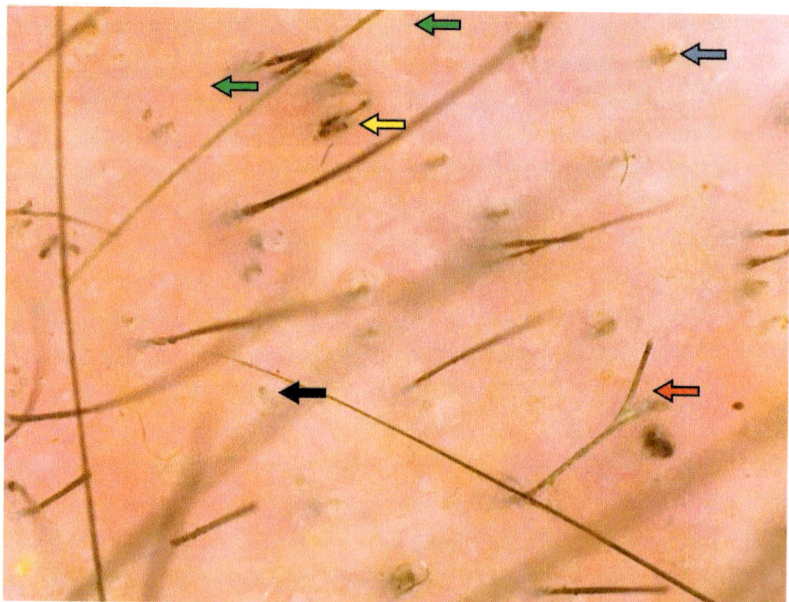

Fig. 8.18A to C: (A) A 27-year-old male presented with loss of hair over the entire scalp for past 6 years. Patient was known case of alopecia totalis for which he had previously taken OMP and reported partial regrowth which relapsed on stopping the therapy. At present there were only few patchy tufts of hair present on central scalp. (B) Overall, trichoscopic evaluation showed presence of yellow dots (red arrows), black dots (yellow arrows), and cadeverized hair (white arrows) hair suggestive of alopecia areata. However, the central tuft of hair (C) showed presence of longitudinal splitting hair shaft (red arrow), unequal length of hair, black dots (black arrow), V sign (yellow arrow), perifollicular haemorrhage (blue arrow) and hair powder (green arrows) suggestive of concomitant presence of trichotillomania. The patient did come up with history of repeated manipulation of the remnant tuft of hair and wearing cap for a prolonged time. Histopathology, confirmed the suspicion in which features suggestive of trichotillomania were present

3. **Fungal infection:** Infections of the scalp, especially fungal infections, can be highly inflammatory and therefore may lead to cicatricial alopecia. Favus is a specific type of tinea capitis characterized by yellowish scales (scutula), which are sulfuric-yellow concretions of hyphae and skin debris in the follicular orifices and exhibit a distinct malodorant smell. A kerion is a deep, highly inflammatory fungal infection of the scalp (Figs 8.19 and 8.20). It presents as a highly suppurative, boggy, nodular, deep folliculitis with fistulas and pus secretion. Both favus and kerion may lead to scarring hair loss and should therefore are to be treated aggressively.

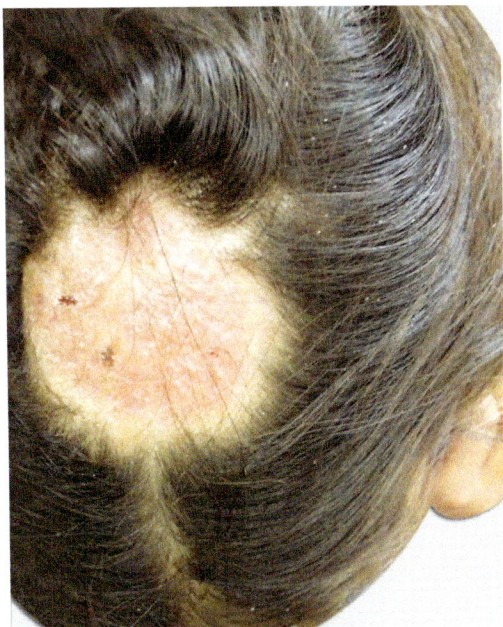

Fig. 8.19: Cicatricial alopecia consequent to a kerion infection

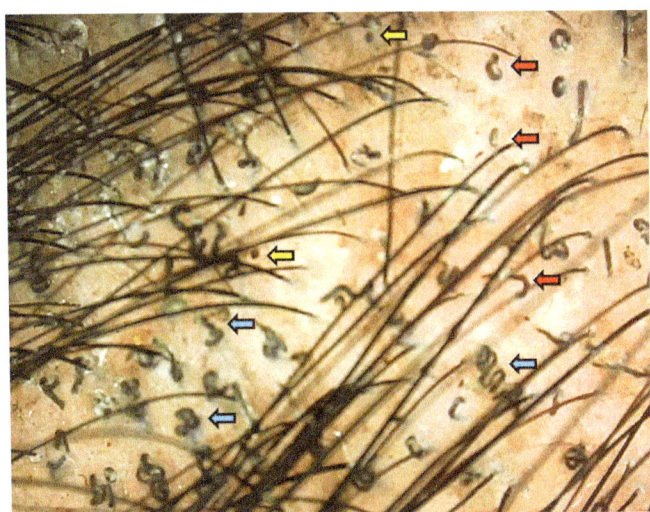

Fig. 8.20: An 8-year-old boy presented with a localized patch of hair loss associated with a painful boggy swelling and cervical lymphadenopathy. Hairs at the margins of the patch were easily pluckable. Trichoscopic evaluation showed presence of black dots (yellow arrows), comma hair (red arrows) and coiled hairs (yellow arrows). KOH evaluation was positive for ectothrix. Patient was started on oral anti-inflammatory and oral griseofulvin with topical ketoconazole lotion

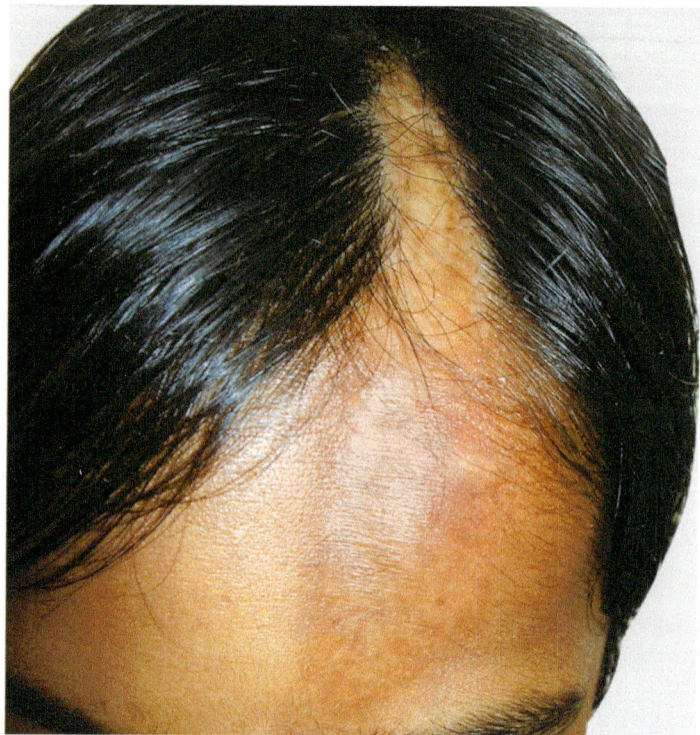

Fig. 8.21: A case of frontoparietal linear morphea with scarring alopecia

4. **Morphea:** Atrophic patches can occur on any body site and scalp involvement leads to cicatricial alopecia. A linear variant of morphea affecting the frontal scalp has been termed linear scleroderma en coup de sabre (Fig. 8.21).

Bibliography

1. Amato L, Mei S, Massi D, Gallerani I, Fabbri P. Cicatricial alopecia; a dermatopathologic and immunopathologic study of 33 patients (pseudopelade of Brocq is not a specific clinicopathologic entity). Int J Dermatol 2002;41:8–15.

2. Beckett N, Lawson C, Cohen G. Electrosurgical excision acne keloidalis with secondary intention healing. J Clin Aesthet Dermatol 2011;4(1):36–39.

3. Bolduc C, Sperling LC, Shapiro J. Primary cicatricial alopecia: Other lymphocytic primary cicatricial alopecias and neutrophilic and mixed primary cicatricial alopecias. J Am Acad Dermatol Dec 2016;75(6):1101–17.

4. Brandt HR, Malheiros AP, Teixeira MG, Machado MC. Perifolliculitis capitis abscedens et suffodiens successfully controlled with infliximab. Br J Dermatol 2008;159:506–7.

5. Cevasco NC, Bergfeld WF, Remzi BK, de Knott HR. A case-series of 29 patients with lichen planopilaris: The Cleveland Clinic Foundation experience on evaluation, diagnosis, and treatment. J Am Acad Dermatol 2007; 57:47–53.

6. Chinnaiyan P, Tena LB, Brenner MJ, Welsh JS. Modern external beam radiation therapy for refractory dissecting cellulitis of the scalp. Br J Dermatol 2005;152:777–9.

7. Cotsarelis G, Sun TT, and Lavker RM. Label-retaining cells reside in the bulge area of pilosebaceous unit: Implications for follicular stem cells, hair cycle, and skin carcinogenesis. Cell 1990; 61(7):1329–37.

8. Housewright CD, Rensvold E, Tidwell J, Lynch D, Butler DF. Excisional surgery (scalpectomy) for dissecting cellulitis of the scalp. Dermatol Surg. 2011;37:1189–91.

9. Inui S. Trichoscopy: A new frontier for the diagnosis of hair diseases. Expert Rev Dermatol 2012;7:1–8.

10. Khaled A, Zeglaoui F, Zoghlami A, Fazaa B, Kamoun MR. Dissecting cellulitis of the scalp: response to isotretinoin. J Eur Acad Dermatol Venereol 2007;21:1430–31.

11. Kossard S. Lymphocytic mediated alopecia: Histological classification by pattern analysis. Clin Dermatol 2001;19(2):201–10.

12. Layton AM, Yip J, Cunliffe WJ. A comparison of intralesional triamcinolone and cryosurgery in the treatment of acne keloids. Br J Dermatol. 1994;130(4):498–501.

13. Maranda EL, Simmons BJ, Nguyen AH, Lim VM, Keri JE. Treatment of acne keloidalis nuchae: a systematic review of literature. Dermatol Ther (Heidelb) 2016;6:363–78.

14. Messenger AG, Sinclair RD, Farrant P, David AR de Berker. Acquired Disorders of Hair. Rook's Textbook of Dermatology, Ninth Edition. Edited by Christopher Griffiths, Jonathan Barker, Tanya Bleiker, Robert Chalmers and Daniel Creamer. 2016 John Wiley & Sons, Ltd.

15. MillianCayetano JF, RepisoJimenez JB, Del Boz J, de TroyaMartin M. Refractory acne keloidalis nuchae treated with radiotherapy. Aust J Dermatol, 2015.

16. Mirmirani P, Willey A, Price VH. Short course of oral cyclosporine in lichen planopilaris. J Am Acad Dermatol 2003;49:667–71.

17. Navarini AA, Trueb RM. Three cases of dissecting cellulitis of the scalp treated with adalimumab: control of inflammation within residual structural disease. Arch Dermatol 2010;146:517–20.

18. Nguyen JV, Hudacek K, Whitten JA, Rubin AI, Seykora JT. The HoVert technique: A novel method for the sectioning of alopecia biopsies. J Cutan Pathol 2011;38:401–6.

19. Nic Dhonncha E, Foley CC, Markham T. The role of hydroxychloroquine in the treatment of lichen planopilaris: A retrospective case series and review. Dermatol Ther 2017 Feb 6.

20. Obermoser G, Sontheimer RD, Zelger B. Overview of common, rare and atypical manifestations of cutaneous lupus erythematosus and histopathological correlates. Lupus 2010;19:1050–70.

21. Ogunbiyi A. Acne keloidalis nuchae: prevalence, impact, and management challenges. Clin Cosmet Investig Dermatol Dec 2016;14;9:483–9.

22. Okoye GA, Rainer BM, Leung SG, et al. Improving acne keloidalis nuchae with targeted ultraviolet B treatment: a prospective, randomized splitscalp study. Br J Dermatol 2014;171(5):1156–63.

23. Olsen EA, et al. Summary of North American Hair Research Society (NAHRS)-sponsored workshop on cicatricial alopecia, Duke University Medical Center, February 10 and 11, 2001. J Am Acad Dermatol 2003:48(1):103–10.

24. Olsen EA. Cicatricial alopecia. In disorders of hair growth: Diagnosis and treatment, Bergfeld WF (editor). New York: McGraw-Hill 2003; p. 363–98.

25. Pasquali P. Cryosurgery in dermatologic surgery. Step-by-Step. 2005;46(4):257–60.

26. Price VH. The medical treatment of cicatricial alopecia. Semin Cutan Med Surg 2006;25(1):56–59.

27. Scott DA. Disorders of the hair and scalp in blacks. Dermatol Clin 988;6(3):387–95.

28. Sellheyer K, Bergfeld WF. Histopathologic evaluation of alopecias. Am J Dermatopathol 2006;28(3):236–59.

29. Sukhatme SV, Lenzy YM, Gottlieb AB. Refractory dissecting cellulitis of the scalp treated with adalimumab. J Drugs Dermatol 2008;7:981–83.

30. Tietze JK, Heppt MV, von Preuben A, Wolf U, Ruzicka T, Wolff H, Sattler EC. Oral isotretinoin as the most effective treatment in folliculitis decalvans: a retrospective comparison of different treatment regimens in 28 patients. J Eur Acad Dermatol Venereol. Sep 2015;29(9):1816–21.

31. Tosti A, Piraccini BM. Scarring alopecias; in Tosti A, Piraccini BM (eds). Diagnosis and Treatment of Hair Disorders. London, Taylor and Francis, 2006.

32. Vañó-Galván S, Molina-Ruiz AM, Fernández-Crehuet P, Rodrigues-Barata AR, Arias-Santiago S, Serrano-Falcón C, Martorell-Calatayud A, Barco D, Pérez B, Serrano S, Requena L, Grimalt R, Paoli J, Jaén P, Camacho FM. Folliculitis decalvans: a multicentre review of 82 patients. J Eur Acad Dermatol Venereol. Sep 2015;29(9):1750–7.

33. Whiting DA. Cicatricial alopecia: Clinicopathological findings and treatment. Clin Dermatol 2001;19(2):211–5.

34. Yu M, Bell RH, Ross EK, et al. Lichen planopilaris and pseudopelade of Brocq involve distinct disease associated gene expression patterns by microarray J Dermatol Sci 2010;57:27–36.

9

Pediatric Hair Disorders

Samipa S Mukherjee,
Ananta Khurana, Kabir Sardana

INTRODUCTION

Pediatric hair disorders encompass a variety of conditions ranging from the benign and easily manageable infectious conditions like tinea capitis and pediculosis to the rare and difficult to manage genotrichoses. Hair disorders in children could be found as an isolated phenomenon or could reflectan underlying systemic disorder or syndrome. The various groups of hair disorders encountered in pediatric age group include genotrichosis, autoimmune hair disorders, infective conditions, acquired conditions due to mechanical or chemical trauma to the hair shaft and disorders owing to mental and emotional stress. This chapter focuses predominantly on the diagnosis and management of genotrichoses, and hair disorders.

GENETIC HAIR DISORDERS (GENOTRICHOSES)

Genotrichosis is a broad spectrum of genetic disorders associated with hair abnormalities that manifest as alopecia, abnormalities of hair color, texture or hair shaft abnormalities. Hair abnormalities can present at birth or later in life as an isolated disorder or with a constellation of other cutaneous and systemic features.

Although several genes have been identified in the pathogenesis of various hair shaft disorders, the actual etiopathogenesis still remains elusive. Genotrichoses present with mendelian trait of inheritance, but some may show non-mendelian phenotypes representing lethal mutations, surviving only by mosaicism, as described by Happle and Konig. The exact pathomechanism of most of the hair shaft disorders remain unknown.

The major genetic hair defects commonly encountered in clinical practice are as follows.

1. Silvery Grey Hair Syndromes (Table 9.1)

Silvery hair is a common presentation of a rare group of autosomal recessive disorders called *silvery hair syndromes* including **Griscelli syndrome (GS), Chédiak-Higashi syndrome (CHS),** and **Elejalde syndrome (ES).** They share many common features like pigmentary dilution, silvery hair, neurological problems and immunological defects.

CHS is a rare autosomal recessive disorder. It is characterized by mild pigment dilution (partial oculocutaneous albinism), silvery blond hair, severe phagocytic immunodeficiency, bleeding tendencies, recurrent pyogenic infections and progressive sensory or motor neurological defects. It is a unique lysosomal disease that causes the gross enlargement of lysosomes in all tissues (generally demonstrated in leucocyte and bone marrow for the purpose of diagnosis). GS has three subtypes with different underlying genetic aberrations. The main signs of dermatological interest in CHS and GS are generalized skin hypopigmentation at birth with tanning capacity after sun exposure, hairs with a unique silvery sheen, and more rarely, pigmentary dilution of the iris. This phenotype has been described as partial albinism. The exact cause of pigment dilution is not known. Destruction of the giant melanosomes may dilute skin color. However, abnormal packing of normal sized melanosomes into large lysosome like structures in the epidermal cells may be a more likely basis. CHS usually enters an accelerated phase in childhood, with pancytopenia, hepatosplenomegaly, and lymphohistiocytic infiltrates in various organs.

Elejalde disease has recently been considered to be the same as GS type 1. In addition to hypopigmentation and silvery hair, there is early onset profound neurological dysfunction. Immunological function is normal.

To make correct diagnosis and to differentiate between CHS and GS (Table 9.1), light microscopic examination of skin and hair shafts, immunological and peripheral blood smear evaluation are needed. The light microscopy of hair shaft in GS shows unevenly large melanin granules, mostly located in vicinity of the medullary zone and polarized light microscopy shows bright shaft with a monotonously whitish appearance. Histopathological examination of skin biopsy shows hyperpigmented oval melanocytes with poorly pigmented keratinocytes. Electron microscopic evaluation of skin specimens shows epidermal melanocytes filled with numerous stage IV melanosomes.

Table 9.1: Distinguishing features of the three silvery grey hair syndromes

Characteristics	Chédiak-Higashi syndrome	Griscelli syndrome	Elejalde syndrome
Neurological dysfunction	Less severe	Less severe	More severe
Defects in immunity	Present	Present	Absent
Melanin clumps	Small	Large	Irregular
Accelerated phase	Present		
Microscopy	Small clumps of melanin	Larger clumps of melanin	Irregular clumps of melanin

2. Disorders with Hypotrichia and Atrichia (Fig. 9.1)

Generalized congenital hypotrichia/atrichia: There is a very long list of conditions that present with hypotrichosis, but not complete alopecia, in infancy (Table 9.2). Many classification systems have been proposed but none is universally accepted. Hypotrichosis can be secondary to follicular hypoplasia or to a faulty hair shaft production and breakage. Some of the common disorders are depicted in Fig. 9.2.

Hypotrichosis simplex is a group of rare autosomal dominant and autosomal recessive nonscarring alopecias in which patients are usually born with normal hair. Hair loss can begin in the first few months or even as late as the first decade and can progress to almost complete loss of scalp hair by adulthood. Graying has been reported to coincide with hair loss. Some individuals show sparse, fine, short hairs, especially at the crown, but hair on sites other than the scalp is normal.

Individuals with autosomal recessive *localized hypotrichosis* (scalp hair, largely sparing secondary sexual hair) may have sparse hair at birth that regrows poorly or not al all: This may be related to either a mutation in the LIPH (607365) gene on chromosome 3q27, desmoglein 4 on chromosome 18q12 or P2RY5 on chromosome 13q14.12–q14.2. Many of the *ectodermal dysplasias* (Fig. 9.1) are associated with hypotrichosis but, unfortunately, most of the hair shaft abnormalities have not been well characterized; the abnormal hair is generally described clinically only as 'brittle', 'sparse' or 'lusterless. Other non-ectodermal dysplasia syndromes present in infancy with sparse, lustreless hair as one part of multiorgan abnormalities (e.g. cartilage–hair hypoplasia (mutation in the *RMRP* gene), hypomelia–hypotrichosis–facial haemangioma and regional choroidal atrophy and alopecia.

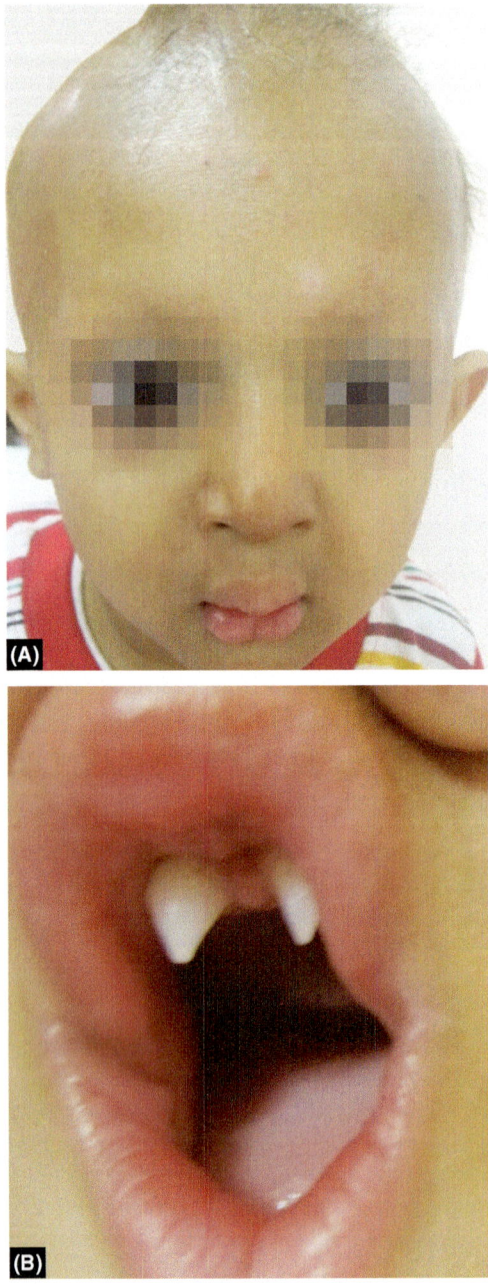

Fig. 9.1A and B: (A) Sparse scalp hair and absence of eyebrows in a child with ectodermal dysplasis; (B) Demonstrates the associated abnormal dentition (*Courtesy:* Ananta Khurana)

Table 9.2: Conditions associated with hypotrichosis (as proposed by Camacho et al)

1 Genodermatosis with nonscarring hypotrichosis

1.1 *With escheletical alterations*
- McKusich disease or condrodysplasia
- Moynahan disease (hypotrichosis, syndactylia, retinitis)
- Trichorhinophalangeal syndromes
- Pierre Robin syndrome
- Cardiofacial cutaneous syndrome
- Alopecia contractures dwarfism (ACD) syndrome with mental retardation
- Oculodental digital syndrome
- Dubowitz syndrome
- Noonan syndrome
- Hallermann-Streiff syndrome

1.2 *With ectodermic alterations*
- Ectodermal dysplasias

1.3 *With neuroectodermal alterations*
- Tricothiodystrophy

1.4 *With chromosomal alterations*
- Down syndrome
- Klinefelter syndrome
- Turner syndrome

1.5 *With amino acid metabolism alterations*
- Citrullinemia
- Hartnup disease
- Homocystinuria
- Tirosinemia I and II

1.6 *Other genodermatosis with hypotrichosis*

1.6.1 *Progeria Werner syndrome or pangeria*
- Hutchinson-Gilford or childhood progeria
- Other progerias

1.6.2 *Others*
- Netherton syndrome
- Tay syndrome
- Rud syndrome
- KID syndrome
- Rothmund-Thomson disease
- Poikiloderma, alopecia, retrognathism, cleft palate syndrome
- Zinsser-Cole-Engman disease
- Kallin syndrome or epidermolysis bullosa simplex

(Contd.)

Table 9.2: Conditions associated with hypotrichosis (as proposed by Camacho et al) (*Contd.*)

1.7 Genodermatosis with hypotrichosis and tumors
- Rombo syndrome
- Bazex-Dupré-Christol's syndrome
1.8 Hereditary simple hypotrichosis
2 Genodermatosis with scarring hypotrichosis
2.1 Darier disease
2.1 Ichthyosis X
2.3 Dystrophic epidermolysis bullosa
2.4 Incontinentia pigmenti
2.5 Polyostotic fibrous dysplasia
2.6 Conradi syndrome
2.7 Happle's syndrome

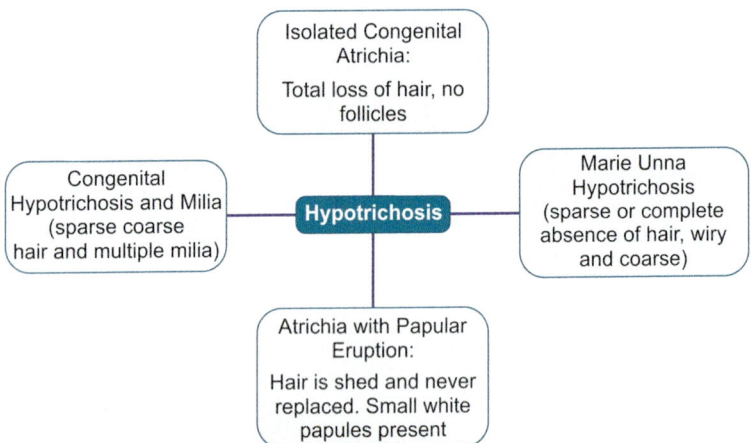

Fig. 9.2: Syndromes presenting with hypotrichosis alone

Trichorhinophalangeal syndrome (TRPS) type I is an autosomal dominant disorder characterized by a distinctive facies with pear-shaped nose, elongated philtrum, thin upper lip, supernumerary incisors, receding chin and skeletal abnormalities including brachydactyly, deviation of the middle phalanges, hip malformation, and short stature. Most patients show fine, sparse, slow-growing hair, but almost normal hair to complete baldness have been described.

Marie Unna hereditary hypotrichosis (MUHH) is a rare autosomal dominant genodermatoses characterized by progressive non-scarring hair loss. Clinically affected individuals are born with sparse or absent hairs at birth, later there is regrowth of coarse, unruly hair in childhood and progressive, nonscarring loss of hair again at or nearing puberty.

There are few cases reported where there is normal to adequate hairs at birth that eventually develops into progressive hair loss. There is receding of hairline with increasingly sparse hair on the vertex, parietal and occipital region resembling androgenetic alopecia. Eyebrows, eyelashes, body hair and secondary sexual hair are sparse or absent. Eyebrow loss and presence of wiry, twisted hair is important for diagnosis. Other ectodermal structures are normal. Diffuse follicular hyperkeratosis with milia-like facial lesions may be present. Some have reported association of MUHH with Ehlers-Danlos syndrome and juvenile macular degeneration, which could be incidental findings.

Hallermann-Streiff, Sensenbrenner, Coffin-Siris, and growth retardation, alopecia, pseudoanodontia, and optic atrophy (GAPO) syndromes all show hypotrichosis in association with facial dysmorphism and other physical signs.

Atrichia congenita (congenital atrichia) is a rare genodermatoses characterized by a mutation of the human hairless (HR) gene on chromosome 8p22. There is loss of scalp hair between one and six months of age, after which no growth occurs. Eyebrow, eyelash, and body hair may also be sparse or absent; patients may have a few pubic and axillary hairs. The condition may present in isolation or along with other defects. *Atrichia congenita with papular lesions* (APL) represents a complex and heterogenous group of genodermatoses characterized clinically by complete and irreversible hair loss shortly after birth, and is associated with the development of keratin-filled cysts over the body resulting from homozygous mutations in the hairless gene (HR) (Fig. 9.3). The patients have normal development, hearing, teeth and nails. There are no abnormalities of sweating. Heterozygous

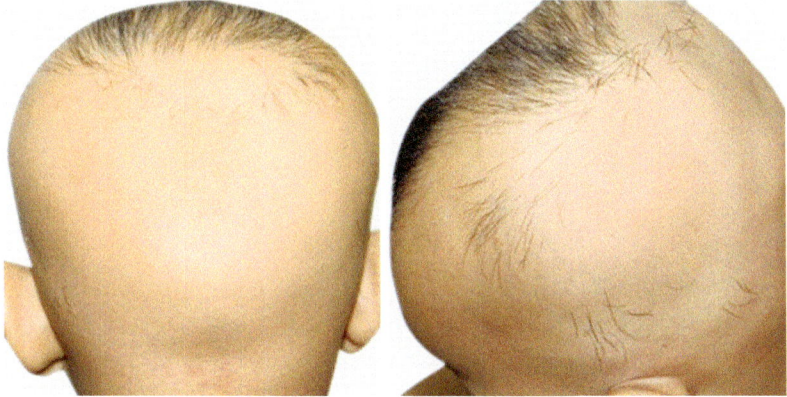

Fig. 9.3: Congenital atrichia

individuals have normal hair and are clinically indistinguishable from genotypically normal persons.

Localized congenital alopecia occurs in congenital triangular alopecia (Brauer's nevus; unilateral or bilateral alopecic patch in frontotemporal region appearing between 3 and 5 years of age), aplasia cutis congenita (Fig. 9.4), Adams-Oliver syndrome (aplasia cutis with digital abnormalities), aplasia cutis congenita, high myopia, and cone-rod dysfunction syndrome and nevus sebaceous.

3. Hair Shaft Disorders

Conditions with hair shaft defects are usually not amenable to treatment but can provide clues to other abnormalities (Box 9.1). The diagnosis is based on light microscopy (LM) and trichoscopy. The disorders can be conveniently classified into those with increased fragility and those without increased fragility and the common disorders are depicted in Fig. 9.5.

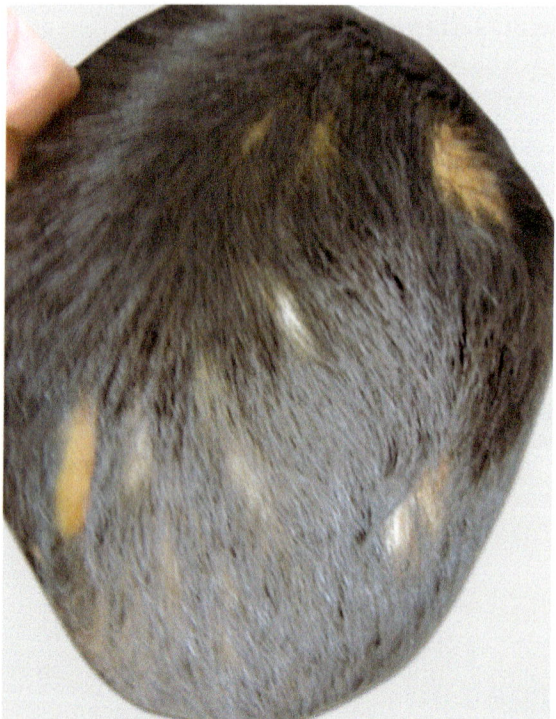

Fig. 9.4: A case of aplasia cutis congenita on the scalp, the discrete patches of cicatricial alopecia since birth are a consequence of tissue defects at birth. (*Courtsey:* Kabir Sardana)

Box 9.1: Classification of hair shaft disorders

With increased fragility	*Without increased fragility*
Pili torti	Pili annulati
Monilethrix	Pili trianguli et canaliculi
Trichorrhexis invaginata	Trichonodosis
Trichorrhexis nodosa	Trichostasis spinulosa
Trichothiodystrophy	Trichoptilosis
Trichoschisis	Loose anagen hair
	Woolly hair

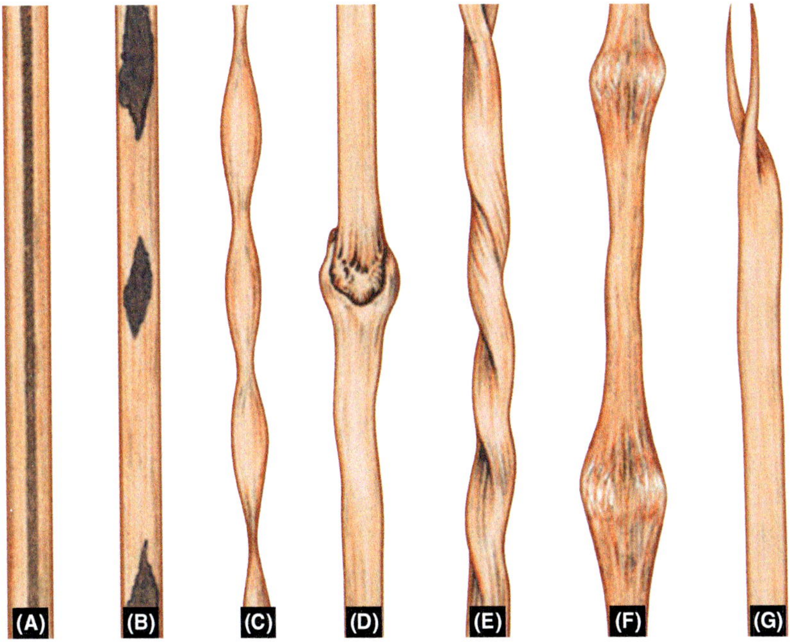

Fig. 9.5A to G: A figurative depiction of the common hair shaft defects. (A) Normal hair, (B) Pili annulati, (C) Monilethrix, (D) Trichorrhexis invaginata, (E) Pili torti, (F) Trichorrhexis nodosa, (G) Trichoptilosis

Trichorrhexis Nodosa (TN)

TN is the most common defect of the hair shaft leading to hair breakage. The primary abnormality is a focal loss of the cuticle, which leads to exposed and eventually frayed cortical fibers (Fig. 9.5B). Minute grayish nodes appear along the hair shaft, where cuticular cells gets disrupted, allowing the cortical cells to splay out, giving the appearance of two paint brushes thrust into one another. It is *most commonly* an **"acquired"** disorder and is without any other issues and is consequent to **trauma** to the hair. This is consequent to use of hot combs, hot hairdryers, hair straighteners, other chemical treatments, or from the cumulative cuticular damage from vigorous combing and brushing, repeated salt-water bathing, prolonged sun exposure, and frequent shampooing. Cream rinses and protein conditioners are helpful. If the causative factors are discontinued, the acquired form of trichorrhexis nodosa generally improves within 2 to 4 years.

TN can however also present at **birth** as an isolated problem or with teeth and/or nail abnormalities, but its presence in an infant or young child should trigger a search for an underlying metabolic problem. Associated metabolic disorders may be citrullinemia, arginosuccinic aciduria, Netherton syndrome (NS), Trichothiodystrophy (TTD), Menkes' syndrome and oculodental digital dysplasia.

Trichorrhexis Invaginata (TI)

TI, also called **bamboo hair**, is a distinctive hair shaft abnormality (Fig. 9.5D) that occurs due to intermittent keratinizing defect of the hair cortex, and is characteristic of **Netherton syndrome (NS)**. NS is a result of mutation in the LEKT1 gene and is characterized by a *triad* of ichthyosis linearis circumflexa, TI and an atopic diathesis. Neonates with Netherton syndrome present with generalized exfoliative erythroderma and failure to thrive, often associated with hypernatremic dehydration, recurrent infections, and sepsis. Severely affected neonates may show extremely sparse and even absent hair, making the diagnosis based on hair shaft examination difficult. However, the eyebrows are almost always short and broken. After infancy, many affected individuals show the characteristic skin finding of ichthyosis linearis circumflexa, with walls of scale surrounding red patches, in addition to their dry, lusterless hair that breaks easily.

Trichorrhexis invaginata can rarely occur in traumatized, otherwise normal hair or with other congenital hair shaft abnormalities.

Trichoschisis

Trichoschisis presents as clean **transverse fracture** across the hair shaft through cuticle and cortex (Fig. 9.6). It is a manifestation seen in **trichothiodystrophy** where low cysteine content in the hair leads to easy breakability. Clinically, patients with trichothiodystrophy have, since early infancy, short brittle hair on the scalp, eyelashes or eyebrows. Polariscopic examination of affected hairs characteristically shows alternating dark and light bands presumably secondary to the alternating sulfur content. Sulfur and/or amino acid analysis of the hair is diagnostic.

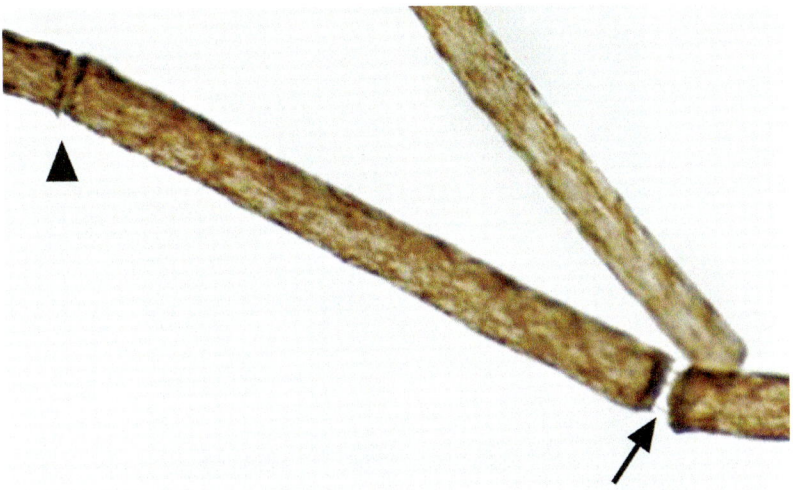

Fig. 9.6: Trichoschisis; the area of fracture is associated with localized absence of the cuticle

Trichoclasis

Trichoclasis is transverse fracture of the hair shaft seen in many congenital fragile hair disorders.

Monilethrix

Monilethrix is usually an autosomal dominant disorder characterized by small node-like defects in the hair shaft producing beaded appearance (Fig. 9.7C). These nodes are elliptical and placed at regular intervals with intervening, nonmedullated tapered fragile constrictions. On dermoscopy, these look like a 'regularly bended ribbon' (Fig. 9.7A). The hair tends to break at these weak internodes leasing to short sparse dry hair on examination.

The cause is a defect in the hard keratins, with mutations in KRT81 and KRT86 being the most common. *Autosomal recessive monilethrix* has been linked to mutations in DSG4, which encodes desmoglein 4. In this there is atrichia, but no beaded appearance on microscopy.

In individuals with this disorder, normal neonatal lanugo hairs are shed during the first few weeks of life. The regrowing hair, which generally appears at about the second month of life, is dry, lusterless, and brittle and fails to grow. The clinical picture, can be very distinctive with the appearance of extremely short brittle hairs emerging through keratotic follicular papules (Fig. 9.7B). In severe cases, the infant may remain bald or the scalp hair may be sparse, easily

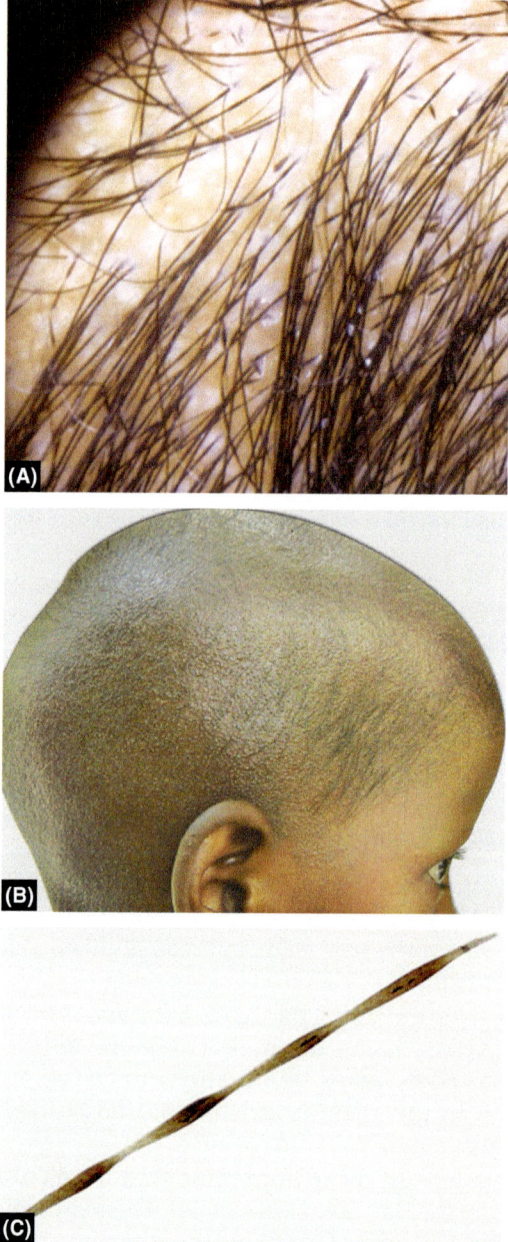

Fig. 9.7A to C: (A) Monilethrix on trichoscopy demonstrating "nodes"; (B) Short stubbles of hair with diffuse keratotic papules; (C) The nodes correspond to the normal caliber of the hair and the defective portion resides in the constrictions

fractured, and stubble-like with follicular prominences, seen markedly on the scalp (occiput and nape of neck being specifically affected) but rarely it may also involve the body.

Treatment: Administration of oral retinoids or 2% minoxidil has been reported to improve the alopecia. Protection against trauma such as excessive brushing, styling and braiding is essential.

Woolly Hair Disease

Woolly hair presents as tight curly or wiry hair that does not form locks (simply stated as the presence of Negroid hair on the scalp of persons of non-Negroid descent). Hairs are fine, dry, light-colored and corrugated at intervals that look almost woolly in appearance. Woolly hair usually occurs as an isolated defect with AD/AR pattern of inheritance but has been reported with other anomalies. Both the AD/AR variants result from abnormalities of the inner root sheath of the hair follicles.

The aberrant hair growth begins at birth or infancy. Hair length may be decreased secondary to brittleness. Woolly hair may go from curly to wavy as the child ages. The entire scalp tends to be affected, but nonscalp hair is normal (Fig. 9.8A and B).

Light microscopy shows grooves, twists and irregularities. Woolly hair is a part of *syndromes* like Nexos disease (arrhythmogenic right

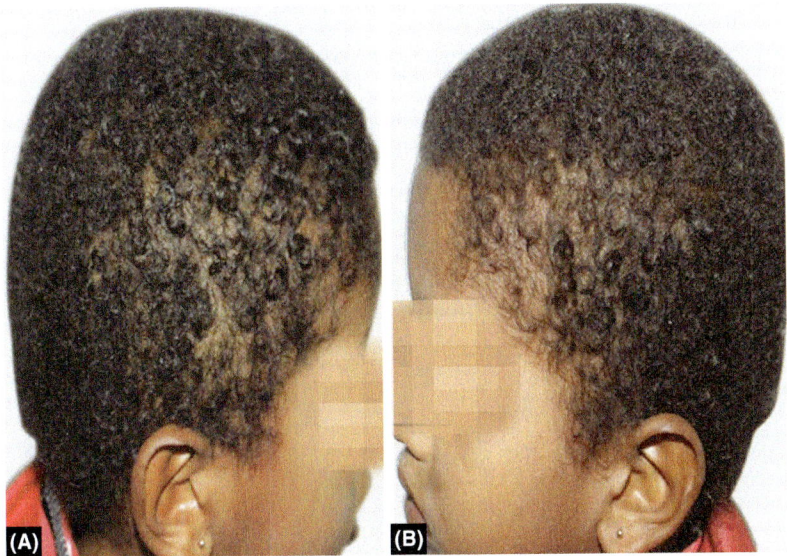

Fig. 9.8A and B: Woolly hair: Tightly curled, short "Negroid" hair over the scalp. The hair length is decreased due to hair shaft brittleness

ventricular cardiomyopathy, nonepidermolytic diffuse PPK) and Carvajal syndrome (left ventricular cardiomyopathy, striate type of epidermolytic PPK).

The woolly hair nevus is a sporadic condition characterized by the development of one or more patches of hair different in color, shape, and consistency from the normal surrounding scalp hair.

Pili Annulati (PA)

PA is a rare disorder presenting as alternating light and dark bands at birth or infancy, that can be seen both on clinical and microscopic examination (Fig. 9.5B). This disorder is thought to be due to formation of hair cavities in the hair shaft. It is nowadays seen commonly in patients who use hot and cold temperature for styling the hair.

Pili Torti (PT)

PT is an autosomal dominant disorder, where the hair shaft is flattened and twisted at angles of about 180° with multiple twists at irregular intervals in the same direction (Fig. 9.5E). The affected hair generally fracture through the twists. The dry, fragile hair is often lighter in color than expected and shimmers in reflected light with a "**spangled**" appearance because of the hair twisting. The hair tends to be short, especially in areas subject to trauma, and may extend out from the scalp.

Pili torti, can occur in the presence of other hair shaft abnormalities, as either an inherited or an acquired finding and is also present in many different syndromes. It has been reported to occur in association with monilethrix, pseudomonilethrix, woolly hair, longitudinal grooving, trichorrhexis nodosa and trichorrhexis invaginata. Menkes' syndrome is an X-linked recessive disorder characterized by skin and hair hypopigmentation with the characteristic presence of pili torti, progressive neurological degeneration with mental retardation, bone and connective tissue alteration, soft doughy skin, joint laxity and vascular abnormalities. The hair stands on end and looks and feels like **steel wool**.

Uncombable Hair Syndrome

It is a condition that starts early in life. Parents typically complain that the hair never flattens after combing.

The hair of the affected child is generally straw-colored, dry and frizzy (Fig. 9.9). The clinical appearance of the spun-glass hair requires a sizable proportion of abnormal hairs, and at least 50% of hairs are abnormal by scanning electron microscopy. The hair tends to become

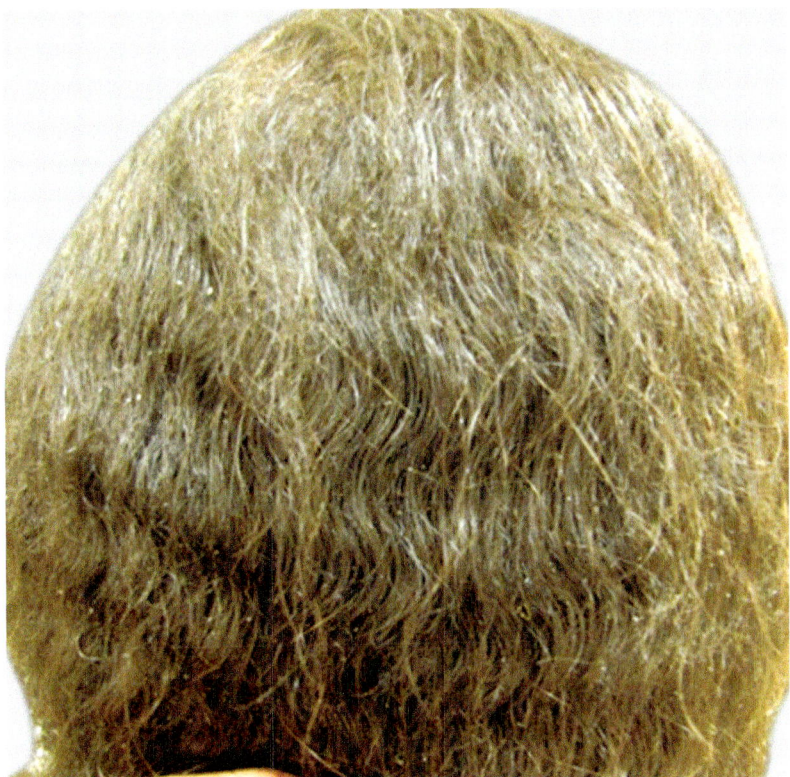

Fig. 9.9: An Indian patient with blonde to light brown hair; dry, frizzy, and spangled hair texture; and slow to normal growth rate. The hair is disorderly, stands out from the scalp, and cannot be combed (*Courtsey:* Kabir Sardana)

progressively more manageable by adolescence, and some patients have responded to biotin administration (Boccaletti V).

The syndrome is thought to be autosomal dominant with variable penetrance, although no associated gene mutations have been identified. The onset is usually during infancy or early childhood, and eyebrows, lashes, and body hair are normal. Affected children may have minor nail abnormalities and some show both uncombable hair and loose anagen hair. Microscopy of the cross section shows grooved or triangular appearance.

Uncombable hair syndrome must be distinguished from *extremely unruly hair*, which is seen in 2% of individuals. Extremely unruly hair tends to stand up from the area of the posterior parietal whorl towards the frontal hairline may be associated with microcephaly and is a potential indicator of abnormal brain growth and morphogenesis.

Acquired Progressive Kinking of Hair

It is a condition generally affecting the adolescent age group, characterized by extreme curliness of hair with coarse and unruly texture. Generally the males are more commonly affected than females. Microscopy of the cross section shows an ellipse or irregular configuration.

Trichothiodystrophy (TTD)

TTD is a heterogeneous group of autosomal recessive disorders in which patients have dry, brittle, cysteine-deficient hair as an isolated finding or in association with a multi-systemic disease. To date, **four genes** have been linked to TTD: ERCC2 (XPD), ERCC3 (XPB), p8 or GTF2H5 (TTDA), and C7Orf11 (TTDN1).

Light microscopy of TTD hairs shows a wavy, irregular outline and a flattened shaft that twists like a folded ribbon. Two types of fracture may be seen: Trichoschisis (clean transverse fracture) or an atypical trichorrhexis nodosa with only slight splaying of the cortical cells. Polarizing microscopy is critical to show the characteristic alternating lights and dark bands, the "tiger-tail" appearance (Fig. 9.10).

There are associated clinical findings in TTD (Faghri S), that include, ichthyosis—ARCI and IV (65%), photosensitivity (24%), xerosis, palmoplantar keratoderma, atopic dermatitis, and/or follicular keratosis. Nail abnormalities (63%) may develop including dystrophy with thickening or yellow discoloration. Systemic findings include developmental delay/intellectual impairment (86%), short stature and low weight (73%), ocular abnormalities (51%, especially cataracts) and facial dysmorphism (66%).

TTDs have now been *reclassified* based on the mutations into 3 groups (Morice-Picard F,) as **group I** (mutations in genes encoding subunits of TFIIH: XPD, XPB, p8), **group II** (TTDN1), and **group III** (no known molecular basis). **Group I** includes patients with photosensitivity (either clinical or *in vitro*) and is the most common subtype. Most individuals in **group II** are not photosensitive and show an increased risk of delayed bone age, seizures, and autistic behavior. Currently unclassified but nonphotosensitive patients (such as those with Pollitt and Sabinas syndromes) are in **group III**. Using this classification, ichthyosis and the collodion-baby phenotype are most highly correlated with group II/III.

Loose Anagen Hair Syndrome

The classic presentation is of a **blonde** preschooler with lusterless, fine, and sparse hair that does not grow long and with easy extractability of the abnormal anagen hair.

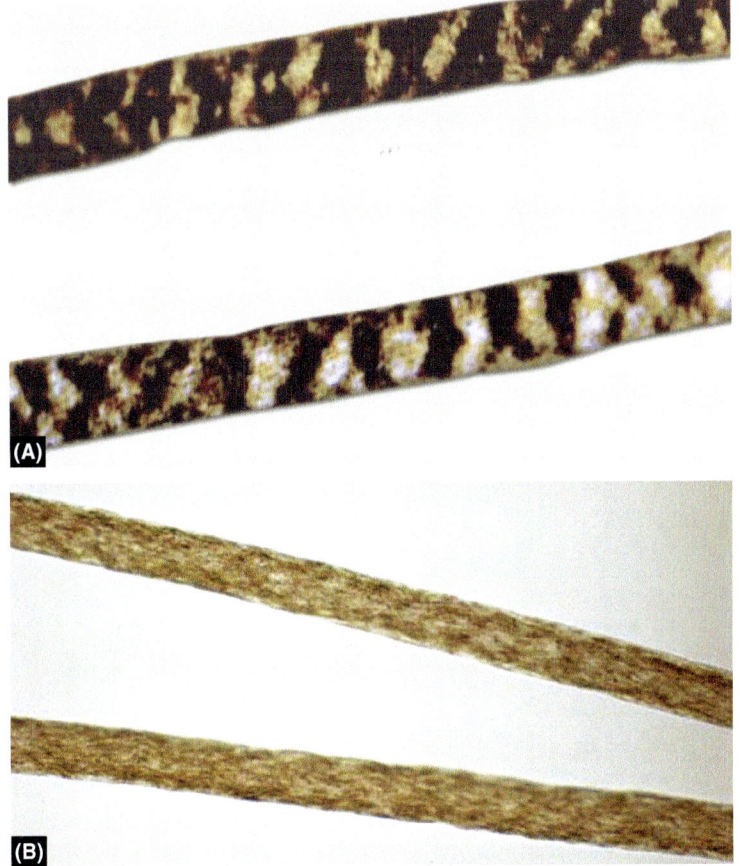

Fig. 9.10A and B: Alternating light and dark banding ("tiger tail phenomenon") in a patient with trichothiodystrophy. The image B is using cross-polarized microscopy with the filters in the "crossed" position (*Courtesy:* Dr EA Knopp)

Most patients are first diagnosed at the age of 2–5 years when they are brought to a physician with the complaint of thin, uneven hair with an abnormal texture. Parents often state that the child's hair "will not grow." LAHS is most frequently diagnosed in girls. The hair loss may be diffuse or patchy but there is no increase in hair fragility. In some cases, the hair has a "sticky" or "tacky" feel. Usually the hair is thin, dry, somewhat unmanageable with a windblown appearance. (Fig. 9.11). The degree of unruliness is generally mild, but cases resembling uncombable hair syndrome have been reported.

Though believed to be AD, most cases are sporadic and occur in girls. A mutation in a hair keratin (KRT75, formerly called K6hf) has been found in some families. Of the actively growing anagen hairs,

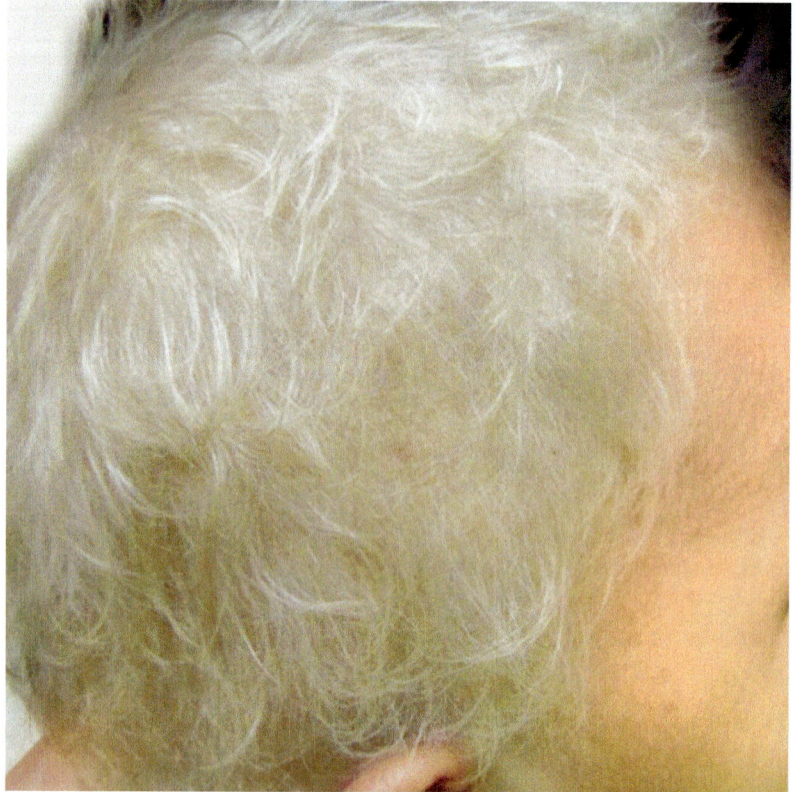

Fig. 9.11: An Indian patient with blonde hair, history of easy pluckability and a general "wind blown appearance" (LAHS)

more than 80% show ruffled cuticles and pigmented misshapen bulbs. The underlying abnormality is a structural defect in the inner root sheath that normally anchors the anagen hair.

Although no treatment is available for this disorder, it is reassuring for patients and their families to know that other abnormalities are not associated with this disorder and individuals with this condition tend to improve with time.

4. Disorders Associated with Poliosis

Poliosis circumscripta is defined as a localized patch of white hair in a group of hair follicles (Fig. 9.12). Although traditionally known as the "white forelock" secondary to the involvement of the central frontal scalp, poliosis may affect various regions of the body including the eyelashes, eyebrows, and beard. On histopathology, poliosis demonstrates either decreased or absent melanin and/or melanocytes

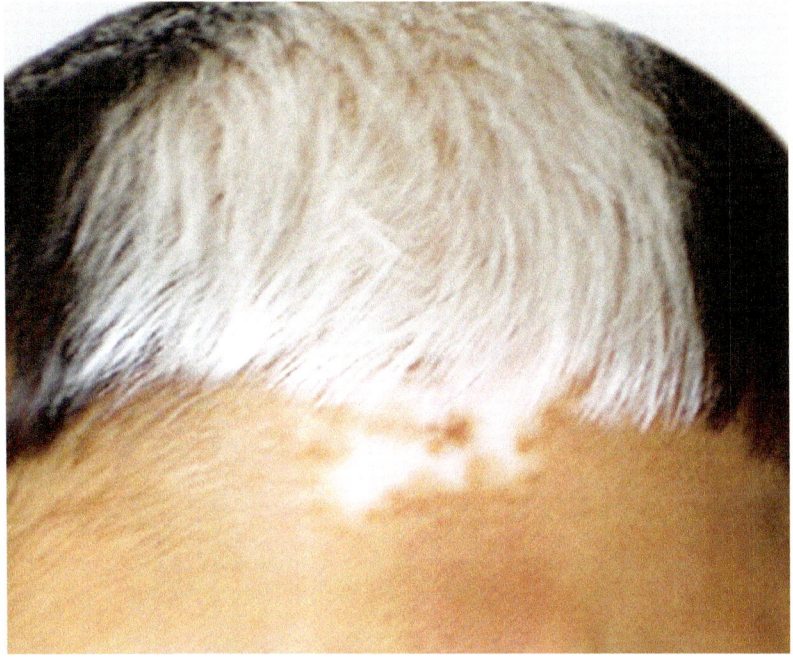

Fig. 9.12: Poliosis circumscripta

in the hair bulbs of the affected hair follicles. The presentation is associated with a variety of genetic and non-genetic disorders.

1. **Genetic conditions** associated with poliosis include tuberous sclerosis, piebaldism, Waardenburg syndrome, neurofibromatosis type 1, Marfan syndrome and prolidase deficiency.

2. **Nongenetic causes** include vitiligo, Vogt-Koyanagi-Harada syndrome, Alezzandrini syndrome, alopecia areata, sarcoidosis, blepharitis, melanocytic lesions, neurofibroma, medications, trigeminal autonomic cephalalgia, postherpetic, trauma/repetitive plucking.

Waardenburg syndrome is characterized by sensorineural deafness and pigmentary abnormalities (typically a white forelock and possible poliosis of eyebrows, and eyelashes). **Piebaldism** is characterized by cutaneous depigmentation ranging from white forelock to almost the entire body and hair depigmentation (Fig. 9.13). Poliosis may be the only manifestation in 80 to 90% of piebaldism cases, or both the hair and the underlying forehead may be involved. Eyebrows and eyelashes may also be involved. Irregular depigmented patches, usually in a symmetric distribution, may also be observed on the face, trunk, and extremities. Repigmentation may occur spontaneously or after injury in some patients, either partially or completely.

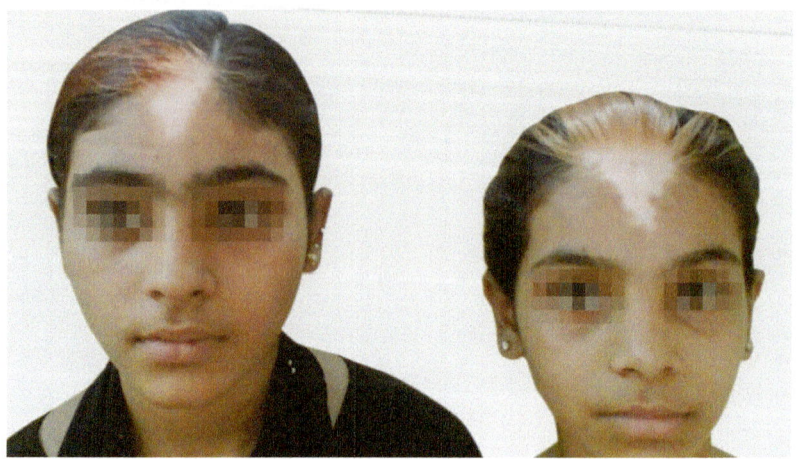

Fig. 9.13: Two sisters with piebaldism, which classically involves the midline (*Courtesy:* Kabir Sardana)

Tietze syndrome is an autosomal dominant disorder characterized by congenital deafness and stable congenital hypopigmented patches of the skin and poliosis.

Amongst nongenetic causes, **vitiligo** is a prominent one. Poliosis has been commonly associated with vitiligo with a frequency reaching up to 25%, especially in patients with segmental vitiligo (Hannet et al; Cho et al; Schallreuter et al). One study on 208 patients with segmental vitiligo revealed poliosis in 101 (48.6%) patients (Hann et al, 1996). The eyebrows were most commonly affected. Eyelash involvement has also been reported.

Graying of human hair **(canities)** is caused by a reduction in the activity of melanocytes within hair follicles. Premature graying of hair, termed premature canities, refers to a loss of color, especially of scalp hair, at an age earlier than that generally accepted as physiologic (before the age of 20 in Caucasians and 30 in African-Americans). In the pediatric age group, premature canities like presentation can occur in the setting of vitiligo or AA. Canities have also been described in children with pernicious anemia, hyperthyroidism and other thyroid disorders, progeria, Werner syndrome, ataxia-telangiectasia, Rothmund-Thomson syndrome, tuberous sclerosis, neurofibromatosis, and the Waardenburg and Vogt-Koyanagi syndromes.

5. Hypertrichosis

Hypertrichosis, refers to a generalized or localized pattern of non-androgen-dependent excessive hair growth in a male or female without evidence of masculinism or menstrual abnormality.

Various Genetic Disorders Associated with Hypertrichosis are

- Hypertrichosis lanuginosa
- Nevoid hypertrichosis
- Hypertrichosis with gingival hyperplasia
- X-linked dominant hypertrichosis
- Ambras syndrome
- Coffin-Siris syndrome
- Cornelia de Lange syndrome
- Craniofacial dysostosis
- Cantu syndrome (hypertrichosis with osteochondrodysplasia)
- Lipodystrophies (Donohue syndrome)
- Mucopolysaccharidoses (Hunter syndrome/Hurler syndrome)

Congenital Hypertrichosis Lanuginosa

The original fine, soft, unmedullated, and usually unpigmented lanugo hairs are shed *in utero* during the seventh or eighth month of gestation. Premature infants, however, commonly display this fine coat of lanugo hair, particularly on the face, limbs, and trunk. In these infants the fine lanugo hairs are shed during the first 3 months of life and replaced by normal terminal hair growth, generally before the first 6 months.

Acquired generalized hypertrichosis

- Drug related (cyclosporin, diazoxide, phenytoin, PUVA, acetazolamide, streptomycin)
- POEMS syndrome (peripheral neuropathy, organomegaly, endocrine dysfunction, monoclonal gammopathy and skin changes)
- Celiac disease
- Juvenile dermatomyositis
- Infantile steatorrhea

Localized hypertrichosis

Congenital localized hypertrichosis may be seen in the following conditions: Congenital hair on the elbows (hypertrichosis cubiti), anterior cervical area (anterior cervical hypertrichosis) (Fig. 9.14) and external ears as an isolated phenomenon; congenital trichomegaly as an isolated finding or as part of syndromes; "hair collar" around congenital alopecic scalp lesions; nevoid hypertrichosis (single/ multiple patches); hypertrichosis overlying primary cutaneous meningiomas, congenital smooth muscle hamartomas or plexiform neurofibromas; congenital hairy nevi (Fig. 9.15); "faun tail" nevus (Fig. 9.16).

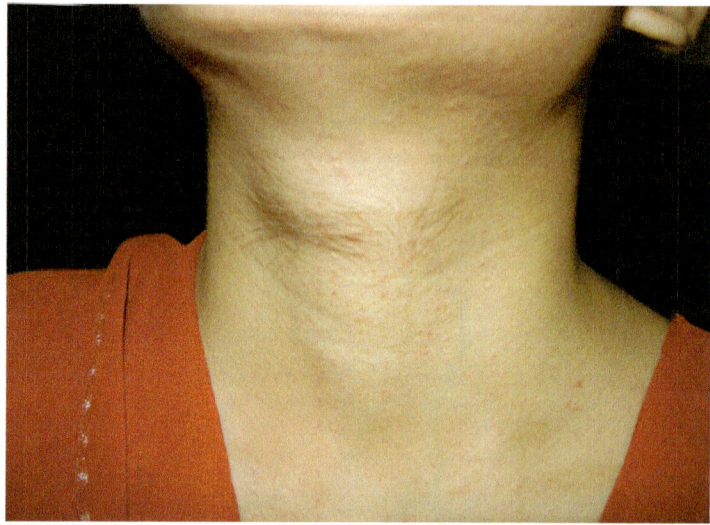

Fig. 9.14: Anterior cervical hypertrichosis (*Courtesy:* Kabir Sardana)

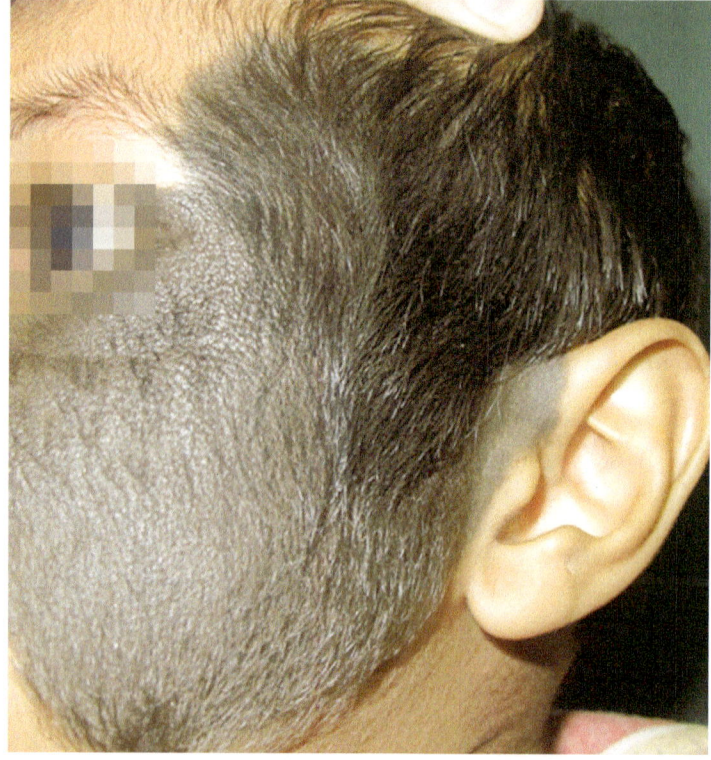

Fig. 9.15: Hairy congenital nevomelanocytic nevus (*Courtesy:* Ananta Khurana)

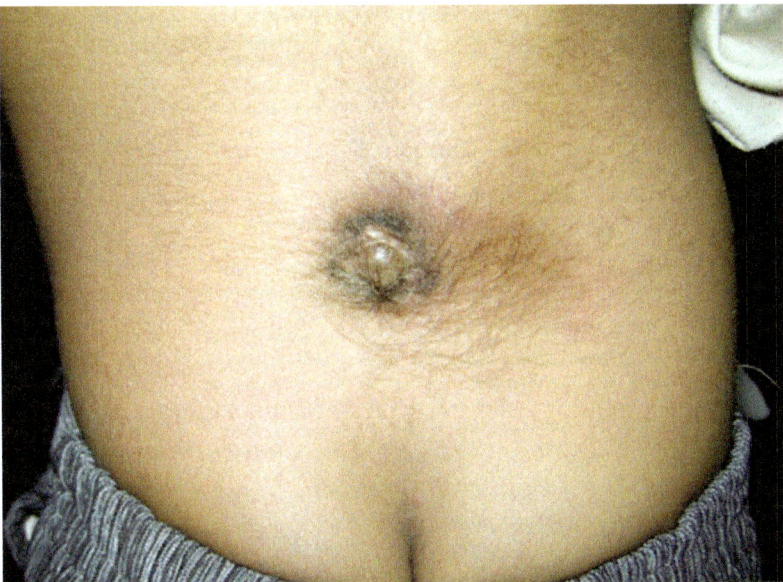

Fig. 9.16: Faun tail nevus with a hair collar sign around a visible spinal defect (*Courtesy:* Kabir Sardana)

Acquired localized hypertrichosis may be seen with repeated irritation, inflammation or trauma (like under the plaster casts); scrotal hair (as a sign of virilization or uncommonly without it with hair appearing at 2–7 months of age and regressing by 18 months); localized hyper-trichosis of eyelashes with interferon and cyclosporin treatment; Becker's nevus.

Nevoid hypertrichosis: Growth of hair abnormal in length, shaft diameter, or color may occur in association with other nevoid abnormalities or as isolated circumscribed developmental defects. Abnormal tufts of hair in the lumbosacral and, at times, the posterior cervical or thoracic areas maybe associated with associated features of spinal dysraphism (Fig. 9.16).

APPROACH TO A CASE OF GENOTRICHOSIS

When to Suspect a Genotrichosis?

Genotrichosis is suspected based on complaints, history, clinical evaluation findings and confirmed by investigations like light microscopy, dermatoscopy and polarized microscopy.

The points to be considered while eliciting history include:
1. History of onset
2. History of consanguinity

3. Family history of similar complaints
4. Complications during pregnancy or at birth
5. Associated features and findings

Points to be Considered During Clinical Evaluation

These include:

1. **Hair and scalp examination**

   - *Hair color:* Evaluation of hair color includes looking into characteristics like nature and color of pigment, pigment dilution, clumping of pigment, distribution of pigment, absence of pigment. The conditions to be borne in mind while evaluating the hair color include albinism, Menkes' kinky hair disease, isolated pili torti, phenylketonuria, homocystinuria, silvery hair syndromes and localized patch of white hair.

   - *Length and fragility:* The most common complaints encountered in case of hair shaft related disorders include that hair does not grow beyond a certain point or hair have never been cut or the hair is brittle and breaks easily. This may be a pointer to any of the hair shaft disorders like monilethrix, trichorrhexis nodosa, trichorrhexis invaginata, pili torti, Menke's kinky hair disease, etc.

   - *Texture:* Texture is commonly defined as feel of the hair to the hand or by visual appearance. The **texture** of **hair** is determined by the thickness of **hair** strand or its circumference or the condition of the cuticle. In conditions affecting the hair texture, parents typically complain of extreme curliness and roughness of hair or inability to flatten the hair while combing. Conditions to be considered include uncombable hair syndrome, woolly hair conditions and acquired progressive kinking of hair.

   - *Atrichia/hypotrichia/hypertrichosis:* These conditions present with reduced hair, complete loss of hair or at times in association with other findings like papular eruptions or milia. They may present at birth or shortly there afterwards and the condition is generally progressive. The conditions to be considered when one evaluates a case of hypotrichosis include atrichia with papular eruption, congenital hypotrichoses, Marie Unna hypotrichoses and isolated congenital atrichia.

   - *Other hair bearing areas affected:* The importance of evaluating other hair bearing areas cannot be understated while examining a patient of hair disorder. It may provide important clues in the diagnosis with certain conditions showing higher specificity and probability of finding hair defects in certain areas. For example: Monilethrix conditions are better diagnosed by evaluating eyebrow hair from the lateral end of the eyebrow. Total loss of body hair could be a pointer towards ectodermal dysplasias or alopecia areata universalis.

2. **Systemic examination**
   - *Presence or absence of ichthyosis:* The association of ichthyoses with hair shaft disorders is a pointer towards the more complex syndromes like ichthyosis follicularis, alopecia and photophobia (IFAP), keratitis ichthyosis and deafness (KID) syndrome or peeling skin syndrome.
   - *Oral, dental, ocular defects and features of ectodermal dysplasias:* Evaluation of the eyes, hearing and dentition along with characteristic dysmorphic facies can be a marker for the more complex and multisystem involved as in syndromes like ectodermal dysplasias and more rare conditions like hypotrichosis with juvenile macular dystrophy.
   - *Neurological manifestations*
   - *Associations with palmoplantar keratodermas*
   - *Photosensitivity*

3. **Developmental milestones:** Developmental delay may be a manifestation of various syndromes like Menkes' kinky hair disease, trichothiodystrophy, silvery hair syndromes, etc.

4. **Microscopy findings**
   - Chédiak-Higashi syndrome: Small melanin clumps
   - Griscelli syndrome: Large melanin clumps
   - Elejalde syndrome: Irregular melanin clumps
   - Monilethrix: Beaded appearance
   - Pseudomonilethrix: Indented appearance
   - Trichorrhexis nodosa: Interlocking paint brush
   - Trichorrhexis invaginata: Telescoping appearance
   - Pili torti: Spangled appearance
   - Trichothiodystrophy: Tiger tail appearance
   - Uncombable hair: Triangular on cross section
   - Acquired progressive kinking of hair: Ellipsoid or irregular configuration.

The need for establishing the diagnosis

Genotrichosis is a diverse group of hair disorders that may be a mirror towards systemic conditions. Establishing the diagnosis and confirmation helps the family in charting out a roadmap for further managing the condition. Few of these genotrichoses are associated with mental, physical and developmental delay of the child, which may be due to the disorder per se or due to the psychiatric comorbidities associated with these conditions. Not only are these conditions difficult to diagnose but also pose a therapeutic challenge to the treating physician and most often can be alleviated predominantly by symptomatic therapy and repeated counseling. The involvement of a specialized multidisciplinary team comprising of a pediatrician, pediatric neurologist, pediatric endocrinologist, pediatric cardiologist serves beneficial towards managing these conditions.

What can we do After Diagnosing a Condition of Genotrichoses?

- **Molecular diagnostics:** Molecular diagnostic is an essential step in confirming the diagnosis of genotrichoses and helps in diagnosing asymptomatic carriers in the family which further helps in prenatal counseling of the parents. It also has the advantage of diagnosing asymptomatic family members at risk in the family and appropriate pre-conception counseling. With recent developments in the prenatal and implantation diagnosis, molecular diagnostics help in gene splicing of the single gene disorders with known gene loci. The above thus helps in not only optimizing patient care but provides holistic therapy to the entire family involved.
- **Standard genetic testing and multigene panel assay:** These tests can be done in various laboratories and the specific centers can be searched on (http://www.ncbi.nlm.nih.gov/gtr/) and (www.genetests.org).

  The specific tests can be searched by the disease name, gene symbol or protein name.

  The sample dispatch can be arranged as per the specifications of the laboratory and a few centers offer these tests at minimal cost or low cost for convenience of the patients.
- **Counseling:** The following points need to be borne in mind while counseling a patient of genotrichoses:
  - It must be done in a language that is understandable to the patient and his caregivers
  - Basic terminologies require to be explained
  - Type of gene variants that can be detected needs to be explained and stressed upon regarding the need for genetic testing and family screening
  - Possibilities of false positive and false negative findings during a particular test must be borne in mind
  - Possibility of incidental finding while screening of family members must be discussed with
  - Privacy issues and genetic information nondiscrimination act 2008 must be abided by.

- **Specific management:** Management of genotrichoses poses a challenge to the treating physician since there are very few reports of specific management modalities for these conditions owing to the paucity of cases and clinical trials.

  Treatment of the underlying conditions as in trichorrhexis nodosa occurring due to citrullinemia, biotinidase deficiency and arginosuccinic academia with specialized diets have resulted in improvement.

  Subcutaneous supplementation of copper along with biotin if deficient have reported improvement in Menkes' kinky hair disease.

  Topical minoxidil 2% solution has shown variable results in the management of genotrichoses with initial improvement. However, the improvement has not been sustained on discontinuation of minoxidil solution.

  In cases of conditions with abnormality in the texture of hair symptomatic improvement has been achieved by using gentle cleansing agents, deep conditioning treatment and leave on hair serums for reducing frizziness and unruliness of the hair.

  Off late, newer therapies using hair peptides are being tried to improve the quality and texture of the hair but reassurance still remains the main stay of therapy.

- **Follow-up:** Regular follow ups by the patient not only helps in charting out a treatment and approach plan for the patient but also helps in monitoring the disease condition.

TINEA CAPITIS

Tinea capitis is one of the most common dermatophytoses of the school-going age group with an increasing incidence. This dermatosis tends to affect more of pediatric age group and poses a community health issue, since it has a tendency to spread through contact and fomites. Therefore, early recognition and complete treatment becomes imperative. As the pediatric age group is affected, invasive investigations are difficult owing to the anxiety of the parents and children and the non cooperative nature of children. Dermoscopy as a noninvasive diagnostic tool in such a scenario is of immense importance for detecting, treating and explaining to the parents.

The varied presentations of tinea capitis include grey patch type, kerion, black dot and favus type.

Kerion

This is an inflammatory variant of tinea capitis. Inflammation may be mild or severe. Clinically it is characterized by erythematous, boggy areas with pustule formation, matting of hair, easy pluckability and fragility of hair. Deep boggy red areas characterized by a severe acute inflammatory infiltrate with pustule formation. This presentation is generally caused by the zoophilic species, typically *Trichophyton verrucosum* or *T. mentagrophytes,* though occasionally a geophilic species may be isolated.

Grey Patch

It clinically presents as well defined areas of grey scaly patch with loss of hair. There is easy pluckability and fragility of hair (Fig. 9.17). Dermatoscopic evaluation reveals broken hair, black dots, comma hair and hook hair. It leads to nonscarring alopecia and the inflammation is not severe. Grouping of cases in families is often observed. *Microsporum audouini* and *M. ferrugineum* are most commonly implicated.

Favus

It is another variant of tinea capitis less commonly noted in Indian subcontinent. Scalp lesions are characterized by the presence of yellow cup-shaped crusts termed scutula, which surround the infected hair follicles.

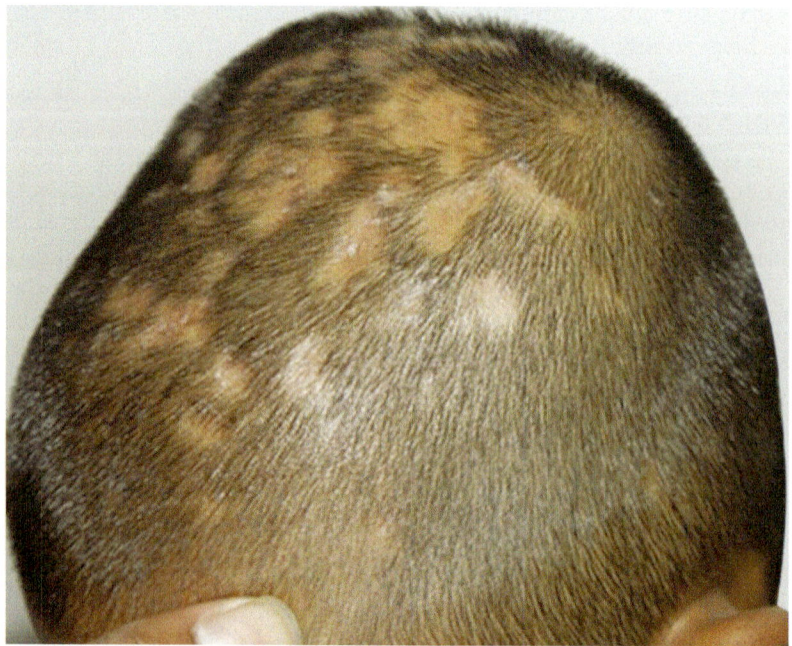

Fig. 9.17: Grey patch tinea capitis

Black Dot

This type presents as well circumscribed patchy areas of hair loss with black dots on the skin surface and is most commonly caused by *T. tonsurans* and *T. violaceum*. The appearance is caused by broken ends of hair on the surface of the scalp skin. It does not lead to scarring alopecia unless there is secondary infection.

Lymphadenopathy of the cervical lymph nodes may be noted in a few cases.

Management

General measure like regular washing of hair and hygiene measures in school and home is advocated. Disinfection of fomites and screening of family members forms one of the pillars of treatment. Topical medications in the form of rinses with antifungals like oxiconazole, sertaconazole, clotrimazole and cimbazole can be used. Griseofulvin (10–20 mg/kg/day, depending on the preparation, in divided doses) remains the mainstay of systemic treatment followed by terbinafine (dose of 62.5 mg for <10 kg, 125 mg for 10–20 kg and 250 mg for >20 kg) and itraconazole (2–4 mg/kg/day). Treatment should continue for 4–6 weeks. Itraconazole 5 mg/kg in weekly pulses for 2–3 rounds may be used as a second-line of treatment.

PEDICULOSIS CAPITIS

Head lice (*pediculosis capitis*) is a common, highly contagious infection/ infestation of the scalp hair that often occurs in nurseries, daycare centers, and schools. It is caused by infestation with the human head louse, *Pediculus humanus capitis*, and it is usually very itchy.

Most commonly the lice (since they remain on the scalp to suck blood) may not be visible and the patient may only present with itchy scalp. However, the lice lay eggs which are visible on the hair shaft as nits which clinches the diagnosis (Fig. 9.18). Many a times, the nits may have mimicker known as pseudonits like scales/hair casts which may confuse the treating physician.

Treatment includes oral ivermectol at 200 µg/kg as a stat dose. Permethrin 1% as a topical solution is given as rinse where it is allowed to be applied as a root to shoot application for ten minutes followed by rinsing of hair. Topical ivermectol shampoo is also now available as a rinse. In the prevalence of coexisting secondary bacterial infection, it needs to be treated with systemic antibiotics. Disinfection of fomites by soaking in warm water, treatment of contacts and nit removal by dipping comb in warm water and wet combing forms the important steps of treatment.

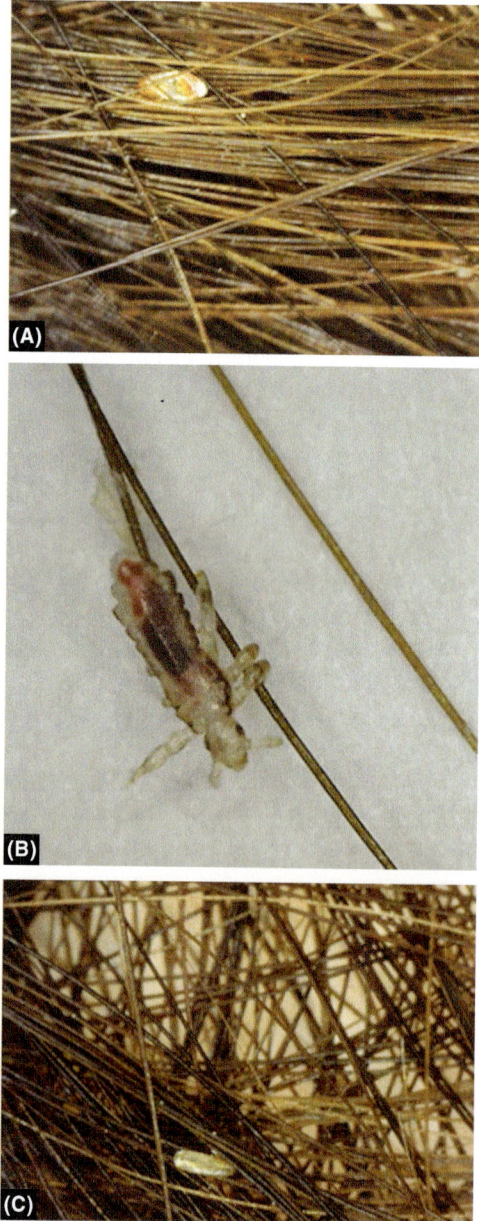

Fig. 9.18A to C: The lifecycle of *Pediculus humanus capitis* on the scalp of an infested 5-year-old girl, with dermoscopy (A and C at 200X; B at 50X). (A) Vital nit, filled with an embryo, seen as a brown, ovoid structure with a convex end; (B) Adult louse following a blood meal; (C) The empty, hatched nit seen as a translucent structure with a planar end

Bibliography

1. Cahali JB, Fernandez SA, Oliveira ZN, Machado MC,Valente NS, Sotto MN. Elejalde syndrome: Report of a case and review of the literature. Pediatr Dermatol 2004;21:479–82.

2. Camacho F. Genodermatosis with hyptrichosis. In: Camacho F, Montagna W, eds. Tricology. Madrid: Aula Médica, 1996: 219–36.

3. Cho S, Kang HC, Hahm JH. Characteristics of vitiligo in Korean children. Pediatr Dermatol 2000;17:189–93.

4. Delamere FM, Sladden MM, Dobbins HM, Leonardi-Bee J. Interventions for alopecia areata. Cochrane Database Syst Rev 2008;2:CD004413

5. Dominant inheritance. Am J Med Genet 1994;52:487–90.

6. Fishtel JC, Richards JA, Davis LS. Trichorrhexis nodosa secondary to argininosuccinic aciduria. Pediatr Dermatol 2007;24:25–7.

7. Gaikwad RP, Mukherjee S, Saha A, Naphade P. Waardenburg syndrome type 2. Indian J Paediatr Dermatol [Epub ahead of print] [cited 2017 Mar 14].

8. Grover C, Arora P, Manchanda V. Tinea capitis in the pediatric population: A study from North India. Indian J Dermatol Venereol Leprol 2010;76:527–32.

9. Hann SK, Lee HJ. Segmental vitiligo: clinical findings in 208 patients. J Am Acad Dermatol 1996;35:671–4.

10. Happle R, Konig A. Familial naevus sebaceous may be explained by paradominant transmission. Br J Dermatol 1999;144:377.

11. Indelman M, Bergman R, Lestringant GG, Peer G, Sprecher E. Compound heterozygosity for mutations in the hairless gene causes atrichia with papular lesions. Br J Dermatol 2003;148:553–7.

12. Kumar TS, Ebenazar S, Moses PD. Griscelli syndrome. Indian J Dermatol 2006;51:269–71.

13. Madke B, Khopkar U. Pediculosis capitis: An update. Indian J Dermatol Venereol Leprol 2012;78:429–38.

14. Mallon E, Dawber RP, De Berker D, Ferguson DJ. Cheveux incoiffables-diagnostic, clinical and hair microscopic finding and pathogenic studies. Br J Dermatol 1994;131:608–14.

15. Mansur AT, Elcioglu NH, Redler S, Serdar ZA, Cetinel S, Betz RC, et al. Marie Unna hereditary hypotrichosis: A Turkish family with loss of eyebrows and a U2HR mutation. Am J Med Genet A. 2010;152A:2628–33. [PubMed: 20814945].

16. Marren P, Wilson C, Dawber RP, Walshe MM. Hereditary hypotrichosis (Marie Unna type) and juvenile macular degeneration (Stargardt's maculopathy) Clin Exp Dermatol 1992;17:189–91. [PubMed: 1451298].

17. Mende B, Kreysel HW. Hypotrichosis congenita hereditaria Marie Unna with Ehlers-Danlos syndrome and atopy. Hautarzt 1987;38:532–5.

18. Meschede IP, Santos TO, IzidoroToledo TC, Gurgel Gianetti J, Espreafico EM. Griscelli syndrome type 2 in twin siblings: Case report and update on

RAB27A human mutations and gene structure. Braz J Med Biol Res 2008;41:839–48.

19. Olsen EA. Hair Disorders. In Irvine A, Hoeger P, Yan A (eds). Harper Textbook of Pediatric Dermatology. 3rd edition. Wiley Blackwell, 2011, UK.

20. Rapelanoro R, Taieb A, Lacombe D. Congenital hypotrichosis and milia: report of a large family suggesting X-linked.

21. Reddy RR, Babu BM, Venkateshwaramma B, Hymavathi Ch. Silvery hair syndrome in two cousins: Chédiak-Higashi syndrome vs Griscelli syndrome, with rare associations. Int J Trichology 2011;3:107–11.

22. Roberts JL, Whiting DA, Henry D, Basler G, Woolf L. Marie Unna congenital hypotrichosis: Clinical description, histopathology, scanning electron microscopy of a previously unreported large pedigree. J Investig Dermatol Symp Proc 1999;4:261–7.

23. Rudnicka L, Rakowska A, Olszewska M, Slowinska M, Czuwara J, Rusek M, et al. Hair shafts. Atlas of Trichoscopy. London: Springer-Verlag: 2012.p11–46.

24. Sahana M Srinivas,Ravi Hiremagalore. Marie Unna Hereditary Hypotrichosis. Int J Trichology. 2014 Oct–Dec;6(4):182–84.

25. Sahana M, Sacchidanand S, Hiremagalore R, Asha G. Silvery grey hair: Clue to diagnose immunodeficiency. Int J Trichology 2012;4:835.

26. Schallreuter KU, Lemke R, Brandt O, Schwartz R, Westhofen M, Montz R, et al. Vitiligo and other diseases: coexistence or true association. Hamburg study on 321 patients. Dermatology 1994;188:269–75.

27. Sleiman R1, Kurban M, Succaria F, Abbas O. Poliosis circumscripta: overview and underlying causes. J Am Acad Dermatol 2013 Oct;69(4):625–33.18:741–9.

28. Steijlen PM, Neumann HA, der Kinderen DJ, Smeets DF, van der Kerkhof PC, Happle R. Congenital atrichia, palmoplantar hyperkeratosis, mental retardation, and early loss of teeth in four siblings: a new syndrome. J Am Acad Dermatol 1994;30:893–98.

29. Sun JD, Linden KG. Netherton syndrome: A case report and review of the literature. Int J Dermatol 2006;45:693–7.

30. Valente NY, Machado MC, Boggio P, Alves AC, Bergonse FN,Casella E, et al. Polarized light microscopy of hair shafts aids in the differential diagnosis of Chédiak-Higashi and Griscelli-Prunieras syndromes. Clinics (Sao Paulo) 2006;61:327–32.

31. Yan KL, He PP, Yang S, Li M, Yang Q, Ren YQ, et al. Marie Unna hereditary hypotrichosis: Report of a Chinese family and evidence for genetic heterogeneity. Clin Exp Dermatol 2004;29:460–3. [PubMed: 15347323]

32. Zlotogorski A, Panteleyev AA, Aita VM, Christiano AM. Clinical and molecular diagnostic criteria of congenital atrichia with papular lesions. J Invest Dermatol 2002;118:887–90.

10

Hair Loss in Women

Ananta Khurana, Kabir Sardana

INTRODUCTION

A good head of hair is a sign of youth, health and beauty in women and any amount of loss leads to anxiety. Thus, hair loss is one of the commonest concerns amongst female patients visiting dermatology clinics. The conditions in this regard have been discussed individually in different chapters. Here, we attempt to summarize and consolidate literature related to the previously discussed conditions from the point of view of female patients only.

Firstly two concepts, which have added to our understanding of the common causes of female alopecias, are discussed.

1. **Exogen/teloptosis:** Much attention has now been given to the process of loss of club hair from the hair follicle. What was previously thought of as a passive process which follows the re-entering of the follicle into anagen, has now been shown to be a precisely controlled active event in the hair cycle. The term exogen was first used by Stenn et al in 1998. Pierard-Franchimont and Pierard later proposed the term teloptosis (meaning *falling off* in Greek), remarking that exogen suggests a biological exogenous process as opposed to an endogenous one. The anchorage of telogen hairs to the follicular epithelium is due to desmosomes between the keratinocytes surrounding the hair club and the basal layer of the outer root sheath. Desmoglein 3 reactivity has been demonstrated in this area. And it is now believed that the shedding of hair shaft is a proteolytic process, wherein these anchors are broken. Premature teloptosis may underlie chronic telogen shedding.

2. **Kenogen** (meaning empty in Greek) is the latent period between teloptosis and emergence of a new anagen. Guarerra et al (1986) had observed, by phototrichograms, that the sequence of anagen–catagen–telogen does not recur regularly in women with

androgenetic alopecia and there are periods when the follicle is free of a hair shaft. Later, Courtis et al observed the same phenomenon in men. Later, kenogen was observed in a normal prepubertal child, suggesting that the phenomenon maybe physiological. It is believed that kenogen may be the true resting phase of hair cycle in contrast with telogen, during which, the epithelial remnants (distal outer sheath, secondary hair germ, bulge) are still engaged in biochemical activity and even some degree of proliferation takes place. In 2 women with progressing FPHL, studied for 2 years with photo-trichogram, kenogen involved 22% of the hair follicles, lasting a variable time in the same patient (from 3 months to 1 year). Both frequency and duration are greater in patients with more severe alopecia.

TELOGEN EFFLUVIUM AND FEMALE PATTERN HAIR LOSS

The two disorders are considered together as there is often a co-association.

Headington's classification of telogen effluvium has stood the test of time and is still widely accepted. The five functional types described by Headington and the associated disorders are detailed in **Chapter 5**.

Chronic Telogen Effluvium (CTE)

It is a poorly understood condition predominantly affecting women between 30 and 50 years of age, and characterized by diffuse shedding of hair for more than 6 months, without any widening of central parting or follicular miniaturization. CTE has an insidious onset, with no obvious triggering event, and a fluctuating course lasting several years. There is considerable loss according to the patients, who often bring balls of hair lost each day (Fig. 10.1), but they appear to have a full head of hair. This is because it may take at least a reduction of 25% for thinning to be evident on examination. The complaints of patient may be marginalized by the treating doctor who sees no obvious alopecia, adding to their distress. However, there maybe some bitemporal thinning (Fig. 10.2) and a positive hair pull test equally over the vertex and occiput. Short re-growing hair may be seen in the frontal/temporal region.

The condition has been historically confused with 'androgenetic alopecia' in females. Guy and Edmundson (1959) were probably the first ones to describe this diffuse cyclic type of hair loss, affecting middle-aged women. Finally, in 1996, Whiting additionally characterized the histopathologic features of the condition finally delineating it from female 'androgenetic alopecia'.

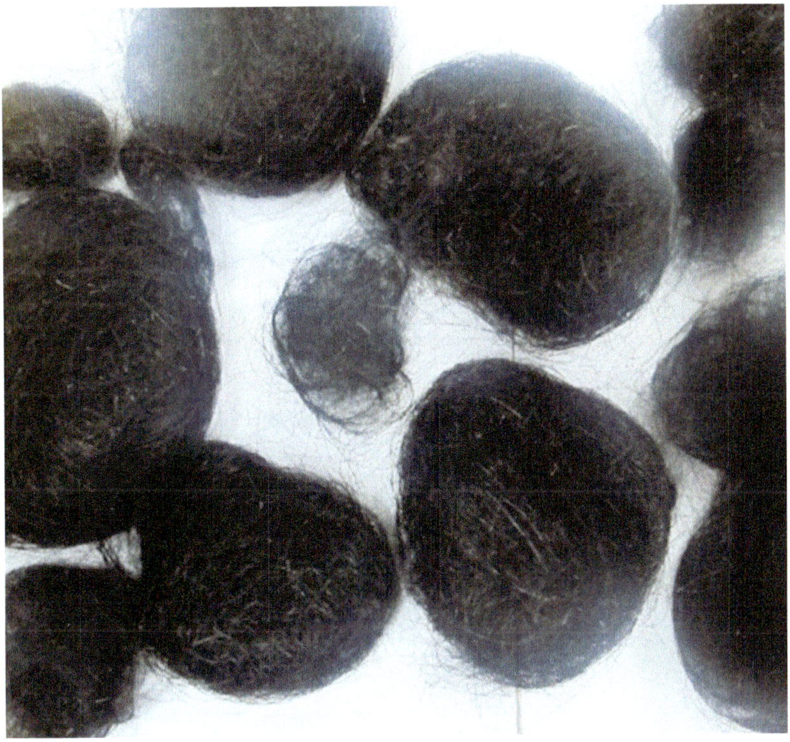

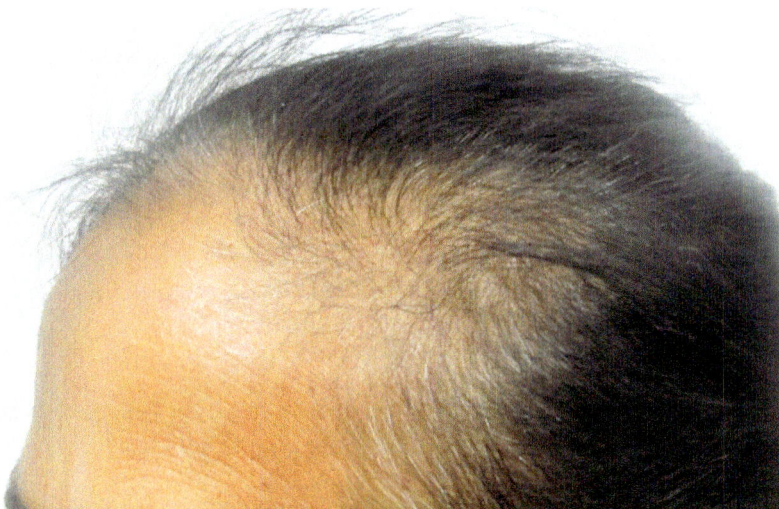

Fig. 10.1: Hair shed each day, brought by a patient with CTE

Fig. 10.2: Bitemporal thinning and short regrowing hair, in the temporal region, in a patient with chronic telogen shedding

Etiology/Diagnosis

A diagnosis of CTE is made after exclusion of other causes of diffuse telogen shedding (Table 5.2, Chapter 5). Chronic diffuse telogen hair loss (CDTHL) is the term used in this regard and refers to telogen hair shedding, longer than 6 months, secondary to a variety of organic causes. Prominent amongst these are profound iron deficiency (as opposed to iron deficiency without anemia or with mild anemia, the association of which is controversial), thyroid disorders (generally reversible with restoration of euthyroid stage except in long-standing cases wherein follicular atrophy ensues), acrodermatitis enteropathica (and not a subclinical zinc deficiency, the correction of which does not lead to improvement in hair fall) and malnutrition (in the form of chronic starvation, hypoproteinemia, and malabsorption disorders).

The mechanism of development of CTE remains obscure. It has been proposed that persistent or intermittent pathologic synchronization phenomena of the hair cycle, shortening of the anagen phase, or premature teloptosis may contribute. However, a reduction of anagen alone, which also underlies FPHL, would suggest that CTE is a mere prodrome of FPHL, although there are long-term follow-up of patients indicating that CTE is a distinct clinical and histological entity. In the 7 year follow-up study on CTE patients, Sinclair et al reported that miniaturization did not occur, except in one patient (which the authors contributed to possible sampling error leading to a misdiagnosis of CTE). Gilmore and Sinclair, using follicular automation, proposed that CTE may instead be due to reduction in the variance of anagen duration and proposed this to be considered as the sixth functional type of telogen effluvium.

Fluctuations in hair loss keep happening over years in all CTE patients. Natural history of CTE has not been studied prospectively; however, it has been suggested that the hair shedding is probably self-limiting over long course of time and that women with this condition do not go bald.

Female Pattern Hair Loss

The other common cause of female alopecia is the female pattern hair loss (FPHL). The pattern of diffuse thinning of the crown area and an intact frontal hairline, as opposed to the male-pattern androgenetic alopecia with its characteristic bitemporal recession of the hair and balding vertex, was originally described by Ludwig in 1977 (Figs 10.3 and 10.4). The concept of frontal accentuation, with a triangular or Christmas tree pattern of alopecia was later described by Olsen in 1994 (Fig. 10.3).

An Australian study showed that FPHL affects 7% of women in their 20s, and more than 55% of the women aged 80 and over. However,

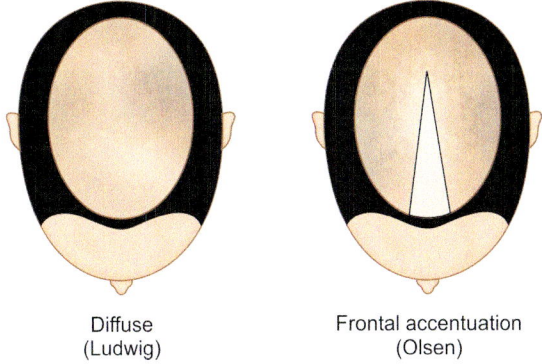

Diffuse
(Ludwig)

Frontal accentuation
(Olsen)

Fig. 10.3: Ludwig and Olsen patterns of hair loss in females

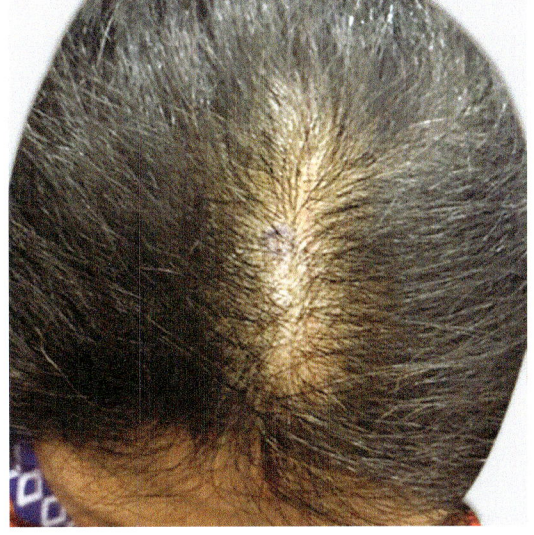

Fig. 10.4: Ludwig pattern frontal thinning in a 32-year-old female patient

it is probably less frequent in Asian women. The mode of inheritance of FPHL remains a grey area. In a large retrospective study including 210 patients of FPHL (Siah et al, 2016), 85% of patients had a positive family history of androgenetic alopecia, and in 51%, the inheritance came from the paternal side.

There are two main ages of onset of FPHL, one in the immediate postpuberty period to the third decade and a second peak in the fifth and sixth decades. The two may have distinct genetic etiologies. The role of **androgens** in FPHL is not completely understood and most women show no clinical or biochemical evidence of androgen excess. **Polycystic ovarian syndrome** is the most common endocrinological abnormality reported with FPHL, though the reported incidence varies widely from 2 to 67% in different populations. The condition may be worsened/unmasked by an episode of telogen effluvium and by use of contraceptive pills containing progestagens with androgenic properties. CTE is the most commonly associated hair disorder amongst FPHL patients. An increased shedding of hair may or may not be reported by FPHL patients as the shedding is often episodic. Based on Sinclair hair shedding scale, 60% of FPHL versus 40% of non-FPHL patients, reported excessive hair shedding on hair washing days (Kovacevic et al, 2017). Without treatment, FPHL is a progressive condition; however, the rate of its progression is highly variable.

Classification of FPHL and its Significance

Unlike authors who believe that FPHL is rarely androgenic, there is a contrarian view that the three patterns of **Ludwig's classification**, represent stages or progressive types of "female androgenetic alopecia" (FAGA) and all have a moderate increase of circulating androgens. (Ludwig, 1987; Olsen 1999). This has been detailed by Camcho-Martinez in his papers. His classification system (severity grading, along with possible etiologies) is described in Fig. 10.5.

FAGA Degree I (Minimal)

It is considered as the beginning of FAGA. There is a perceptible thinning of hair from the anterior part of the crown with minimal widening of the part width. Women hide the frontovertical area of hair loss by combing the hair forward. This type of alopecia is observed in young women with SAHA syndrome (i.e. seborrhea, acne, hirsutism,

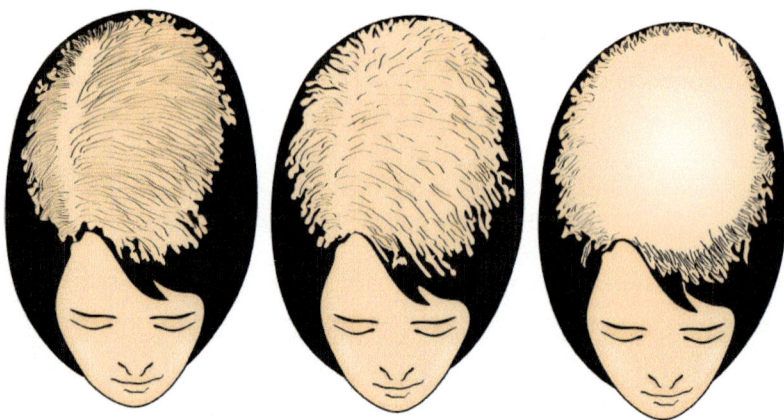

Fig. 10.5: Ludwig classification: Three progressive stages of hair loss

alopecia), generally of ovarian origin. It is accompanied by other manifestations of hyperandrogenism such as seborrhea, acne, hirsutism, seborrheic dermatitis, and slight menstrual alterations. Because SAHA syndrome is *constitutional*, there are *no* associated *biochemical alterations*.

FAGA Degree II (Moderate)

Herein, the thinning of the crown area is more evident. This makes it more difficult, although still possible, to camouflage the alopecia with combing the hair forward. This pattern of alopecia is a marker of excess androgens, generally of *ovarian* origin. The stage of SAHA syndrome has passed. Blood biochemical studies can demonstrate an excess of androstenedione, free testosterone, and androstanediol glucuronide.

FAGA Degree III (Intense)

Finally, in some perimenopausal or menopausal women, the crown becomes practically totally alopecic, with significant widening of the part width, but the frontal hairline is still maintained. Although women comb their hair forward trying to cover the alopecia, it will always be possible to see the alopecia.

This type of alopecia can be seen in women with *adrenal diseases*, tumoral or not, with very high levels of androstenedione, DHEAS, free testosterone, sometimes of prolactin, and always of androstanediol glucuronide.

Female Androgenetic Alopecia of Male Pattern (FAGA.M)

This type of alopecia was also described by Ludwig in 1977. Women may manifest male pattern hair loss in the form of frontotemporal recession, referred to as female androgenetic alopecia with male pattern (FAGA.M) (Fig. 10.8). In this eventuality, Ludwig's classification system may not be applicable. Ebling's five-level classification (Fig. 10.6) or Hamilton-Norwood's classification should be used in these patients.

FAGA.M may be present in **4 conditions:** Persistent adrenarche syndrome, alopecia caused by an adrenal or an ovarian tumor, post-hysterectomy, and as an involutive alopecia.

In **FAGA.M I**, a *functional* alteration must be suspected. When the alopecia is Ebling's degree IV or V, *laboratory tests* along with *imaging*, including magnetic nuclear resonance or computed tomography, to find the tumor are indicated. Ludwig did not observe cases of **FAGA.M II** and **III**, and he did not write about them in his report. This type of FAGA can be observed in hypoestrogenic alopecia and after hysterectomy. **FAGA.M II** and **III** can also be observed in women with a high production of adrenal or ovarian androgens and can also

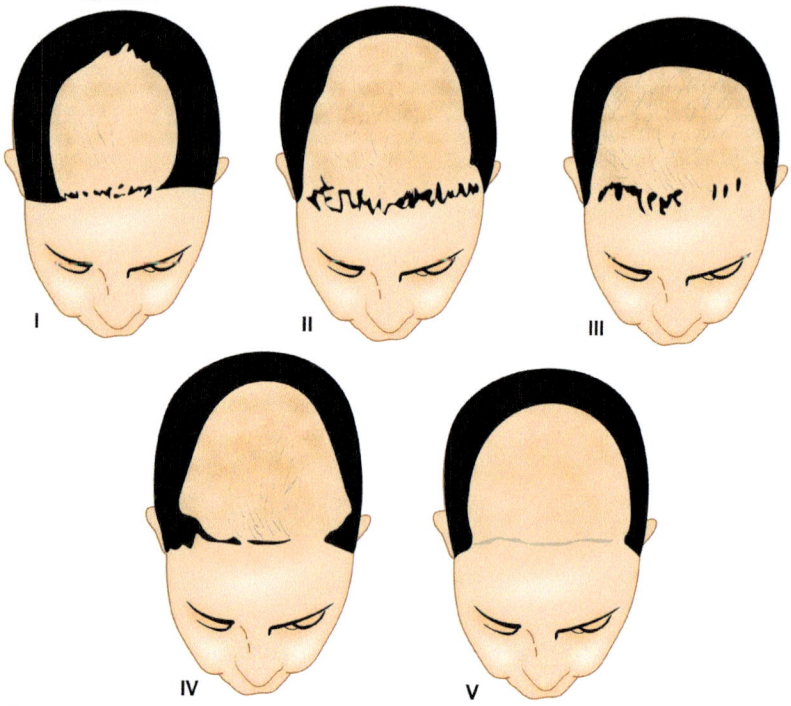

Fig. 10.6: Ebling's classification: 5 progressive stages of hair loss. The first two are the same as Ludwig system. Type III and IV show progressive rarefaction in the same areas along with increasing loss from the frontotemporal hairline as well. The final example is Hippocratic alopecia

be observed in diseases, such as congenital adrenal hyperplasia, Cushing syndrome, and polycystic ovary syndrome (PCOS).

Women with FAGA.M, who progress from **to FAGA.M II** to **V**, producing a gradual loss of the frontal hairline, may develop hair loss because of a genetic predisposition as well as alterations in androgen metabolism at the level of the hair follicle and systemic hormonal changes.

In general, FAGA.M can be observed in 4 circumstances (Camacho et al, 1989):

1. Persistent adrenarche syndrome
2. Adrenal or ovarian tumoral alopecia
3. Posthysterectomy alopecia
4. Involution alopecia.

Differentiation between CTE and FPHL becomes important from the point of view of prognostication and treatment, especially in early FPHL.

a. The most reliable way would be to perform a scalp biopsy. For this purpose, a horizontally sectioned 4 mm punch biopsy specimen taken from the vertex area of scalp is most useful. Sinclair et al (2004) demonstrated that 3 adjacent horizontally sectioned biopsies increase the accuracy of diagnosing early FPHL to 98% vs 79% from a single biopsy. The histologic hallmark of FPHL is miniaturization of hair follicles with a progressive transformation of terminal hair follicles into vellus-like follicles. Vellus-like follicles are defined as hairs with a hair shaft diameter of 0.03 mm or less and thinner than its inner root sheath. The shaft lacks pigment and a medullary cavity. The cut off points for diagnosis are a terminal/vellus (T:V) ratio of 4:1 for FPHL and 8:1 for CTE. However, it is not entirely clear how these cut points have been determined and validated. Further, scalp biopsy is an invasive procedure and women do not always consent for it. There are non-invasive ways to distinguish the two disorders as detailed below.

b. Modified wash test is a simple and easy to perform test, wherein the patient refrains from shampooing for 5 days and collects all the hair shed on shampooing on the sixth day (by covering the drain with a gauze and collecting all hair on the gauze). The hairs are counted in total and the number of hair less than 3 cm is estimated as a percentage of total hair shed. It is assumed that hair less than 3 cm are telogen vellus hair. Interpretation is as follows:

- CTE: >100 hair and <10% shorter than 3 cm
- FPHL: <100 hair and >10% shorter than 3 cm
- FPHL + CTE together: >100 hair and >10% shorter than 3 cm
- CTE in remission: <100 hair and <10% shorter than 3 cm

Rebora et al (2005) validated the method in their study involving 100 patients and found that the cut off of 100 hairs provided best concordance with the clinical diagnosis (better than the values of 80, 150 and 200). It is a simple, non-invasive and non-expensive test which helps to reliably distinguish the two conditions (or show their co-association) and assesses severity and treatment response as well.

c. Trichoscopy has found an important role in differentiating FPHL and CTE. To look for signs of FPHL, it needs to be performed in the frontoparietal area, approximately at the cross between the nose line and ear implantation line. Hair diameter diversity, or anisotrichosis, involving >20% of the hairs, strongly suggests a diagnosis of FPHL (Fig. 10.7). Trichoscopy was demonstrated to be superior to the classical trichogram for the evaluation of early FPHL, showing 75% sensitivity and 61.54% specificity. Rakowska et al (2009) have proposed trichoscopic criteria for diagnosis of FPHL. The major criteria are presence of (1) more than four yellow dots in four images (70-fold magnification) in the frontal area,

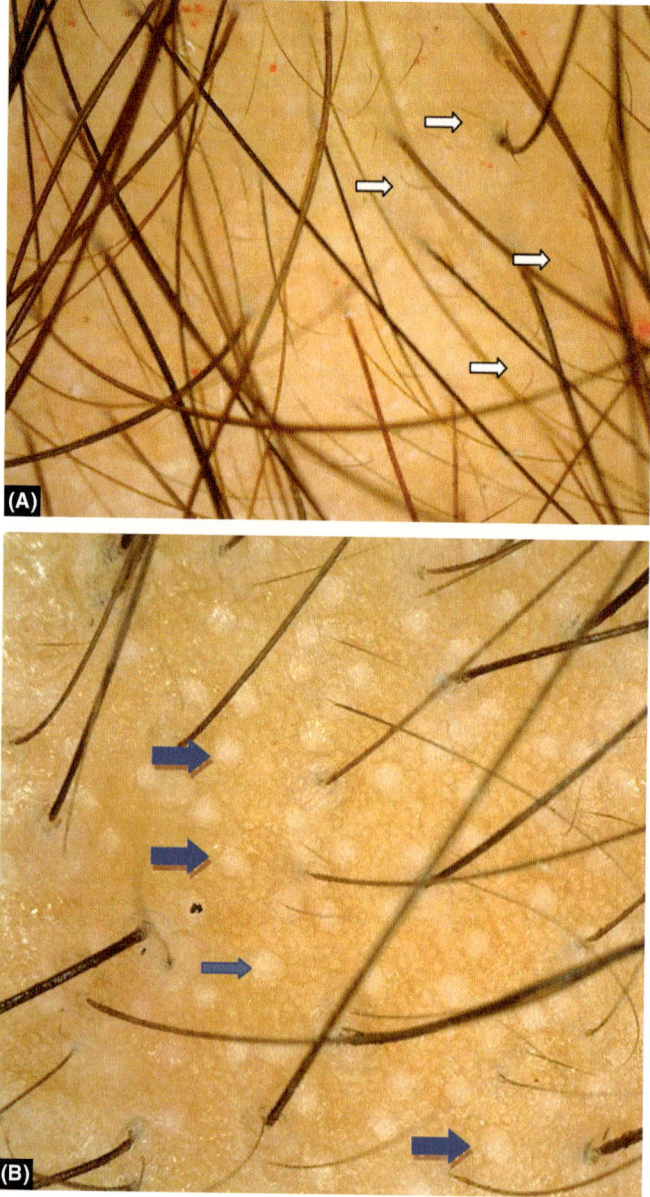

Fig. 10.7A and B: (A) Trichoscopy (50X) from the frontal region of a female patient showing a prominent anisotrichosis and vellus hair (white arrows). Presence of more than 6 vellus hairs in the frontal region in 20X suggests FPHL; (B) Shows prominent yellow dots (blue arrows); Presence of more than four yellow dots in four images (70-fold magnification) in the frontal area is one of the three major criteria to diagnose FPHL as proposed by Rakowska et al (2009)

(2) lower average hair thickness in the frontal area compared to the occiput and (3) more than 10% of thin hairs (below 0.03 mm) in the frontal area. Minor criteria encompass increased frontal to occipital ratio of (1) single-hair pilosebaceous units, (2) vellus hairs and (3) perifollicular discoloration. Fulfillment of two major criteria or one major and two minor criteria diagnoses FPHL with a 98% specificity.

As estimating percentages may be difficult, an attempt has been made to establish absolute number cut offs for vellus hair to diagnose FPHL. Rakowska et al (2009) determined that there are normally only 2 short vellus hair in the frontal area of healthy individuals under 20-fold magnification. Herskovitz et al (2013), on the basis of their findings in 45 women with early FPHL, recommend that presence of more than 6 vellus hairs in the frontal area in 20-fold magnification be considered as an additional diagnostic criteria for FPHL. Predominance of single hair in follicular ostium compared to 2–4 hairs seen in normal people is another sign of early FPHL. Peripilar sign is the presence of a brown halo, roughly 1 mm in diameter, at the follicular ostium and suggests presence of a superficial perifollicular lymphocytic infiltrate. In advanced stages, empty follicular ostia (expression of the kenogen phase), yellow dots and a honeycomb-like pigmented network are seen. CTE has no specific trichoscopic findings but may be suspected when empty hair follicles (sometimes appearing as yellow dots) and short, dark, regrowing hairs of normal thickness are present in the absence of the characteristic features of other scalp disorders.

Biochemical Investigations

Among the laboratory tests, androgenic determination has priority.

A basic protocol consists of investigating for **androgen index or free testosterone, 5α-dihydrotestosterone (DHT), dehydroepiandrosterone (DHEAS), 17α-hydroxyprogesterone, prolactin, and 3α-androstanediol glucuronide.** The last of these is the ideal for assessing end organ cutaneous hyperandrogenism.

For **PCOS**, apart from a transvaginal ultrasound, serum **anti-mullerian hormone (AMH)** is a simple and effective test in females above 25 years of age. The ratio of LH:FSH is now not considered to be an appropriate test as its normal in obese cases of PCOS.

Some authors use **prostate specific antigen (PSA)** as a marker of androgenization but we do not recommend its usage. **Cortisol** levels will be normal in **congenital adrenal hyperplasia (CAH)** and adrenal tumors and increased in Cushing's disease. If CAH is considered, then levels of **17-hydroxyprogesterone** before and after the ACTH stimulation may be investigated. When cutaneous signs of **Cushing's** disease are present, a 24-hour urinary-free cortisol and creatinine excretion must be determined, and the overnight "dexamethasone (Dx) suppression test" can also be performed. When **hyperandrogenism, insulin resistance and acanthosis nigricans (HAIRAN)** syndrome is suspected, serum insulin levels must be also determined.

When androgen levels are *normal*, screening should include TSH, T4, antimicrosomal and antithyroglobulin antibodies, and ferritin or total iron binding capacity.

Treatment

Treatment of FPHL is detailed in Table 10.1. It must be emphasized that if an androgenic source is suspected, a specific intervention targeting the source, adrenal or ovarian, should be addressed as in such cases minoxidil by itself may be of a little use. This is discussed in detail in the chapter of FPHL.

No specific treatment is available for TE. An acute TE will resolve in 3–6 months without any treatment. For CDTHL/CTE, patients need to be reassured that this hair loss will not lead to baldness. If an underlying cause is found, it needs to be treated. There is no proven role for vitamins or supplements. If a measurable deficiency like iron deficiency anemia is found, then replacement will help. Some have claimed benefit with maintaining serum ferritin above 40 ng/dl. Biotin supplementation, although frequently prescribed, has not been shown to affect TE. Potential therapeutic agents for TE would be drugs that inhibit catagen, induce anagen or inhibit exogen. None in these categories are available so far. However, exclusion of catagen inducing drugs (retinoids, anticoagulants) or endocrine disorders (thyroid dysfunction, hyperandrogenism, hyperprolactinemia) may help. Substitution therapy for catagen promoting deficiencies (like iron, zinc, estradiol, proteins) can also be initiated. Topical minoxidil has also been tried and it is a reasonable candidate drug which is known to prolong anagen. The importance of taking a balanced diet and maintaining stable body weight must be explained.

Androgenetic Alopecia in Children

'Androgenetic alopecia' is rarely reported to develop in prepubertal children. Interestingly, a 'female pattern' alopecia develops in both girls and boys, with increase in the width of the central parting. Tosti et al (2005) found normal circulating levels of hormones in their series of 20 children (12 girls and 8 boys) with age at onset ranging from 6 to 10 years. DHEAS levels were within the post adrenarche levels in 12 patients, though none had precocious puberty.

Table 10.1: Treatment of FPHL

Drug	Mechanism of action	Approval status for FPHL	Dosage	Efficacy	Adverse effects
		Androgen independent treatment modalities (topical)			
Minoxidil	Arteriolar vasodilatation by K+ channel opening ↓ Inc cutaneous blood flow, inc VEGF, inc hair growth promoters in dermal papilla	2% solution (approved in 1991), 5% foam (approved in 2014)	Concentrations of 2 and 5% (solution and foam)	High quality evidence, efficacy established in FPHL by several double blind, randomized and placebo controlled trials 5% foam OD has similar efficacy to 2% solution used BD (Blume-Peytavi et al, 2011)	*Contact dermatitis* (mainly due to propylene glycol in vehicle. Foam preparation does not contain propylene glycol, hence better tolerance) *Facial hypertrichosis* (resolves 1–3 months after discontinuation) Transitory increase in hair shedding Teratogenic data lacking in humans, none in animal studies Compatible with lactation
Prostaglandin analogs and antagonists	Balance between different PGs controls hair growth **PGF₂ analogs:** Prolongation of anagen phase	Not approved (Bimatoprost, PGF₂ analog, approved for eyelash hypotrichosis since 2008) Trials in progress	—	Single published case of mesotherapy with 0.03% bimatoprost, showed no improvement (Emer et al, 2011) Setipiprant, a selective	*Erosive pustular dermatosis* following use of latanoprost (PGF₂ analog) for MPHL

(Contd.)

Table 10.1: Treatment of FPHL (Contd.)

Drug	Mechanism of action	Approval status for FPHL	Dosage	Efficacy	Adverse effects
		Androgen independent treatment modalities (topical)			
	PGD_2: Expression increases in AGA scalp, high levels induce miniaturization and alopecia PGE_2: Hair growth promoter, levels higher in normal scalp than AGA scalp	for AGA in men and women		oral antagonist to PGD_2 receptor: Not yet studied for AGA	
		Antiandrogens			
Finasteride	5α-reductase inhibitor	Not approved (off label)	1 mg, 2.5 mg, 5 mg once a day	2 large RCTs in postmenopausal women found no benefit with 1 mg (Price et al, 2000 and Whiting et al, 1999) Cochrane systematic review (2016): No evidence Case reports/case series/uncontrolled	Feminization of male fetus (effective birth control required in reproductive age group) Avoid in those with family history of breast cancer (as estrogen excess may occur due to testosterone conversion to estradiol by aromatase, following inhibition of DHT)

(Contd.)

Table 10.1: Treatment of FPHL (Contd.)

Androgen independent treatment modalities (topical)

Drug	Mechanism of action	Approval status for FPHL	Dosage	Efficacy	Adverse effects
				studies: Positive results with 2.5–5 mg in pre- and post-menopausal women (especially those with hyperandrogenism)	*Libido reduction* *Increase liver enzymes* (uncommon)
Dutasteride	5α-reductase inhibitor	Not approved (off label)	0.5 mg OD 0.15 mg OD	Retrospective analysis: 0.15 mg OD in 60 patients; improvement in 65% (Boersma et al, 2014) One case report demonstrated efficacy of 0.5 mg daily for 6 months, following limited response to finasteride and topical minoxidil (Olszewska et al, 2005)	*Feminization of male fetus* (effective birth control required in reproductive age group) Avoid in those with family history of breast cancer (as estrogen excess may occur due to testosterone conversion to estradiol by aromatase, following inhibition of DHT production) *Libido reduction* *Increase liver enzymes* (uncommon)

(Contd.)

Table 10.1: Treatment of FPHL (Contd.)

Androgen independent treatment modalities (topical)

Drug	Mechanism of action	Approval status for FPHL	Dosage	Efficacy	Adverse effects
Spironolactone (most commonly used systemic agent for FPHL)	A K+ sparing diuretic, reduces testosterone levels and blocks androgen receptors in target tissues	Not approved (off label)	50–200 mg daily	Spironolactone 200 mg/day was equally effective (improvement in 88% of 80 women) as cyproterone acetate at a dose of either 50 mg/day or 100 mg/day given for 10 days every menstrual cycle (Sinclair et al, 2005) Recent study on 166 patients (Famenini et al, 2015): 74.3% of patients receiving spironolactone reported stabilization or improvement of their disease	Postural hypotension, electrolyte disturbances, menstrual irregularities, fatigue, urticaria, breast tenderness, and hematological disturbances Frequent potassium monitoring is not necessary for healthy young women receiving spironolactone

(Contd.)

Table 10.1: Treatment of FPHL (*Contd.*)

Androgen independent treatment modalities (topical)

Drug	Mechanism of action	Approval status for FPHL	Dosage	Efficacy	Adverse effects
				Single report of successful use in prepubertal FPHL (Yazdabadi et al)	
Cyproterone acetate (CPA)	Blocks the binding of DHT to its receptor Decreases release of FSH, LH leading to reduced testosterone levels	Not approved (off label)	Combination therapy of 2 mg in oral contraceptives with ethinyl estradiol 35 μg Or Up to 100 mg/day on days five to 15 of the menstrual cycle	Variable results Few reports Comparison of topical minoxidil 2% with OCP (ethinyl estradiol 30 μg and gestodene 75 μg/day) *vs* CPA 50 mg for 20 days of cycle *plus* OCP containing 2 mg of CPA with ethinyl estradiol 35 μg showed better results in minoxidil group based on phototrichogram data but similar cosmetic effect. CPA did better in presence of other	Hepatotoxicity, weight gain, decreased libido, breast tenderness, and feminization of the male fetus

(Contd.)

Table 10.1: Treatment of FPHL (*Contd.*)

Androgen independent treatment modalities (topical)

Drug	Mechanism of action	Approval status for FPHL	Dosage	Efficacy	Adverse effects
				signs of hyperandro-genism (seborrhea, menstrual irregula-rities, high BMI) (Vesiau et al, 2002) Inc in anagen % after 1 year of OCP with CPA plus CPA 20 mg on days 5 to 15 (Peereboom-Wynia et al) CPA 50 mg in reverse sequential regimen, not effective after 12 months in hyperandrogenic women (Carmina et al)	
Flutamide	Blocks androgen binding to its receptor	Not approved (off label)	62.5 mg, 125 mg, 250 mg	No RCTs Prospective study with 101 patients reported improvement (Paradisi et al) Randomized trial	Hepatotoxicity limits use

(*Contd.*)

Table 10.1: Treatment of FPHL (*Contd.*)

Androgen independent treatment modalities (topical)

Drug	Mechanism of action	Approval status for FPHL	Dosage	Efficacy	Adverse effects
				comparing flutamide, CPA and finasteride showed modest improvement in flutamide 250 mg group at one year, none with other two (Carmina et al) Response in one patient who failed minoxidil and spironolactone (Yazdabadi et al)	

Adjuvant treatments

| Low level laser therapy (655 nm) | Approved (2011) | | 20 minutes/day, 3 times a week | Activation of dormant hair follicles, increased blood flow, upregulated growth factors and adenosine triphosphate, and stimulation of anagen hair | 2 Randomized double blind, sham device controlled trials showed improvement with the laser device (Kin et al, 2013, Lanzafame et al, 2013) | None reported |

(*Contd.*)

Table 10.1: Treatment of FPHL (Contd.)

Drug	Approval status for FPHL	Mechanism of action	Dosage	Efficacy	Adverse effects
		Androgen independent treatment modalities (topical)			
Fractional erbium glass laser (1550 nm)	Not approved	–Same–	5–10 sessions at 2 weekly intervals	Improvement after 10 sessions (Lee et al, 2011)	Thermal hair follicle injury, scarring
Platelet-rich plasma	Not approved	Differentiation of bulge stem cells into hair follicles, prolongation of anagen phase	Variable; sessions at 1 week to 3 months intervals Maintenance treatments likely required to maintain benefit	Recent meta-analysis concluded that evidence in AGA is suggestive but not definitive (Gupta et al, 2016) Variations in preparation and injection protocols, best protocol not established Placebo controlled, double blind, half-headed study including 13 women with FPHL showed increase hair density on treated side after 6 months (Alves et al, 2016)	Minor: Pain, slight bleeding

(Contd.)

Table 10.1: Treatment of FPHL *(Contd.)*

Androgen independent treatment modalities (topical)

Drug	Approval status for FPHL	Mechanism of action	Dosage	Efficacy	Adverse effects
				However, another recent double-blind, multicenter, placebo controlled study in FPHL patients did not show statistically significantly difference in hair mass index or hair count, although 13.3% of the treatment subjects (vs 0% of the placebo subjects) experienced substantial improvement in hair loss, rate of hair loss, hair thickness, and ease of managing/styling hair, and 26.7% (vs 18.2% of the placebo group) reported that hair felt coarser or heavier after the treatment (Puig, 2017)	

(Contd.)

Table 10.1: Treatment of FPHL (*Contd.*)

Androgen independent treatment modalities (topical)

Drug	Approval status for FPHL	Mechanism of action	Dosage	Efficacy	Adverse effects
Scalp microneedling	Not approved	Induces release of platelet-derived growth factor, activation of follicle stem cells, and overexpression of hair growth related genes (VEGF, β-catenin, Wnt3a, Wnt10b)	Variable, sessions at 1–2 weeks intervals	No data in women	Mild pain, bleeding

Potential future treatment options

1. Stem Cells: Culture expanded follicular cells obtained through patient's scalp biopsy, RepliCel™, Adipose derived stem cells
2. Wnt signaling: Topical valproic acid (activates Wnt/β-catenin pathway) induces hair growth by anagen induction: SM04554; hair stimulating complex (HSC), a bioengineered, nonrecombinant, human cell derived formulation containing Wnt7a protein, epidermal growth factors and follistatin
3. JAK-STAT signaling: Topical JAK-STAT pathway inhibitor caused induction of anagen in an *in vitro* study
4. Alfatradiol (17β-estradiol) 0.025%: topical anti-androgen; contradictory results in females so far
5. Fluridil: Topical anti-androgen available in some countries; dissolves in sebum and blocks androgen receptor in hair follicles. One study in FPHL did not show improvement in A/T ratio but halted progression
6. Fulvestrant: Pure estrogen receptor antagonist. Topical treatment did not show encouraging results in FPHL

Camouflage and hair style changes

- Hair fibers, masking lotions, topical shading, scalp spray thickeners, micropigmentation
- Hair extensions and wigs

Hair transplantation

There is a strong genetic predisposition in most of these children. Genetic predisposition may induce an increased androgen sensitivity of scalp follicles due to an abnormal activity of the enzyme 5α-reductase type II or to an excessive expression of the androgen receptor in the scalp. It is, therefore, possible that adrenal androgens may be responsible for AGA in genetically predisposed children. Another possible explanation for the occurrence of AGA in prepubertal children may be that this pattern of hair loss is not necessarily androgen dependent. However, an endocrinological workup and follow-up is essential in these children. Yazdabadi et al reported successful use of spironolactone in a 9-year-old prepubertal girl with FPHL and normal hormonal profile.

POSTPARTUM TELOGEN EFFLUVIUM (PP-TE)/TELOGEN GRAVIDARUM

The incidence of this supposedly common condition has never been defined. However, it has been believed to be a common occurrence since ages. The mechanism proposed is delayed anagen release, wherein some follicles remain in the anagen phase longer than normal before entering the telogen phase. The teloptosis/exogen phase is delayed during pregnancy and hair shedding reduced, increasing hair fullness. After delivery, a synchronous telogen-teloptosis process occurs. The onset of hair loss has been reported to be anywhere between one week postpartum to 2–4 months (more commonly) postpartum. The shedding usually continues for 6 to 24 weeks, occasionally longer. Women at risk of FPHL tend to develop postpartum alopecia. This is because the anagen period is shortened in AGA, hence the number of follicles exposed to prolonged anagen is greater, and thus the number of follicles entering the telogen phase is greater in the postpartum period.

The exact cause of hair cycle changes in pregnancy cannot be pinpointed. Metabolic or endocrine changes related to pregnancy likely play a role. A variety of hormones rise significantly throughout pregnancy, including thyroid hormone, secondary androgen and estrogen hormones. There occurs a 9-time increase in progesterone, 4-times increase in estrone, 8 times increase in estradiol and about 9 times increase in estriol during pregnancy. Prolactin levels reach about 20 times the normal pre-pregnancy levels at term. Prolactin remains high during breastfeeding, but returns to normal levels within a week postpartum in non-breastfeeding women. The changes in hair cycle seen during pregnancy are possibly multifactorial. 17β-estradiol (E_2) probably plays an important role. Topical application of E_2 to the human scalp reduces the rate of telogen, and prolongs the anagen phase. In addition, E_2 slightly elongates the anagen phase both in male and female frontotemporal hair follicles. Further, hyperprolactinemia is known to cause AGA-like hair loss, amenorrhea, infertility, hirsutism and acne vulgaris. This is possibly related to prolactin's incremental effect on adrenal androgen production, though it infact has an inhibitory effect on 5α-reductase. High prolactin levels have been shown to inhibit hair shaft elongation, induce the development of early catagen, reduce proliferation in hair bulb keratinocytes and to induce apoptosis in tissue cultures.

Lynfield (1960) was the first to objectively assess hair cycle changes in pregnant and postpartum women. They reported that the mean values of anagen hair were highest in women at term (94% anagen hair). The levels remained the same at one week postpartum, dropping to 76% at 6 weeks postpartum and remaining at about the same levels at 3 months postpartum. More recently, Gizlenti et al studied 116 women for ratios of anagen and telogen at different times during pregnancy and postpartum period (28 in 24th week of pregnancy, 30 at term, 29 in 4th postpartum month and 29 in the first postpartum year), also recording data separately for breastfeeding and non-breastfeeding women. They found that the mean anagen rate in the 4th postpartum month was significantly lower than in the 6th and 9th month of pregnancy, while the average telogen rate was significantly higher. The 4th month mean anagen rate was significantly higher in breastfeeding group compared to non-breastfeeding group (which is contrary to the expected effect of prolactin on hair growth, discussed above). This difference equalized at the one year postpartum follow-up.

However, how the observed findings convert to noticeable increase in hair shedding is not well studied. Gizlenti et al observed that their findings of a 3% change in telogen rates, suggest that postpartum TE is an infrequent cause of hair shedding. Further they mention that there are not many patients presenting to dermatologists with complains of postpartum shedding, and a significant proportion of those who do may well have AGA as the underlying problem. In the 26 patients reported by Lynfield, there were those who had significant alterations in hair cycle dynamics, but no complaints of hair loss. Rebora et al (2016) also reiterated this fact, mentioning that only 4 of their 20 patients developed a clinically manifest TE. Another 10 had a modest increase of shed telogen hair but it was not enough for them to complain of TE and to be diagnosed as TE according to modified wash test. Mirallas et al (2016) analysed the studies done on PP-TE so far and concluded that the incidence of PP-TE seems to be low and undefined.

The present literature (albeit scanty) thus concludes that postpartum TE is probably not a physiological phenomenon as it does not occur in all women, nor in all the pregnancies of the same woman. Further follow-up studies are needed to understand the mechanisms and clinical implications of the hair cycle changes in pregnancy and postpartum period.

Treatment

Patients who present with the condition need to be explained regarding the self-limiting nature of the disorder in most patients. However, whether normal random asynchrony is regained in all after PP-TE or whether a general or regional loss will continue indefinitely in some patients is not known.

ALOPECIA AND MENOPAUSE

Menopausal women do not necessarily have hair loss. When a menopausal woman develops sudden hair loss, other causes of alopecia must be considered. If there is a genetic predisposition, it is likely that she will develop male pattern alopecia (Fig. 10.8), with 63%

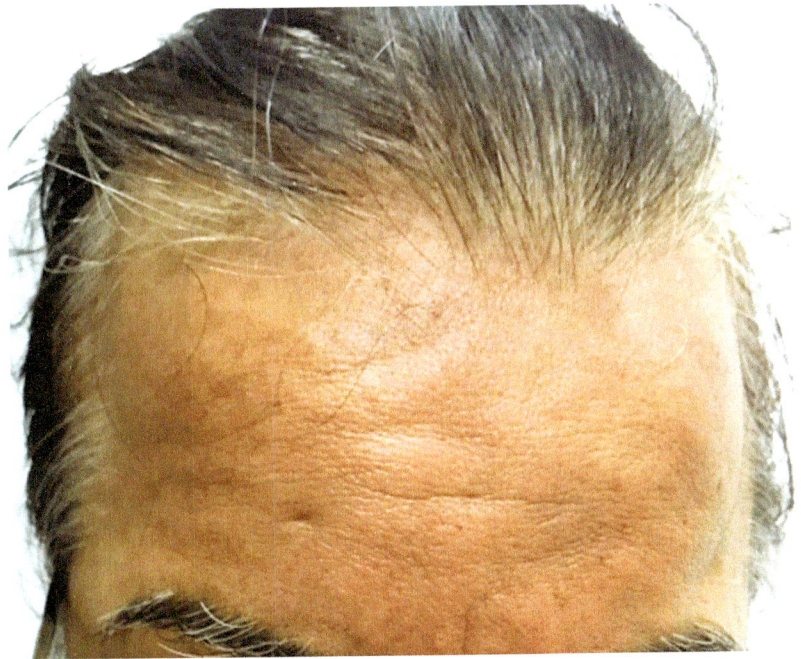

Fig. 10.8: Prominent temporal recession (male pattern alopecia) in a 60-year-old postmenopausal lady. Hormonal evaluation and imaging was normal

showing a Ludwig pattern and 37% an Ebling pattern. Postmenopausal or adrenopausal FAGA 1 can also be produced because of a functional alteration of follicular androgenic receptors without a change in the serum androgen levels. In the UK, 42% of women older than 70 years of age show FAGA (Birch et al, 2002).

TRICHOTILLOMANIA/TRICHOTILLOSIS

Trichotillomania is a psycho-dermatologic disorder characterized by uncontrollable urge to pull one's own hair. Trichotillosis is a more appropriate term, as the condition is probably an obsessive compulsive disorder and is not a 'mania'. When presenting in the adult age group, the disorder is much more common in females than males (4:1). In older age group, the female predominance is even more prominent at about 15:1.

Hair pulling is a very common behavior, but is considered a problem when it is severe and meets the following diagnostic and statistical manual of mental disorders (DSM-5; 2013) criteria:

1. Recurrent pulling out of one's hair, resulting in hair loss.
2. Repeated attempts to decrease or stop hair pulling.
3. The hair pulling causes clinically significant distress or impairment in social, occupational, or other important areas of functioning.
4. The hair pulling or hair loss is not attributable to another medical condition (e.g. a dermatological condition).
5. The hair pulling is not better explained by the symptoms of another mental disorder (e.g. attempts to improve a perceived defect or flaw in appearance in body dysmorphic disorder).

Clinical Features

Scalp is the most common site from where patients pull hair (72.8% of patients) followed by eyebrows (56.4%), and pubic region (50.7%). The symptoms of hair pulling, although waxing and waning in intensity, frequently persist for years without treatment. About 5–20% of patients also report eating hair after pulling it out ("trichophagia"), which can result in gastrointestinal obstruction and the formation of intestinal hair-balls ("trichobezoars"), requiring surgical intervention in extreme cases. 'Rapunzel syndrome' refers to a trichobezoar with a tail that extends farther into the small intestine, producing obstructive symptoms.

On examination, there are single or multiple asymmetrical, occasionally geometrically shaped areas of (partial/incomplete) hair loss on the scalp or other areas of the body (Fig. 10.9). The patches have hair of varying lengths. There may be permanent scarring in between. The pattern of plucking activity is generally centrifugal from a single starting point, or linear in a wave-like pattern. In extreme cases, all hair except the occiput may be removed ('tonsure pattern' or 'Friar Tuck' distribution). A traumatic folliculitis may ensue and keloids may form in predisposed individuals.

As trichotillosis has association with a variety of other disorders such as major depressive illness (39–65%), anxiety (27–32%), and substance use (15–19%) disorders, these must be screened for in all patients.

Diagnosis

Although the diagnosis is usually obvious on examination, difficulties may arise at times when the presentation is not characteristic. Alopecia areata may become a difficult differential in some cases and cicatricial alopecias may need to be ruled out in case prominent scarring is seen. Tinea capitis need to be considered in the pediatric age group. A definite diagnosis may then be established by a scalp biopsy which demonstrates characteristic increase in catagen hair, trichomalacia and pigment casts within the follicular canal secondary to traumatic hair removal (Fig. 10.9).

Many trichoscopic features of trichotillosis have been described and aid diagnosis in difficult cases, avoiding the need for biopsy. A chaotic coexistence of multiple hair shaft abnormalities with no significant changes in the perifollicular area is the usual pattern. Hair shaft abnormalities described include hairs broken at different lengths, short hair with trichoptilosis (split ends), coiled hair, exclamation mark hair, and hair shaft residues (i.e. black dots). Flame hairs are seen in 25% of patients and are highly specific. They are semitransparent, wavy, cone-shaped hair residues that remain attached to the scalp after anagen hair have been pulled out. A V sign is created when >2 hairs emerging from 1 follicular unit are pulled simultaneously and break at the same length above the scalp surface. Tulip hairs are short hair with darker, tulip flower shaped ends. These are diagonally fractured hair shafts. At times, hair shafts may be totally damaged by mechanical manipulation, so that only sprinkled hair residues ("hair powder") remain (Fig. 10.9).

Treatment

Treatment is essentially pshychiatric (summarised in Table 10.2). Treatment of associated folliculitis and keloids needs to be undertaken simultaneously (also *see* Chapter 13).

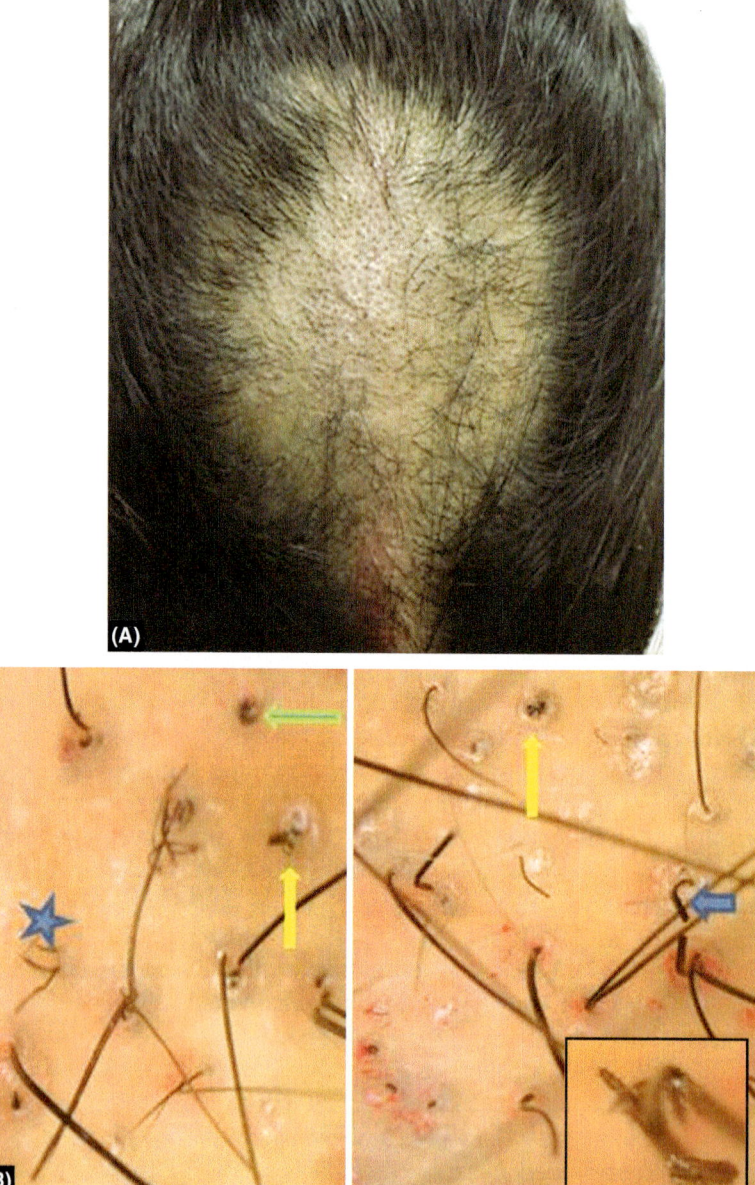

Fig. 10.9A and B: (A) A 35-year-old female presented with a patch of incomplete hair loss with hair of unequal length; (B) Trichoscopy demonstrating shafts broken at different lengths, V sign (blue star), flattened twisted hair (blue arrow), hair dust (green arrow), flame hair (yellow arrows) and fractured hair shafts (inset), suggestive of trichotillomania

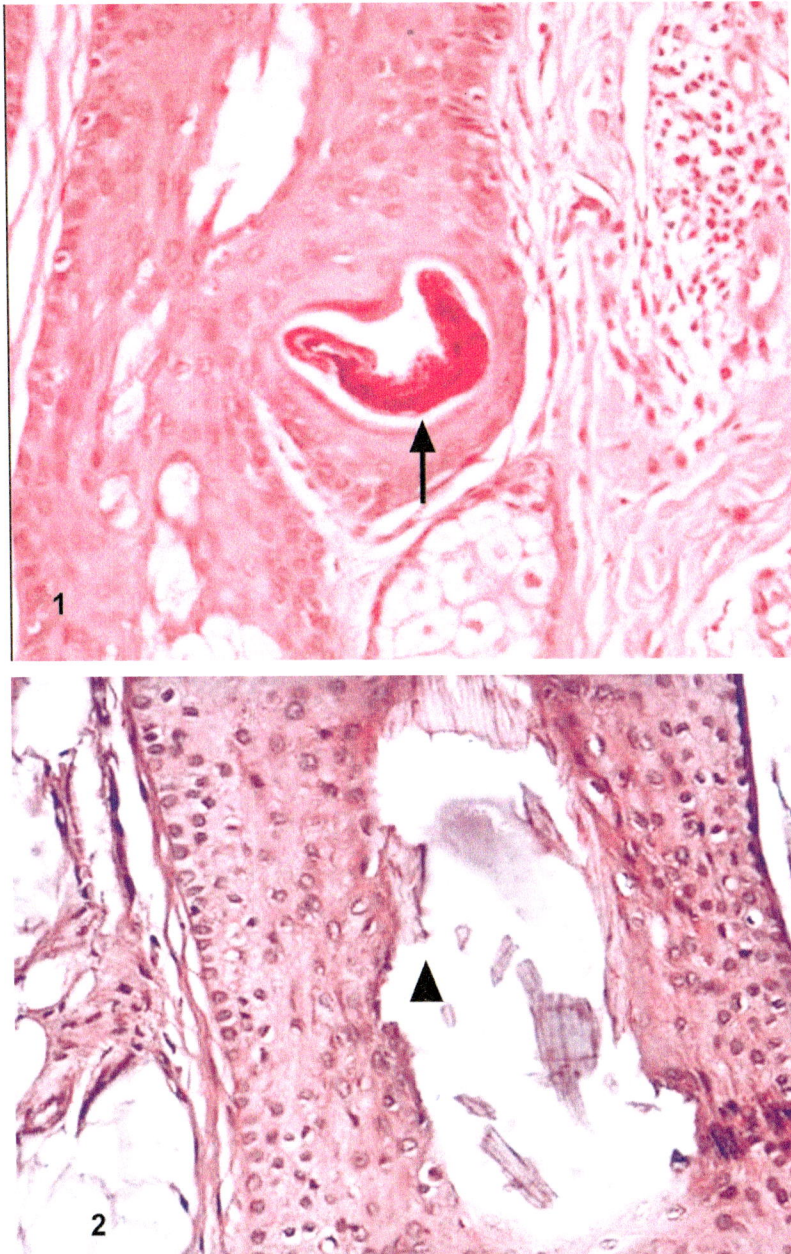

Fig. 10.9C: Histopathology of the above patient demonstrated (1) pigment cast (arrow), with no surrounding inflammation; (2) damaged hair shaft showing loss of the inner root sheath (triangle) (*Courtesy:* Dr Purnima Malhotra)

Table 10.2: Treatment of trichotillosis

Non-pharmacological

Habit reversal therapy (finding someone well trained in habit reversal therapy is essential for appropriate treatment outcomes)

Pharmacological

N-acetylcysteine (NAC) 1200 mg BD:	Glutamate modulator	⎫ Recent Cochrane review (2013)
	Showed good benefit in recent randomized double-blinded trial	⎬ concluded that preliminary evidence suggests effects with
	Onset of action is about 9 weeks	these three agents, albeit with
	Major adverse effects: Flatulence, bloating	⎭ small sample sizes

Olanzapine (antipsychotic): 10 mg OD

Clomipramine (tricyclic antidepressant): 30 mg OD

Selective serotonin reuptake inhibitors (antidepressants) have not demonstrated benefit

Dronabinol (cannabinoid agonist): Successful in open label study; may be a promising agent for future

ALOPECIA AREATA INCOGNITA (AAI) AND ACUTE DIFFUSE AND TOTAL ALOPECIA (ADTA)

These two entities (possibly describing the same spectrum) essentially refer to alopecia areata presenting without well defined bald patches. AAI was first described by Rebora et al in 1987 and the term ADTA was first used by Sato-Kawamura et al in 2002. Both have been reported to have a very prominent female predominance.

AAI mimics acute TE in having an acute onset and producing diffuse telogen shedding and causing severe thinning in a few months, without any known triggers. But, a good response has been observed in most reported patients. According to Rebora, AAI occurs when alopecia areata affects those with high percentages of telogen hairs on the scalp. In these cases, early anagen VI hairs (the ones with the highest mitotic rate and, therefore, vulnerable to damage by a noxious event) are scarce and thus only isolated anagen hairs can be damaged. Dermoscopic features are also consistent with alopecia areata.

Following the report of 9 patients with an 'acute and diffuse total alopecia' by Sato-Kawamura et al, Lew et al described 30 patients (all females in their thirties) who had sudden severe hair loss leading to balding, over the entire scalp, with features of AA on histopathology and re-growth within 6 months, with or without treatment. Tissue eosinophilia was prominent in most patients, nail changes limited to 10% and recurrence rate was low (at about 10%). Choi et al have used the term 'acute alopecia totalis' for a similar presentation. Marked pigment incontinence has been observed in the dermal papilla, matrix, and connective tissue sheath of affected hair follicles in ADTA. This might be due to a redistribution of numerous melanocytes and melanin that results from the immediate loss in the structural integrity of keratinocytes at the center of the supramatrical zone in the upper bulbar area, indicating an extensive and massive destruction of hair follicles.

Treatments tried by various authors are summarized in Table 10.3.

FRONTAL FIBROSING ALOPECIA

The incidence of this primary cicatricial alopecia has been increasing since it was first described about two decades back. A genetic susceptibility, along with an environmental factor is believed to be the underlying cause. The recent interest in this regard has been with the use of leave-on facial cosmetics, particularly sunscreens, although the association has not been conclusively proven so far. The histology is similar to lichen planopilaris, although the clinical presentation is distinct and less than 15% of patients have mucocutaneous lichen planus. The disorder typically presents in postmenopausal women as

Table 10.3: Treatment of AAI/ADTA
No treatment/wait and watch? Untreated ADTA patients reportedly recovered spontaneously within 6 months (Lew et al)

Treatments used in the described patients
- Corticosteroids
  - Oral
  - Intravenous methylprednisolone pulse
  - Intramuscular
  - Topical with occlusion
- Contact immunotherapy with diphenylcyclopropenone (DPCP)
- Anthralin
- Topical PUVA
- Minoxidil

an ear to ear band of alopecia causing receding of the fronto-temporal hairline.

Clinical signs of inflammation in the form of perifollicular erythema, scaling and follicular hyperkeratosis may be evident at the margin of the receding hairline. Eyebrow loss is recorded in 50–83% of cases but body hair loss and loss of eyelash volume occur less commonly. Eyelash loss, facial papules, and body hair involvement are associated with severe FFA, while eyebrow loss as the initial presentation may be associated with milder FFA. FPHL is commonly associated.

Dermoscopy demonstrates follicular hyperkeratosis and perifollicular erythema. Peripilar casts on dermoscopy are a good indicator of disease progression.

On histology, loss of sebaceous glands is an early finding. Early active stage shows a perifollicular lichenoid inflammatory infiltrate involving the isthmus and infundibulum and later stages are characterized by perifollicular fibrosis with follicular drop out and scars.

The course of disease is unpredictable, although slow progression with spontaneous remission is the most frequently reported outcome. Treatment (Table 10.4) is often disappointing. Prolonged treatment (12–18 months) is required to produce results. Loss of transplanted hair grafts can also occur years after the hair restoration surgery.

TRACTION ALOPECIA

Traction alopecia (TA) is a result of prolonged or repeated tension on the hair root, which causes mechanical damage to follicles, ultimately resulting in hair loss. It results with tight braids, ponytails and dreadlocks. TA most commonly presents along the marginal hairline: frontal, temporal, or occipital.

Table 10.4: Treatment of frontal fibrosing alopecia

Topical agents
- Topical steroids: Clobetasol 0.05%, flucinolone acetonide (generally ineffective)
- Intralesional triamcinolone 10 mg/ml
- Minoxidil 2% (benefit in a small study)
- Pimecrolimus 1%
- Tacrolimus 0.1%

Systemic agents
- Finasteride 2.5 mg/day
- Dutasteride 0.5 mg/day
- Hydroxychloroquine 400 mg/day
- Chloroqiune
- Oral steroids
- Intramuscular triamcinolone 40 mg every 3 weeks
- Mycofenolate moefetil 2 g/day
- Cyclosporine 4–5 mg/kg/day
- Acitretin 25 mg/day

Excimer laser 308 nm

The disorder is most common amongst black women, attributed to their unique hairstyling practices. Traction alopecia may have to be differentiated from alopecia areata (especially oophiatic pattern) and FFA in some cases. It may sometimes be unmasked by an episode of telogen effluvium. The hair loss is initially reversible, but follicular atrophy ensues with prolonged traction.

The diagnosis is suspected in a patient presenting with linear, curved or geometric patterns of hair loss. In early disease, there are often perifollicular papules and pustules at the area of maximum tension (Fig. 10.10). A reduced but retained follicular markings and a "fringe" of finer or miniaturized hairs at the margin of the alopecic area provide additional clues. The presence of hair casts is a sign of ongoing or persistent TA.

Patients need to be educated to tie hair loosely during the day and leave them open at night. Hair restoration surgery is successful in advanced cases, provided the hairstyling techniques are modified.

SEASONAL HAIR LOSS

Seasonal hair loss is complained by many women, especially those with an underlying CTE and FPHL. This seasonal variation in hair loss was objectively assessed by Kunz et al (2009). The study included 823 patients (79% had FPHL) followed up with repeated trichograms. Maximal proportion of telogen hairs was seen in July (Fig. 10.11).

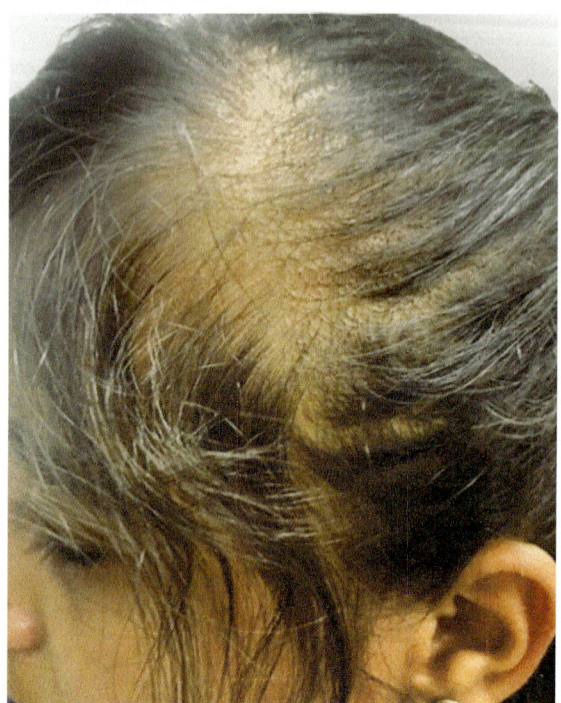

Fig. 10.10: Traction alopecia (follicular and perifollicular papules are seen at the sites of maximal tension). Patient was advised to modify her hairstyling practices

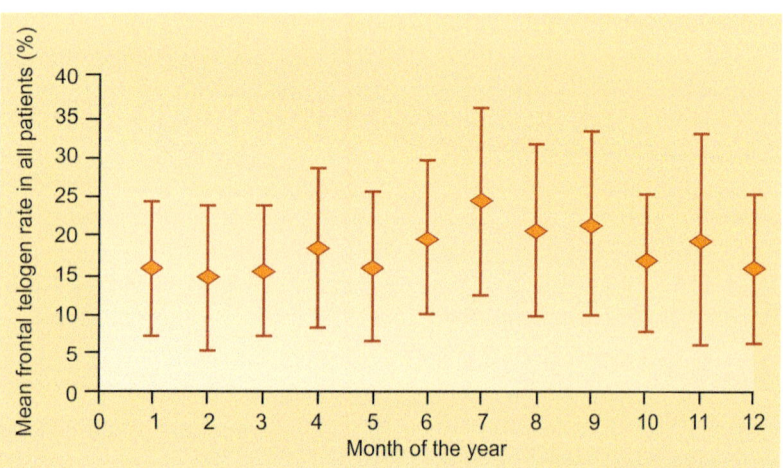

Fig. 10.11: Variation in telogen rates by month of the year (Adapted from Kunz M, Seifert B, Trüeb RM. Seasonality of hair shedding in healthy women complaining of hair loss. Dermatology 2009;219(2):105–10)

Taking a telogen phase duration of approximately 100 days into account, shedding of these hairs would be expected by October/ November. The telogen rate was lowest towards the beginning of February. The fluctuations were similar in FPHL group and the total group. Similar findings have been reported by few other studies as well.

These findings have bearing on patient counseling as well as assessment of treatment response. In the active stage of seasonal telogen effluvium, the involved hair follicles would probably fail to respond to the therapeutic agent, which may cause a false-negative result. In the recovery stage, the increased amounts of spontaneously re-growing hair might be interpreted falsely as a positive result.

Bibliography

1. Adams JU. Raising hairs. Nat Biotechnol 2011;29(6):474–6.

2. Alves R, Grimalt R. Randomized placebo-controlled, double-blind, half head study to assess the efficacy of platelet-rich plasma on the treatment of androgenetic alopecia. Dermatol Surg 2016 Apr;42(4):491–7

3. American Psychiatric Association. Diagnostic and Statistical Manual of Mental Disorders. 5th ed. American Psychiatric Association; Washington, DC: 2013.

4. Bewley A, Taylor RE. Psychodermatology and psychocutaneous disease. In Griffiths CEM, Barker J, Blekler T, Chalmers R, Creamer D (eds). Rook's Textbook of Dermatology. 9th edition. 2016 Blackwell Publishing, Ltd.

5. Bhamla SA, Dhurat RS, Saraogi PP. Is trichoscopy a reliable tool to diagnose early female pattern hair loss? Int J Trichology 2013;5:121–5.

6. Birch MP, Lalla SC, Messenger AG. Female pattern hair loss. Clin Exp Dermatol 2002;27:383–8.

7. Blume-Peytavi U, Hillmann K, Dietz E, Canfield D, Garcia Bartels N. A randomized, single-blind trial of 5% minoxidil foam once daily versus 2% minoxidil solution twice daily in the treatment of androgenetic alopecia in women. J Am Acad Dermatol 2011;65:1126–34.

8. Blume-Peytavi U, Kunte C, Krisp A, Garcia Bartels N, Ellwanger U, Hoffmann R. Comparison of the efficacy and safety of topical minoxidil and topical alfatradiol in the treatment of androgenetic alopecia in women. J Dtsch Dermatol Ges 2007;5:391–5.

9. Boersma IH, Oranje AP, Grimalt R, et al. The effectiveness of finasteride and dutasteride used for 3 years in women with androgenetic alopecia. Indian J Dermatol Venereol Leprol Nov–Dec 2014;80(6):521–5.

10. Camacho F, Sanchez-Pedreño P: Alopecia androgenética. Monogr Dermatol 1989;2:107–17.

11. Camacho F. Acnéen el síndrome SAHA: in Piquero Martin J (ed): Acné: Manejoracional. Caracas, Venezuela, Mediciencia Editora CA, 1995; pp 19–34.

12. Camacho F. Hirsutism: In Blume-Peytavi U, Tosti A, Whiting DA, Trüeb R (eds): Hair Growth and Disorders. Berlin, Germany, Springer-Verlag, 2008; pp 357–77.

13. Bolduc C, Sperling LC, ShapiroJ. Primary cicatricial alopecia: Lymphocytic primary cicatricial alopecias, including chronic cutaneous lupus erythematosus, lichen planopilaris, frontal fibrosing alopecia, and Graham Little syndrome. J Am Acad Dermatol Dec 2016;75(6):1081–99.

14. Carmina E1, Lobo RA. Treatment of hyperandrogenetic alopecia in women. Fertil Steril Jan 2003;79(1):91–5.

15. Cela E, Robertson C, Rush K, Kousta E, White DM, Wilson H, et al. Prevalence of polycystic ovaries in women with androgenetic alopecia. Eur J Endocrinol 2003;149:439–42.

16. Choi HJ, Ihm CW. Acute alopecia totalis. Acta Dermatovenereol Alp Panonica Adriat 2006;15:27–34.

17. Conrad F, Ohnemus U, Bodo E, Bettermann A, Paus R. Estrogens and human scalp hair growth-still more questions than answers. J Invest Dermatol 2004;122:840–2.

18. Courtois M, Loussouarn G, Hourseau C, Grollier JF. Ageing and hair cycles. Br J Dermatol 1995;132:86–93.

19. Daily versus 2% minoxidil solution twice daily in the treatment of androgenetic alopecia in women. J Am Acad Dermatol 2011;65(1126–34):e2.

20. Emer JJ, Stevenson ML, Markowitz O. Novel treatment of female-pattern androgenetic alopecia with injected bimatoprost 0.03% solution. J Drugs Dermatol 2011;10(7):795–8.

21. Famenini S, Slaught C, Duan L, et al. Demographics of women with female pattern hair loss and the effectiveness of spironolactone therapy. J Am Acad Dermatol Oct 2015;73(4):705–6.

22. Fertig R, Tosti A. Frontal fibrosing alopecia treatment options. Intractable Rare Dis Res. Nov 2016;5(4):314–5.

23. França K, Lotti T. N-acetylcysteine in the treatment of trichotillomania. Dermatol Ther Nov 27:2016.

24. Gan DC, Sinclair RD. Prevalence of male and female pattern hair loss in Maryborough. J Investig Dermatol Symp Proc 2005;10:184–9.

25. Gilmore S1, Sinclair R. Chronic telogen effluvium is due to a reduction in the variance of anagen duration. Australas J Dermatol 2010 Aug; 51(3): 163–7. doi: 10.1111/j.1440–0960.2010.00654.x.

26. Gizlenti S, Ekmekci TR. The changes in the hair cycle during gestation and the postpartum period. J Eur Acad Dermatol Venereol Jul 2014;28(7): 878–81.

27. Grant JE, Odlaug BL, Chamberlain SR, Kim SW. Dronabinol, a cannabinoid agonist, reduces hair pulling in trichotillomania: a pilot study. Psychopharmacology (Berl) Dec 2011;218(3):493–502.

28. Grant JE, Odlaug BL. Clinical characteristics of trichotillomania with trichophagia. Compr Psychiatry 2008;49(6):579–84.

29. Guarrera M, Cipriani C, Rebora A. Delayed telogen replacement in a boy's scalp. Dermatology 1998;197:335–7.

30. Guarrera M, Ciulla MP. A quantitative evaluation of hair loss: the phototrichogram. J Appl Cosmetol 1986;4:61–66.

31. Guarrera M, Rebora A. Anagen hairs may fail to replace telogen hairs in early androgenetic alopecia. Dermatology 1996;192:28–31.

32. Gupta AK, Carviel JL. Meta-analysis of efficacy of platelet-rich plasma therapy for androgenetic alopecia. J Dermatolog Treat Feb 2017;28(1):55–58.

33. Gurvich N, Klein PS. Lithium and valproic acid: parallels and contrasts in diverse signaling contexts. Pharmacol Ther 2002;96(1):45–66.

34. Guy WB, Edmundson WF. Diffuse cyclic hair loss in women. Arch Dermatol 1960;81:205–27.

35. Drake L, Hordinsky M, Fiedler V, Swinehart J, Unger WP, Cotterill PC, Thiboutot DM. Gynecol Endocrinol 2007 Mar;23(3):142–5. PubMed PMID:17454167.2.

36. Hamilton JB. Patterned loss hair in man. Types and incidence. Ann NY Acad Sci 1951;53:708–28,

37. Haskin A, Aguh C. All hairstyles are not created equal: What the dermatologist needs to know about black hairstyling practices and the risk of traction alopecia (TA)? J Am Acad Dermatol Sep 2016;75(3):606–11.

38. Headington JT. Transverse microscopic anatomy of the human scalp. Arch Dermatol 1984;120:449–56.

39. Headington JT. Telogen effluvium. New concepts and review. Arch Dermatol Mar 1993;129(3):356–63.

40. Herskovitz I, de Sousa IC, Tosti A. Vellus hairs in the frontal scalp in early female pattern hair loss. Int J Trichology Jul 2013;5(3):118–20.

41. Hoffmann R, Niiyama S, Huth A, Kissling S, Happle R. 17α-estradiol induces aromatase activity in intact human anagen hair follicles *ex vivo*. Exp Dermatol 2002;11:376–80.

42. Hordinsky M, Donati A. Alopecia areata: an evidence-based treatment update. Am J Clin Dermatol Jul 2014;15(3):231–46.

43. Jimenez F1, Harries M2, Poblet E. Frontal fibrosing alopecia: a disease fascinating for the researcher, disappointing for the clinician and distressing for the patient. Exp Dermatol Nov 2016;25(11):853–4.

44. Kelly Y, Blanco A, Tosti A. Androgenetic Alopecia: An update of treatment options. Drugs Sep 2016;76(14):1349–64.

45. Kim H, Woong Choi J, Young Kim J, Won Shin J, Lee S, Huh C. Low level light therapy for androgenetic alopecia: a 24-week, randomized, double-

blind, sham device-controlled multicenter trial. Dermatol Surg 2013;39(8):1177–83.

46. Koch PJ, Mahoney MG, Cotsarelis G, Rothenberger K, Lavker RM, Stanley JR. Desmoglein-3 anchors telogen hair in the follicle. J Cell Sci 1998;111:2529–37.

47. Kohler C, Tschumi K, Bodmer C, Schneiter M, Birkhaeuser M. Effect of finasteride 5 mg (Proscar) on acne and alopecia in female patients with normal serum levels of free testosterone.

48. Kovacevic M, Goren A, Shapiro J et al. Prevalence of hair shedding among women. Dermatol Ther Jan 2017;30(1).

49. Kucerova R, Bienova M, Novotny R. Current therapies of female androgenetic alopecia and use of fluridil, a novel topical antiandrogen. Scr Med (Brno) 2006;79:35–48.

50. Kunz M, Seifert B, Trüeb RM. Seasonality of hair shedding in healthy women complaining of hair loss. Dermatology 2009;219(2):105–10.

51. Lanzafame RJ, Blanche RR, Bodian AB, Chiacchierini RP, Fernandez-Obregon A, Kazmirek ER. The growth of human scalp hair mediated by visible red light laser and LED sources in males. American Society for Laser Medicine and Surgery Annual Conference; 3–7 Apr 2013; Boston [Poster].

52. Lee GY, Lee SJ, Kim WS. The effect of a 1550 nm fractional erbium-glass laser in female pattern hair loss. J Eur Acad Dermatol Venereol 2011;25(12):1450–4.

53. Lew BL, Shin MK, Sim WY. Acute diffuse and total alopecia: a new subtype of alopecia areata with a favorable prognosis. J Am Acad Dermatol 2009; 60:85–93.

54. Liu C, Yang J, Qu L, Gu M, Liu Y, Gao J, Collaudin C, Loussouarn G. Changes in Chinese hair growth along a full year. Int J Cosmet Sci Dec 2014;36(6):531–6.

55. Ludwig E. Classification of the types of androgenetic alopecia (common baldness) occurring in the female sex. Br J Dermatol 1977;97:247–54.

56. Mirallas O, Grimalt R. The postpartum telogen effluvium fallacy. Skin appendage disord May 2016;1(4):198–201.

57. Lynfield YL. Effect of pregnancy on the human hair cycle. J Invest Dermatol 1960;35:323–7.

58. Mubki T, Rudnicka L, Olszewska M, Shapiro J. Evaluation and diagnosis of the hair loss patient: part II. Trichoscopic and laboratory evaluations. J Am Acad Dermatol Sep 2014;71(3):431.e1–431.e11.

59. Olsen EA. Androgenetic alopecia. In: Olsen EA, editor. Disorders of Hair Growth: Diagnosis and Treatment. New York: McGraw-Hill? 1994;pp. 257–83.

60. Olsen EA. Female pattern hair loss. J Am Acad Dermatol 2001;45(3 Suppl):S70–80.

61. Olsen EA. The midline part: An important physical clue to the clinical diagnosis of androgenetic alopecia in women. J Am Acad Dermatol 1999; 40:106–9.

62. Olszewska M, Rudnicka L. Effective treatment of female androgenic alopecia with dutasteride. J Drugs Dermatol 2005;4:637–40.

63. Otberg N, Shapiro J. Hair Growth Disorders in Goldsmith LA, Katz AI, Gilchrest BA, Paller AS, Leffell DJ, Wolff K (eds) in Fitzpatrick Dermatology in Internl Medicine. 8th ed, 2012. The McGraw-Hill Companies, Inc.

64. Moftah N, Moftah N, Abd-Elaziz G, et al. Mesotherapy using dutasteride-containing preparation in treatment of female pattern hair loss: photographic, morphometric and ultrastructural evaluation. J Eur Acad Dermatol Venereol 2013;27(6):686–93.

65. Paradisi R, Porcu E, Fabbri R, Seracchioli R, Battaglia C, Venturoli S. Prospective cohort study on the effects and tolerability of flutamide in patients with female pattern hair loss. Ann Pharmacother Apr 2011; 45(4): 469–75.

66. Peereboom-Wynia JD, van der Willigen AH, van Joost T, Stolz E. The effect of cyproterone acetate on hair roots and hair shaft diameter in androgenetic alopecia in females. Acta Derm Venereol 1989;69(5):395–8.

67. Pie´rard-Franchimont C, Pie´rard GE. Teloptosis, a turning point in hair shedding biorhythms. Dermatology 2001;203:115–7.

68. Price VH, Roberts JL, Hordinsky M, Olsen EA, Savin R, Bergfeld W, et al. Lack of efficacy of finasteride in postmenopausal women with androgenetic alopecia. J Am Acad Dermatol 2000;43:768–76.

69. Puig CJ1, Reese R, Peters M. Double-blind, placebo-controlled pilot study on the use of platelet-rich plasma in women with female androgenetic alopecia. Dermatol surg Nov 2016;42(11):1243–47.

70. Rakowska A. Trichoscopy (hair and scalp videodermoscopy) in the healthy female. Method standardization and norms for measurable parameters. J Dermatol Case Rep Apr 2009;3(1):14–9.

71. Rakowska A, Slowinska M, Kowalska-Oledzka E, Olszewska M, Rudnicka L. Dermoscopy in female androgenetic alopecia: method standardization and diagnostic criteria. Int J Trichology Jul 2009;1(2):123–30.

72. Rebora A, Guarrera M, Baldari M, et al. Distinguishing androgenetic alopecia from chronic telogen effluvium when associated in the same patient. Arch Dermatol 2005;141:1243–45.

73. Rebora A. Alopecia areata incognita: A hypothesis. Dermatologica 1987;174:214–8.

74. Rebora A, Guarrera M, Drago F. Postpartum telogen effluvium. J Eur Acad Dermatol Venereol Mar 2016;30(3):518.

75. RepliCel™. Research findings. http://www.replicel.com/ourscience/research findings.

76. Rothbart R , Amos T, Siegfried N, et al. Cochrane Database Syst Rev. Nov 2013;8(11):CD007662. Pharmacotherapy for trichotillomania.

77. Sato-Kawamura M, Aiba S, Tagami H. Acute diffuse and total alopecia of the female scalp. A new subtype of diffuse alopecia areata that has a favorable prognosis. Dermatology 2002;205:367–73.

78. Shin H, Ryu HH, Kwon O, Park BS, Jo SJ. Clinical use of conditioned media of adipose tissue-derived stem cells in female pattern hair loss: a retrospective case series study. Int J Dermatol 2015;54(6):730–5.

79. Siah TW, Muir-Green L, Shapiro J. Female pattern hair loss: A Retrospective study in a tertiary referral center. Int J Trichology Apr–June 2016;8(2):57–61.

80. Sinclair R, Wewerinke M, Jolley D. Treatment of female pattern hair loss with oral antiandrogens. Br J Dermatol Mar 2005;152(3):466–73.

81. Sinclair R. Chronic telogen effluvium: a study of 5 patients over 7 years. J Am Acad Dermatol 2004;51:1–5.

82. Sinclair R1, Jolley D, Mallari R, Magee J. The reliability of horizontally sectioned scalp biopsies in the diagnosis of chronic diffuse telogen hair loss in women. J Am Acad Dermatol Aug 2004;51(2):189–99.

83. Stenn KS. Growth of the hair follicle: a cycling and regenerating biological system. In: Chuong CM, ed. Molecular basis of epithelial appendage morphogenesis. Austin, Tex: Landes Bioscience; 1998:111–24.

84. Stout SM, Stumpf JL. Finasteride treatment of hair loss in women. Ann Pharmacother 2010;44(6):1090–7.

85. Tosti A, Iorizzo M, Piraccini BM. Androgenetic alopecia in children: report of 20 cases. Br J Dermatol Mar 2005;152(3):556–9.

86. Tru¨eb RM, Swiss Trichology Study Group. Finasteride treatment of patterned hair loss in normoandrogenic postmenopausal women. Dermatology. 2004;209:202–7.

87. Trüeb RM. Telogen Effluvium: Is there a need for a new classification? Skin Appendage Disord Sep 2016;2(1–2):39–44.

88. Vaccaro M, Barbuzza O, Borgia F, Cannavo SP. Erosive pustular dermatosis of the scalp following topical latanoprost for androgenetic alopecia. Dermatol Ther 2015;28(2):65–7.

89. van Zuuren EJ, Fedorowicz Z, Carter B. Evidence-based treatments for female pattern hair loss: a summary of a Cochrane systematic review. Br J Dermatol 2012;167:995–1010.

90. Vañó-Galván S, Molina-Ruiz AM, Serrano-Falcón C et al.Frontal fibrosing alopecia: a multicenter review of 355 patients.J Am Acad Dermatol Apr 2014;70(4):670–8.

91. Vexiau P, Chaspoux C, Boudou P, et al. Effects of minoxidil 2% vs. cyproterone acetate treatment on female androgenetic alopecia: a controlled, 12-month randomized trial. Br J Dermatol 2002;146:992–9.

92. Whiting DA, Waldstreicher J, Sanchez M, Kaufman KD. Measuring reversal of hair miniaturization in androgenetic alopecia by follicular counts in horizontal sections of serial scalp biopsies: results of finasteride 1 mg treatment of men and postmenopausal women. J Investig Dermatol Symp Proc 1999;4:282–4.

93. Whiting DA. Chronic telogen effluvium: increased scalp hair shedding in middle-aged women. J Am Acad Dermatol 1996; 35:899–906.

94. Whiting DA. Scalp biopsy as a diagnostic and prognostic tool in androgenetic alopecia. Dermatol Ther 1998;3:24–33.

95. Woods DW, Flessner CA, Franklin ME, Keuthen NJ, Goodwin RD, Stein DJ, Walther MR. TLC-Scientific Advisory Board. The Trichotillomania Impact Project (TIP): exploring phenomenology, functional impairment, and treatment utilization. J Clin Psychiatry 2006;67:1877–88.

96. Wozel GNS, Jackel A, Lutz GA. An effective and safe therapy for the treatment of androgenetic alopecia in women and men. Aktuel Dermatol. 2005;31:553–60.

97. Yazdabadi A, Green J, Sinclair R. Successful treatment of female-pattern hair loss with spironolactone in a 9-year-old girl. Australas J Dermatol May 2009;50(2):113–4.

98. Yazici Y, Smith SR, Swearingen CJ, Simsek I, DiFrancesco A, Hood JD. Safety and efficacy of a topical treatment (SM04554) for androgenetic alopecia (AGA): results from a phase 1 trial [poster]. In: 9th World Congress for Hair Research Nov 2015;18–21: Miami.

99. Zimber MP, Ziering C, Zeigler F, Hubka M, Mansbridge JN, Baumgartner M, et al. Hair regrowth following a Wnt and follistatin containing treatment: safety and efficacy in a first-inman Phase I clinical trial. J Drugs Dermatol 2011;10(11):1308–12.

11

Aging of Hair

Deepashree Daulatabad

INTRODUCTION

The hair follicular unit undergoes an array of changes with increasing age. Each hair follicle is an autonomous structure that undergoes a sequence of cycling independent of the other follicular units. It has been observed that the average number of cycles over a lifespan range from anywhere between 10 and 30 (Harrison S and Sinclair R, 2002). The normal hair biology has been discussed in previous sections. This chapter will deal with the changes associated with aging of hair.

The scalp hair is subject to intrinsic aging and extrinsic aging. Intrinsic factors are related to individual genetic and epigenetic mechanisms; prototypes being familial premature graying and androgenetic alopecia (AGA). Extrinsic factors include ultraviolet radiation, air pollution, smoking, nutrition, and lifestyle (Trueb RM, 2006). The extrinsic factors contribute to weathering of the hair shaft, while the intrinsic factors lead to the aging of the hair follicle. The former involves progressive degeneration of the hair from the root to the tip due to environmental and cosmetic damage (Dawber R, 1996). On the other hand, intrinsic aging manifests as decrease in melanocyte function in canities and decrease in hair production in androgenetic alopecia. In an individual with both loss of melanocyte function and decrease in hair production, it is found that the 2 processes operate independent of each other.

CHANGES DURING AGING

The common changes that occur as a part of hair aging include:
- Loss of pigment production
- Thinning of hair
- Dull, lusterless and brittle hair
- Changes in hair cycle

Decreased Pigment Production (Canities)

The follicular unit has a limited capability of pigment production. Hair graying, scientifically termed as **canities,** is a physiological phenomenon that occurs with chronological aging, regardless of the gender or the race. Though the age of onset varies with the race, the average age for Caucasians is mid 30s, for Asians late 30s and for Africans mid 40s (Lapeere H et al, 2008). The visual impression of graying is due to an admixture of pigmented and white hair.

The normal incidence of physiological hair graying in white races is at the age of 34.2 ± 9.6 years, and by the age of 50 years, 50% of the population have at least 50% gray hair known as the **50/50/50 rule of thumb** (Keogh EV and Walsh RJ, 1965). The validity of this rule of thumb has been questioned by a large population based study which reported that 6–23% of people have 50% gray hair by 50 years of age (Panhard S et al, 2012). The onset in black people is slightly later, at 43.9 ± 10.3 years, while in Japanese graying occurs between 30 and 34 years in men and between 35 and 39 years in women. The beard and moustache areas are reported to gray before scalp or body hair. In men, graying usually begins at the temples and in the sideburns. Women will usually start around the perimeter of the hairline. Gradually, the gray works its wayback through the top, sides, and back of the hair. The graying occurs in individual hair diffusely scattered on the scalp, but majority of the gray hair are limited to the top of the scalp or the temporal areas. The scalp skin essentially remains normal. The rate at which an individual turns gray depends on his genetic makeup (Tobin DJ, 2015).

When graying begins before the usual age of onset, it is termed as premature graying of hair or **premature canities** (Fig. 11.1A and B). Hair is said to gray prematurely if it occurs before the age of 20 in whites, 25 years in Asians and before 30 in Africans (Trueb RM, 2006). Usually the process is progressive and permanent, though there exist occasional reports of re-pigmentation of previously non-pigmented hair (Verbov J, 1981; Shaffrali FC et al, 2002; Comaish S, 1972). **Premature canities** is presumably inherited in an autosomal dominant manner (Trueb RM, 2006).

The whiteness of hair seen when melanin is absent is an **optical effect** resulting from reflection and refraction of incident light from various interfaces at which zones of different refractive index meet. Thus, in general, non-pigmented hair with a broad medulla appears paler than non-medullated hair.

Oxidative stress appears to play a key role in many pathways within the hair follicle (Van Neste D and Tobin DJ, 2004). Melanin synthesis

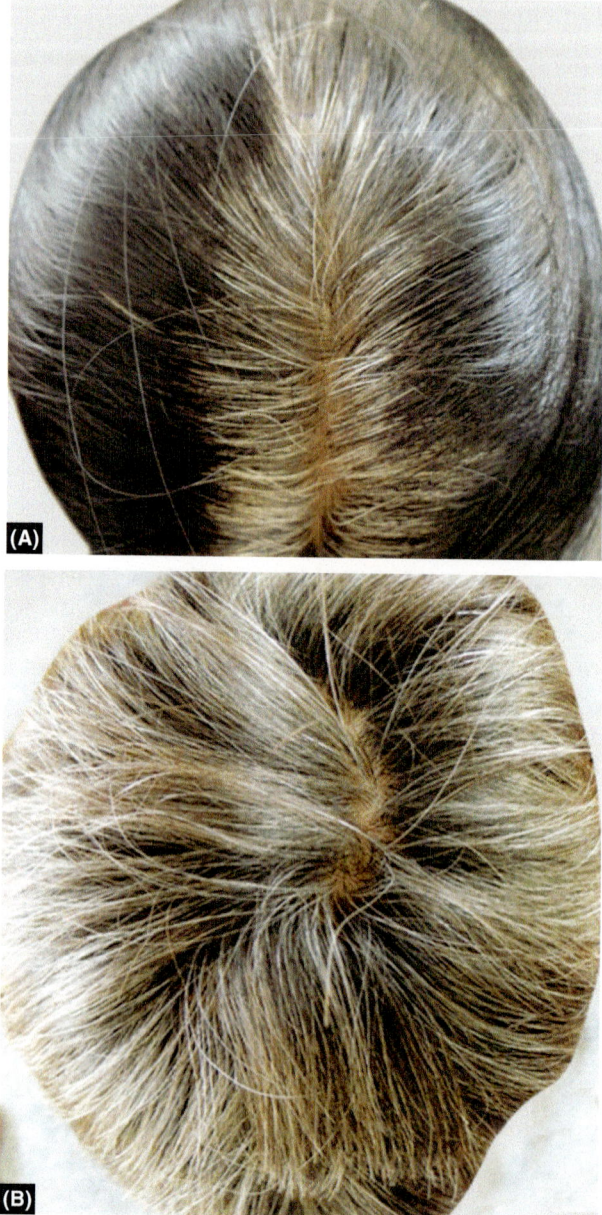

Fig. 11.1A and B: (A) A 12-year-old girl with prominent graying of hair as seen in the midline partition of hair (the hair have been dyed, hence the clear demarcation being visible between the dyed hair and the gray hair). (B) 28-year-old Indian man with aging of hair seen as presence of gray hair diffusely intermixed with colored hair

(which occurs throughout the anagen phase) in hair by itself generates oxidative stress. Several of the steps in melanin production yield hydrogen peroxide (H_2O_2) and other free radicals (Nappi AJ and Vass E, 1996). This places melanocytes under a higher oxidative stress load (Arck PC et al, 2006). Oxidative stress generated outside hair follicle melanocytes, e.g. by UV light induced, psycho-emotional, or inflammatory stress may add to this endogenous oxidative stress, overwhelming the hair follicle melanocyte antioxidant capacity, and speeding up terminal damage accumulating in the aging hair follicle. Free radicals have a capacity to damage cell membranes (lipid peroxidation of membranes), DNA (produces single-stranded breaks in DNA) and proteins (protein fragmentation and degradation of critical enzymes) due to their extreme reactivity. Recent studies have stressed upon the role of H_2O_2-mediated oxidative stress in senile hair graying (Wood JM et al, 2009) as well as premature graying (Daulatabad D et al, 2015). Low H_2O_2 concentrations increase tyrosinase activity, while high concentrations **irreversibly deactivate** the enzyme (Wood JM et al, 2004). This leads to decreased pigment production resulting in hypopigmented hair fibers. Further these free radicals lead to mitochondrial DNA damage that accumulates with age and hampers the process of pigment production. The damage may be severe enough to induce apoptosis of the affected cell. Abundant evidence indicates that many proteins and peptides, including the H_2O_2-reducing enzyme catalase as well as the two repair mechanisms for free and bound methionine sulfoxide, methionine sulfoxide reductases A and B (MSRA and MSRB), are structurally damaged and functionally altered by H_2O_2-mediated oxidation (Wood JM et al, 2009).

Histopathology of canities: In gray hair, the pigmentary unit becomes fuzzy with few round melanocytes. Below Auber's line, lightly pigmented oligodendritic melanocytes become detectable in the proximal hair bulb. Ultrastructurally, these melanocytes contain fewer and smaller melanosomes. Eventually, no melanogenic melanocytes remain in the hair bulb. True gray hairs have some persisting color with aberrantly distributed melanosomes and need to be differentiated from white hair which have no melanocytes or pigmentation. True gray hair shows reduced DOPA reaction (indicator of tyrosinase activity) while white hair bulbs are negative (Tobin DJ and Paus R, 2001).

Thinning of Hair

The apparent visual effect of hair density is a product of two factors: The **number of hair follicles** and the **type of hair fiber**. The number of hair follicles that an individual is born with tends to be constant and does not increase; in fact it decreases, with age. On the other hand, the type of hair fiber undergoes change with aging (Sinclair R et al, 2005; Robbins C et al, 2012). Newborns and infants have fine unpigmented downy hair that is subsequently replaced with vellus hair within a year's time. Finally as the follicles mature, these vellus hairs are replaced by terminal hairs, which are longer, thicker, coarser and pigmented. With further aging the hair follicle has the ability to revert back to production of vellus hair. This transition has been thought as the cause of thinning associated with aging but the precise mechanism of the transition is not known (Tobin DJ, 2010).

During the 2nd and 3rd decades of life, the hair diameter increases, this tends to counter the effect of decreasing hair density with age, hence the effect of aging is not as appreciable by this time. Subsequently, as the hair diameter gradually decreases with age, with the added effect of hair thinning the overall effect may be more apparent (Goodier M and Hordinsky M, 2015).

This thinning of hair is also termed as **senescent alopecia or late onset or age related alopecia**. The following criteria have been proposed for making the diagnosis: (a) Hair thinning that does not become apparent until after approximately 50 years of age and (b) no family history of androgenetic alopecia. The hair thinning in senescent alopecia is diffuse in contrast to the patterned thinning seen in androgenetic alopecia, although both often tend to coexist. However, histologically both the types of alopecia demonstrate miniaturization of the follicle (Mirmirani P, 2015).

Lack of Luster and Increased Brittleness

This is primarily contributed by the extrinsic environmental factors and is termed as **weathering**. With aging, the cuticular layers tend to be appear damaged giving a rough surface to the hair fiber (Jeong KH et al, 2011).

Also with age, the curvature of the hair fiber increases, which further contributes to the lusterless appearance of the hair (Nagase S et al, 2009). This is further added on by the decrease in sebum production seen with increasing age (post-menopause in women and later around 80 years in men) (Pochi PE et al, 1979).

With age, there is a decrease in the keratin and keratin associated protein levels, this also contributes to decline in the mechanical strength of the hair fiber (Giesen M et al, 2011).

Changes in Hair Cycle

With age, the duration of telogen increases and that of anagen decreases, indicating a decreasing ability of hair follicle stem cells to initiate and maintain the anagen phase (Courtois M et al, 1995).

Also the duration of kenogen is found to be raised resulting in longer absence of visible hair on the scalp. These changes are more apparent with the pigmented follicles as compared to the hypopigmented ones.

TREATMENT OF AGING OF HAIR

Aging is an inevitable phenomenon. It may be delayed but cannot be halted. The need for youthful appearance has been well exploited by the pharmaceutical companies, with the market flooding with newer and newer anti-aging cosmeceuticals. Table 11.1 lists the proposed treatment options for hair aging alongwith scientific evidence of their use.

Topical minoxidil and finasteride are currently common forms of treatment for alopecia, especially co-existing androgenetic and age related alopecia. Minoxidil increases the thickness of the hair and prevents further miniaturization of the terminal hairs. Finasteride slows hair loss and increases hair growth, the effect being perceivable after at least 6 months of usage.

Another product promoted for aging hair is coenzyme Q10 (CoQ10) emulsion, which is theorised to have antioxidant effect. This has been previously used for its anti-aging effects in the skin. Experimentally this product has been shown to increase keratins in the hair root which may help in aging (Giesen M et al, 2009). Low level light therapy has also been shown to be effective although the precise mechanism is not known. For repigmentation of hair, many vitamin supplements have been tried but the evidence is poor. Anecdotal reports and case series of repigmentation of gray hair with high doses of para-aminobenzoic acid (12–20 gm per day) do exist. Most of them also suggest that the effect lasts only as long as the supplement is continued (Zarafonetis C, 1950). Similarly, there are reports of repigmentation of hair using calcium pantothenate (Pasricha SJ, 1981). Biotin is also often used as a supplement for treatment of premature canities, but there exist no studies to document its benefit. Melitane, a biomimetic peptide agonist of α-MSH, stimulates melanin synthesis and induces skin pigmentation via the activation of its receptor MC1-R. Melitane also has a preventive action on DNA damage induced by UVA or (UV B) radiations. Based on these features it is postulated to also have beneficial effect on graying of hair (Sehrawat M et al, 2017). Melatonin is another molecule that is postulated to benefit aging hair. It acts as a potent antioxidant, direct radical scavenger, and anti-aging factor protects against damage caused by UV rays (Trüeb RM, 2009). L-methionine is also thought to benefit aging of hair by its antioxidant effects in the hair follicle. Other investigational products of interest include green tea polyphenols, selenium, copper and phytoestrogens. One should avoid heat based treatment of hair.

Table 11.1: Proposed treatment options for hair aging

Treatment options	Level of evidence	Remarks
Minoxidil	None in published literature for graying of hair	Definite role in androgenetic alopecia, telogen effluvium and female pattern alopecia
Finasteride	None in published literature for graying of hair	Used mainly for androgenetic alopecia and female pattern hair loss
Coenzyme Q10 (CoQ10) emulsion	None in published literature	Based on an increase in age-relevant hair keratins in human hair roots treated with coenzyme Q10 used for 4 days in placebo-controlled trial. No evaluation of clinical changes in the study subjects
P-aminobenzoic acid	4	Based on case series with no control subjects
Calcium pantothenate	4	Based on case series with no control subjects
Melitane	None in published literature	A biomimetic peptide agonist of α-melanocyte stimulating hormone
Melatonin	None in graying of hair	Evidence of improvement of hair density in AGA, but no studies in graying of hair
L-methionine	None in published literature	Role is postulated based on the ability to restore the methionine sulfoxide repair mechanism implicated in generating oxidative stress in hair follicle
Hair dyes, Camouflage techniques, cinnamidopropyltrimonium chloride	None in published literature for graying of hair	Proposed to benefit by avoiding UV induced damage to hair

Hair dyes are popular means of covering up the effect of graying. Hair dyes, in particular parmanent ones, can contribute to weathering of the hair fiber but they also provide some added benefit by imparting protection against sun damage (Pande CM *et al*, 2001).

Bibliography

1. Arck PC, Overall R, Spatz K, et al. Towards a "free radical theory of graying": melanocyte apoptosis in the aging human hair follicle is an indicator of oxidative stress induced tissue damage. FASEB J 2006;20: 1567–69.

2. Comaish S. White scalp hairs turning black—an unusual reversal of the aging process. Br J Dermatol 1972;86:513–4.

3. Courtois M, Loussouarn G, Hourseau C, et al. Aging and hair cycles. Br J Dermatol 1995;132:86–93.

4. Daulatabad D, Singal A, Grover C, Sharma SB, Chhillar N. Assessment of Oxidative Stress in Patients with Premature Canities. Int J Trichology 2015; 7: 91–94.

5. Dawber R. Hair: its structure and response to cosmetic preparations. Clin Dermatol 1996;14:105–12.

6. Giesen M, Gruedl S, Holtkoetter O, et al. Aging processes influence keratin and KAP expression in human hair follicles. Exp Dermatol 2011; 20: 759–61.

7. Giesen M, Welss T, Zur Wiesche ES, et al. Coenzyme Q10 has anti-aging effects on human hair. Int J Cosmetic Sci 2009; 31:154–55.

8. Goodier M, Hordinsky M. Normal and aging hair biology and structure 'aging and hair'. Curr Probl Dermatol 2015;47:1–9.

9. Harrison S, Sinclair R: Telogen effluvium. Clin Exp Dermatol 2002;27: 389–95.

10. Jeong KH, Kim KS, Lee GJ, et al. Investigation of aging effects in human hair using atomic force microscopy. Skin Res Technol 2011;17:63–68.

11. Keogh EV, Walsh RJ. Rate of graying of human hair. Nature 1965;207: 877–78.

12. Lapeere H, Boone B, De Schepper S, et al. Hypomelanoses and Hypermelanoses. In: Goldsmith LA, Katz SI, Gilchrest BA, Paller AS, Leffell DJ Wolff K (eds). Fitzpatrick's Dermatology in General Medicine. 7th ed. New york, McGraw-Hill, 2008;p.630.

13. Mirmirani P. Age-related hair changes in men: mechanisms and management of alopecia and graying. Maturitas 2015;80:58–62.

14. Nagase S, Kajiura Y, Mamada A, et al. Changes in structure and geometric properties of human hair by aging. J Cosmet Sci 2009;60:637–48.

15. Nappi AJ, Vass E. Hydrogen peroxide generation associated with the oxidations of the eumelanin precursors 5,6-dihydroxyindole and 5,6-dihydroxyindole-2-carboxylic acid. Melanoma Res 1996;6:341–9.

16. Pande CM, Albrecht L, Yang B. Hair photoprotection by dyes. J Cosmet Sci 2001;52:377–78.

17. Panhard S, Lozano I, Loussouarn G. Graying of the human hair. A worldwide survey, re-visiting the "50" rule of thumb. Br J Dermatol, 2012.

18. Pasricha SJ. Successful treatment of gray hairs with high dose calcium pantothenate. Indian J Dermatol Venereol Leprol 1981;47:311–3.

19. Peters EM, Imfeld D, Graub R. Graying of the human hair follicle. J Cosmet Sci 2011;62:121–5.

20. Pochi PE, Strauss JS, Downing DT. Age related changes in sebaceous gland activity. J Invest Dermatol 1979;73:108–11.

21. Robbins C, Mirmirani P, Messenger AG, et al. What women want quantifying the perception of hair amount: An analysis of hair diameter and density changes with age in caucasian women. Br J Dermatol 2012; 167:324–32.

22. Sehrawat M, Sinha S, Meena N, Sharma PK. Biology of hair pigmentation and its role in premature canities. Pigment Int 2017;4:7–12.

23. Shaffrali FC, McDonagh AJ, Messenger AG. Hair darkening in porphyria cutanea tarda. Br J Dermatol 2002;146: 325–29.

24. Sinclair R, Chapman A, Magee J. The lack of significant changes in scalp hair follicle density with advancing age. Br J Dermatol 2005;152:646–49.

25. Tobin DJ, Paus R. Graying: gerontobiology of the hair follicle pigmentary unit. Exp. Gerontol 2001;36:29–54.

26. Tobin DJ. Age-related hair pigment loss. Curr Probl Dermatol. 2015;47:128–38.

27. Tobin DJ. Gerontobiology of the hair follicle; in Trüeb RM, Tobin DJ (eds): Aging Hair. Heidelberg, Springer, 2010.

28. Trueb RM. Pharmacological interventions in aging hair. Clin Interv Aging 2006;1:122.

29. Trüeb RM. Oxidative stress in aging of hair. Int J Trichol 2009;1:6–14.

30. Van Neste D, Tobin DJ. Hair cycle and hair pigmentation: dynamic interactions and changes associated with aging. Micron 2004;35: 193–200.

31. Verbov J. Erosive candidiasis of the scalp, followed by the reappearance of black hair after 40 years. Br J Dermatol 1981;105:595–98.

32. Wood JM, Chavan B, Hafeez I, et al. Regulation of tyrosinase by tetrahydropteridines and H_2O_2. Biochem Biophys Res Commun 2004;325: 1412–17.

33. Wood JM, Decker H, Hartmann H, et al. Senile hair graying: H_2O_2-mediated oxidative stress affects human hair color by blunting methionine sulfoxide repair. FASEB J 2009;23:2065–75.

34. Zarafonetis C. Darkening of gray hair during para-aminobenzoic acid therapy. J Invest Dermatol 1950;15:399–401.

12

Seborrheic Dermatitis

Anamika Bhattacharyya,
Ranjeet Singh Patel, Shamik Ghosh

INTRODUCTION

Seborrheic dermatitis (SD) is a common disorder of the skin that affects the seborrheic areas of the human body. A chronic and relapsing inflammatory condition, it presents with symptoms of scaling and poorly defined erythematous patches. It primarily affects sebum-rich areas, such as the scalp, face, upper chest, and back and is often associated with pruritus. The pathogenesis of SD may involve various intrinsic and environmental factors, such as, skin surface fungal colonization, deregulated sebaceous secretions, individual susceptibility, epidermal barrier defects, host immune response, genetic factors, neurogenic factors, stress and nutrition, etc. Dandruff is the mild variant of seborrheic dermatitis which is restricted to the scalp, and involves itchy, flaking skin without visible inflammation. Multiple species belonging to *Malassezia* genus are implicated as important role players in the development of dandruff and SD based on the observation of their presence in affected areas of the skin and therapeutic response to antifungal agents. Dandruff and SD, combined, affect approximately half of the adult population. An even higher incidence can be found amongst patients with HIV infection, Parkinson's disease, and several other medical conditions.

EPIDEMIOLOGY

The lack of valid diagnostic criteria allows only tentative estimation of the prevalence of seborrheic dermatitis. Yet, it is clear that SD is prevalent among a wide range of age groups from newborn infants to the people of 60 years of age. In infants up to three months of age, seborrheic dermatitis mainly involves the scalp and is termed "cradle cap", but sometimes it also affects the face, and diaper area. Incidence in this age group can be up to 42%. In adolescents and adults, seborrheic dermatitis affects the scalp and other seborrheic areas on the face, upper chest, axillae, and inguinal folds. One to three percent of the general adult population is affected and the incidence increases in patients older than 50 years of age. It is more prevalent in men than in women in all age groups suggesting a distinct correlation with sex hormones such as androgens. The hormonal link is further substantiated through the observation that the condition appears in infancy (cradle cap), resolves spontaneously and in most affected individuals re-appears more prominently post puberty. Immune compromised patients such as HIV/AIDS patients, organ transplant recipients, patients with lymphoma and those with chronic alcoholic pancreatitis are more susceptible to seborrheic dermatitis than the general population. SD has been suggested to be associated with immune alteration based on the observation of the marked severity of SD in AIDS patients and the direct correlation of worsening SD with progressive worsening of AIDS in such patients. SD also appears to be more common in people with neurologic disorders like Parkinson's disease as well as in patients with genetic disorders such as Down syndrome and Hailey-Hailey disease. The incidence among HIV patients ranges from 30 to 83%. From an etiological point of view, dandruff is considered a milder version of the condition where the spread of the disease is limited to the scalp with no visible inflammation. Dandruff is almost omnipresent and its manifestation is highly correlated with winter condition.

PATHOGENESIS OF SEBORRHEIC DERMATITIS AND DANDRUFF

Multiple predisposing factors have been identified in the pathogenesis of SD and dandruff. Amongst them, three factors that immensely influence the development of seborrheic dermatitis are rapid expansion of *Malassezzia* colonies, presence of generous amounts of epidermal lipids and host inflammatory response. These factors are partially controlled by some independent means but fortunately some of the regulation of these predisposing factors are interdependent as well. These interdependences can further be exploited by carefully choosing the treatment options.

Role of Malassezia

Lipophilic yeasts of the genus *Malassezia* (formerly *Pityrosporum*), capable of metabolizing the fatty components of sebum, are commensals in the skin microbiota of healthy individuals. Currently there are at least 14 recognized species of *Malassezia*. Most of the species under *Malassezia* genus are generally dependent on lipids from external sources except *Malassezia pachydermatis*, a predominantly veterinary pathogen. It is lipophilic but not lipid-dependent. *Malassezia* species involved in skin diseases in humans, including dandruff and seborrheic dermatitis, are *M. globosa* and *M. restricta*. The dependence of *M. globosa* on external sources of lipid for survival is explained by the absence of a fatty acid synthase gene in its genome. But this inability to synthesize fatty acids has been complemented by the presence of multiple secreted lipases. Besides, an array of genes encoding secreted hydrolases like phospholipases, acid sphingomyelinases, etc. are also found in the *M. globosa* genome to further bolster its ability to degrade lipids from its milieu as needed.

Sebum lipids are essential for *Malassezia* proliferation, so a certain amount of sebum is always required in order to provide permissive conditions for **seborrheic dermatitis** development. **Seborrheic dermatitis** is most common in puberty and adolescence, during periods of highest sebum production and multiple studies have shown that a higher distribution of *M. globosa, M. furfur* and *M. restricta* colonies correlates with skin of lipid-rich anatomic locations and with greater disease severity.

Role of Sebaceous Secretion

Dysregulation of sebum production plays a pivotal role in the progression of seborrheic dermatitis. Not only there is a change in quantity of sebum released but also the quality of sebum changes. This sebum enriched condition of skin provides a conducive ambience for *Malassezia* to grow. Several reports suggest that triglycerides and squalene are reduced in the skin of patients with SD, but free fatty acids and cholesterol are present in copious amounts. Lipase enzymes released by *Malassezia* degrade sebum lipids and produce saturated and unsaturated fatty acids by degrading triglycerides. The saturated fatty acids are utilized as proliferative fuel for *Malassezia* while many of the remaining unsaturated fatty acids penetrate the skin and induce inflammation. It is very important to understand the key components of this unique niche to comprehend strategies on how to manage this vicious cycle.

Role of Host Inflammatory Responses

Lipases secreted from colonizing *Malassezia* can initiate inflammatory response by releasing oleic and arachidonic acid from the sebum lipids. Both of these unsaturated fatty acids have direct irritative and desquamative effects on keratinocytes. Furthermore, arachidonic acid metabolized by cyclooxygenase, serves as a source of pro-inflammatory eicosanoids (particularly prostaglandins), leading to inflammation and subsequent damage of stratum corneum. In addition, these metabolites induce keratinocytes to produce pro-inflammatory cytokines such as IL-1α, IL-6, IL-8 and TNF-α, thus prolonging the inflammatory cycle.

Other Factors

Apart from *Malassezia* colonization, excessive sebum production and host immune response, various other factors also contribute to the pathogenesis of **seborrheic dermatitis** like epidermal barrier integrity, neurogenic factors, emotional stress, genetic factors and nutritional factors. Understanding the interplay between these factors is very crucial to determine an individual's susceptibility to SD and dandruff. Moreover, it may hold the key to the unresolved issue of how a commensal *Malassezia* turns into a pathogenic colonizer.

Structural abnormalities in the barrier have been detected in dandruff infested scalp by electron microscopy. In a likely scenario, there may be aberrant epidermal barrier function due to genetic predisposition, and excessive or altered sebum composition would exacerbate this condition and provide a favorable ambience for *Malassezia* colonization. Disrupted barrier function facilitates entry of more number of *Malassezia* and its metabolites, irritates the epidermis and elicits host's immune response. The host inflammatory response further disturbs epidermal differentiation and barrier formation, and pruritus and subsequent scratching damages the barrier even further, leading to a never-ending cascade of immune stimulation, abnormal epidermal differentiation, and barrier disruption.

CLINICAL MANIFESTATIONS OF SEBORRHEIC DERMATITIS

Seborrheic dermatitis produces flaking, and redness of the affected skin and in certain severe cases pruritus and burning. Seborrheic dermatitis scales are yellow red and greasy in appearance, unlike the dry scales of dandruff. *M. globosa* and *M. restricta* are capable of generating oleic acid through lipase activity and interestingly, oleic acid has been reported to produce desquamation as seen on dandruff affected skin.

Clinical Phenotypes

Infantile SD is often a self-limited condition that presents in the 2nd to 10th week of life, peaks at 3 months and resolves by 5 to 6 months. In patients with a family history of atopy, a significant proportion (30–40%) go onto develop atopic dermatitis. Most infants with SD have mild disease (dandruff, cradle cap, involvement of the eyebrows, paranasal areas and intertriginous areas). The differential diagnoses to consider include infantile atopic dermatitis, infantile psoriasis, neonatal acne, Langerhans' cell histiocytosis, food allergies manifesting as worsening dermatitis and inherited or acquired zinc deficiency.

In rare instances, when infants present with SD-like erythroderma and failure to thrive, one has to consider other differential diagnoses including genodermatoses, primary immune deficiency (Leiner's disease), metabolic disease or infection. These infants require specialized investigations and management.

Adult SD affects areas with high sebaceous gland activity. Mild SD on the scalp can present with dandruff. In severe cases of scalp SD, thick scales with matted hairs typical of pityriasis amiantacea can occur (Fig. 12.1). On the face, SD typically presents with persistent scaly erythema, thin pink papules and plaques on the medial aspects of the eyebrows, nasolabial folds and periauricular areas, with overlying *yellowish oily scales* (Fig. 12.2). On the trunk (presternal and interscapular areas), SD presents with thin pink papules and plaques with fine scaling in *a petaloid* (described as circinate patches with a light-red scaling area in the center and darker red papules at their margin, Fig. 12.3) or *pityriasiform* pattern (Figs 12.4 and 12.5). SD may also affect the axilla, submammary area, umbilicus and anogenital area.

Other dermatological conditions that can mimic SD include psoriasis (Fig. 12.6), eczema, contact dermatitis and superficial fungal infections. In patients with HIV infection, SD is often more inflammatory and extensively distributed.

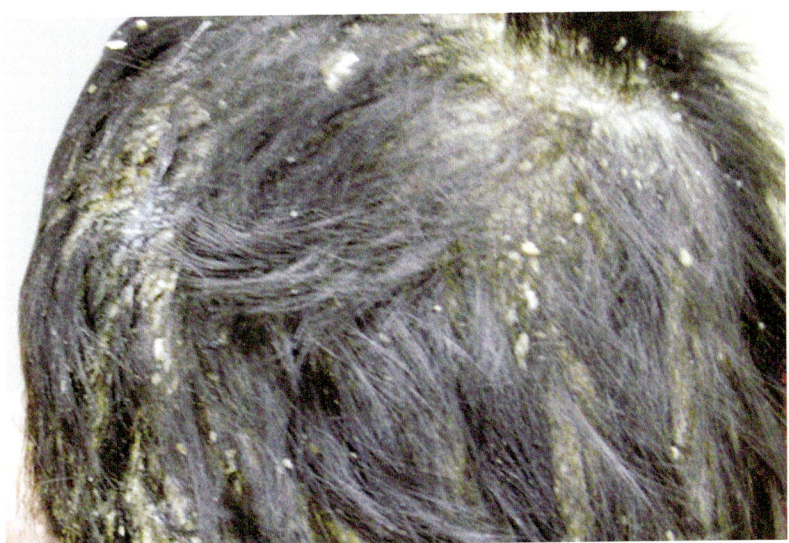

Fig. 12.1: Thick scales in a case of pityriasis amiantacea

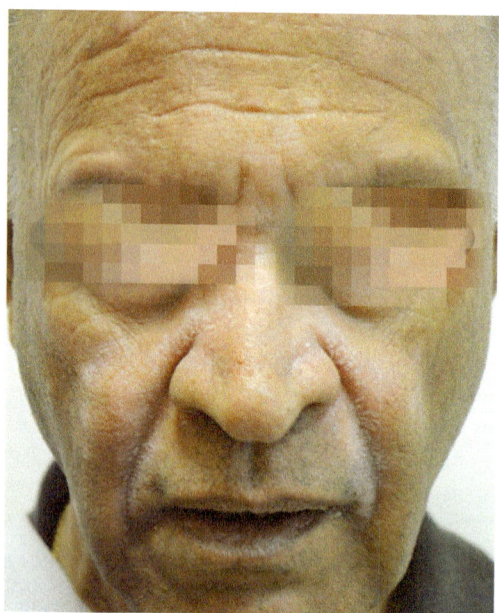

Fig. 12.2: Seborrheic dermatitis affecting the nasolabial folds and medial corners of the eyebrows

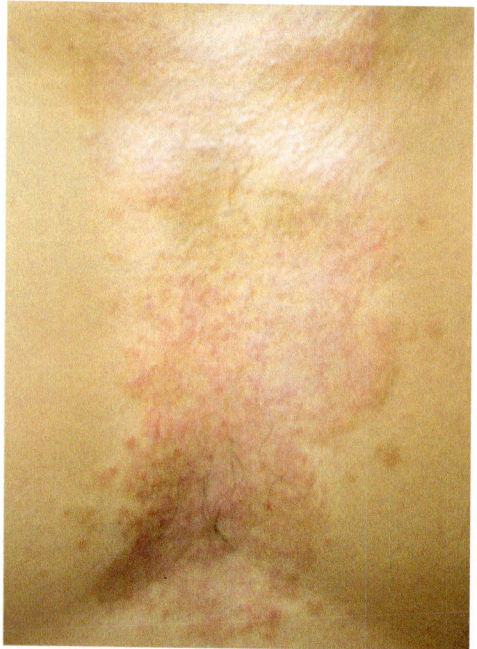

Fig. 12.3: Seborrheic dermatitis affecting the presternal area in a petaloid pattern

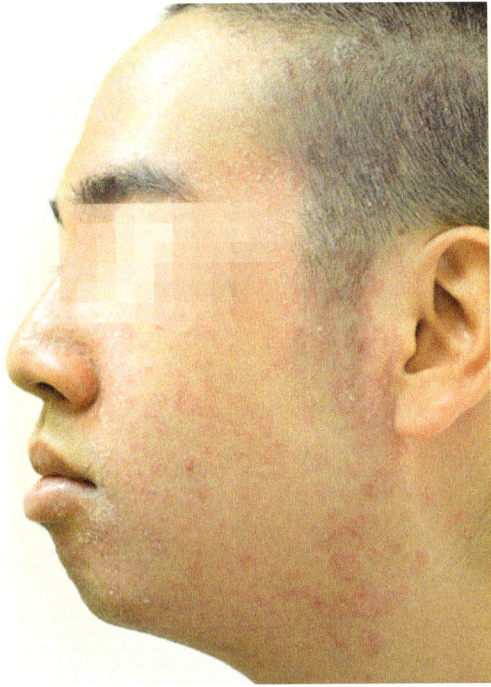

Fig. 12.4: Severe seborrheic dermatitis involving the scalp and face

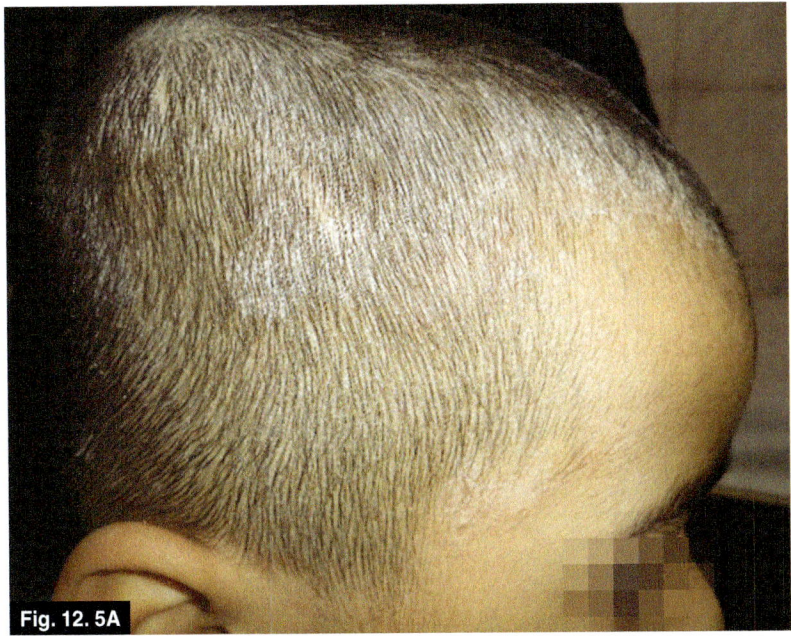

Fig. 12. 5A

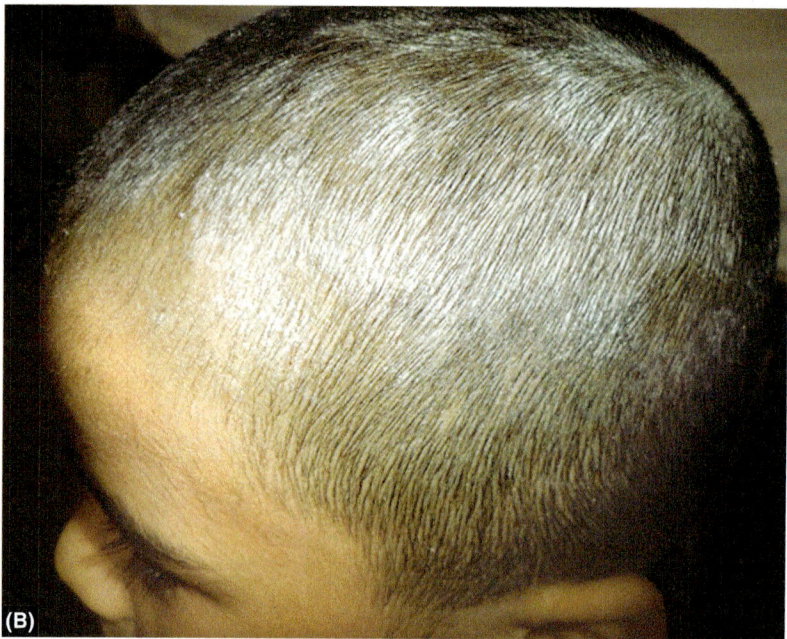

Fig. 12.5A and B: A child with dry scaly lesions without hair loss, this is also called pityriasis sicca. The patient had been labelled as a case of psoriasis by a practitioner of alternative medicine

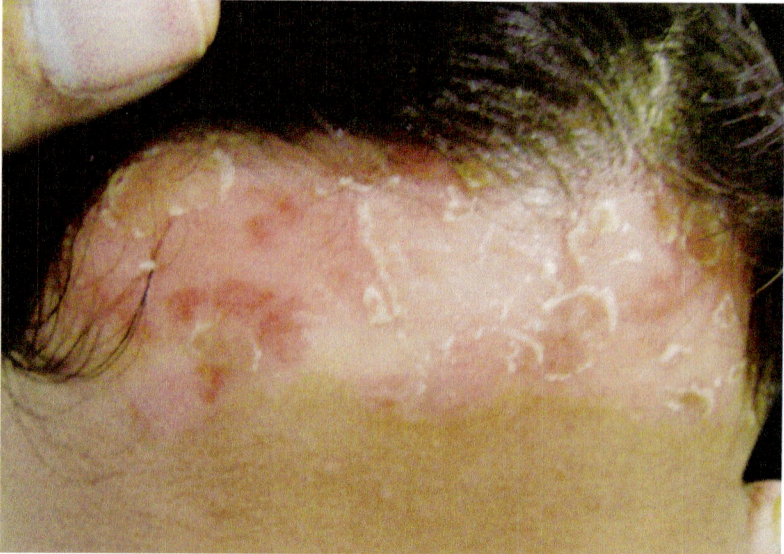

Fig. 12.6: Well defined plaque extending beyond the scalp margin with silvery scales, an unmistakable morphology of psoriasis

In rare instances, genodermatoses (Darier's disease and Hailey-Hailey disease), immunobullous disease (pemphigus foliaceus) and infections (secondary syphilis) can mimic adult SD on the trunk and flexures while acute lupus and rosacea can mimic adult facial SD. Patients should be assessed carefully if atypical features (photosensitivity, erosive lesions, persistent disease despite adequate treatment) are present.

DIAGNOSIS

Diagnosis of seborrheic dermatitis can occasionally be tricky due to overlapping symptoms with other skin conditions including psoriasis, dermatophytosis, atopic dermatitis, contact dermatitis, candidiasis, erythrasma, Langerhans' cell histiocytosis, systemic lupus erythematosus, etc. In children, sometimes the clinical features mimic tinea capitis. During examination, superficial skin scraping prepared with potassium hydroxide can be used to confirm the diagnosis.

The clinical diagnosis of seborrheic dermatitis is usually based on the characteristic distribution and appearance of lesions. In infants, it may present as thick white or yellow greasy scales on the scalp which are usually benign, non-pruritic and resolve spontaneously. In adolescents and adults, seborrheic dermatitis typically presents as flaky, greasy, erythematous patches on the scalp, nasolabial folds, ears, eyebrows, anterior chest, or upper back. Physicians often rely strongly on patient history. In case of HIV patients, the eruption can be sudden, widespread. Recently, dermoscopic features of scalp SD have been defined and mainly include twisted red loops and comma vessels. These may help to differentiate it from its close clinical differential scalp psoriasis, which shows atypical red vessels, red dots and globules, signet ring vessels, structureless red areas and hidden hairs.

PATHOLOGY

Histologically, SD shows superficial perivascular inflammatory infiltrates, composed mainly of lymphocytes and histiocytes, with associated spongiosis and psoriasiform hyperplasia, and parakeratosis.

TREATMENT (Table 12.1)

Treatment of seborrheic dermatitis primarily aims to ameliorate the symptoms associated with the disease, especially pruritus, and preventing relapse with long-term therapy. The mechanism of action of most common treatments includes inhibition of fungal growth, reduction of pruritus and erythema, loosening of crusts and scale

Table 12.1: Summary of treatment

Site	First-line	Second-line
Scalp and beard region	2% ketoconazole shampoo or Selenium sulphide shampoo (twice a week for a month, then once or twice a week for symptom control)	• Coal tar/salicylic acid-based shampoos • Zinc pyrithione shampoos • Topical steroid lotion for short-term use
Face and body	Ketoconazole 2% cream Bifonazole 1% cream, Miconazole 2% cream Clotrimazole 1% cream (for four weeks, then less frequently)	Mild topical steroid for a short period of time Topical calcineurin inhibitors (tacrolimus and pimecrolimus) for control of disease Twice weekly tacrolimus 0.1% ointment may be considered for prevention of recurrence Ketoconazole shampoo as body wash

Systemic agents: Itraconazole, terbinafine, fluconazole, ketoconazole, isotretinoin, systemic steroids

and reduction of inflammation. So the therapies consist of antifungal agents, corticosteroids, immunomodulators and keratolytics. Most treatments are topical but systemic therapy is given in unresponsive cases.

Topical Anti-fungal Therapy

Azoles

Azole class of antifungal agents is the most effective in growth inhibition of *Malassezia* species. Among the azoles, ketoconazole applied in various vehicles showed superior effects, and hence it is the first-line treatment for seborrheic dermatitis. Ketoconazole is available in different over-the-counter topical preparations, such as shampoos, creams and gels.

Ketoconazole shampoo 2% is effective in treating scalp seborrheic dermatitis, used twice weekly. Intermittent use of ketoconazole 2% shampoo (once weekly) has been shown to have a significant prophylactic effect. Ketoconazole 2% cream significantly improves seborrheic dermatitis lesions of the face and chest used twice daily.

Bifonazole 1% cream, used once daily, is usually effective in the treatment of seborrheic dermatitis of the scalp and face. Miconazole can also be used in the treatment of seborrheic dermatitis as a monotherapy or in combination with hydrocortisone.

Ciclopirox

Ciclopirox olamine is a synthetic antifungal agent with a high affinity for trivalent metal cations.

Ciclopirox has both antifungal and anti-inflammatory properties. Ciclopirox 1% cream, is effective and provides a reduction of symptoms when used twice daily. Combinations of ciclopirox 1.5% shampoo with salicylic acid 3% or zinc pyrithione 1% are also effective.

Zinc Pyrithione

Zinc pyrithione is a common active ingredient in most of the over-the-counter anti-dandruff shampoos and has antifungal effects. Its antifungal effect is thought to derive from its ability to disrupt membrane transport by blocking the proton pump that energizes the transport mechanism. Zinc pyrithione is available in concentrations of 1% and 2% in shampoos as well as a 1% cream formulation.

Selenium Sulfide

Selenium sulfide is a cytostatic agent, slowing the growth of hyperproliferative cells in seborrheic dermatitis. Selenium sulfide acts by an antimitotic action resulting in a reduction in the turnover of epidermal cells. It also has local irritant, antibacterial, and mild antifungal activity, which may contribute to its effectiveness. Selenium sulfide 1% and 2.5% strengths are used on the scalp to help control the symptoms of dandruff and seborrheic dermatitis.

Tea Tree Oil

Tea tree oil is also known as *Melaleuca alternifolia* and it has broad-spectrum antimicrobial activity. Tea tree oil has been used as a natural alternative for treating scalp seborrheic dermatitis. The topical use of tea tree oil is generally regarded as safe.

Corticosteroids

In severe cases of seborrheic dermatitis, low to mild potency topical corticosteroids are effective in fast clearing of visible signs and associated symptoms. Most commonly used are hydrocortisone and beclomethasone dipropionate which can be used alone or in combination with antifungal agents. However, frequent and prolonged use of topical corticosteroids is not recommended because of their well-known side effects. They have been found to be associated with the potential development of undesirable conditions like skin atrophy, telangiectasias, folliculitis and hypertrichosis. Hence, antifungal agents are the first choice in the treatment of seborrheic dermatitis because antifungal agents are superior in reducing symptoms and lowering the load of *Malassezia* spp.

Calcineurin Inhibitors

Topical calcineurin inhibitors, decrease cutaneous inflammation by inhibiting T-lymphocyte driven cytokine production. Pimecrolimus 1% cream and tacrolimus 0. 03% and 0. 1% ointment, twice daily therapy, is effective and well tolerated in the treatment of seborrheic dermatitis.

Metronidazole

Metronidazole has anti-inflammatory activity via inhibition of free radical species. It is an effective treatment for facial seborrheic dermatitis.

Lithium Gluconate/Succinate

Lithium gluconate/succinate 8% gel is used for the treatment of facial seborrheic dermatitis. It has anti-inflammatory action via increased IL-10 and decreased TLR2 and TLR4 in keratinocytes.

Coal Tar

Coal tar belongs to a class of drugs known as keratoplastics. It works by causing the skin to shed dead cells from its top layer and slow-down the growth of skin cells. Coal tar can decreases itching from these skin conditions. The beneficial effects of tar in seborrheic dermatitis may be attributed to its antiproliferative activity, anti-inflammatory properties, antifungal action, and inhibition of sebum secretion.

Molecular Replacement Therapy

The fungal membrane has the fundamental role of maintaining cell order and integrity and hence most antifungal treatments target the fungal membrane. But prolonged use of antifungal compounds, along with suboptimal delivery into relevant layers of skin, make the fungus recalcitrant to treatment and the patient a non-responder to the therapy. Careful analysis of functional genomics data of the pathogen show that some of the excipients being supplied with the antifungal agents as part of the topical formulation inadvertently act as nutrient source for the lipid starved fungus. This further leads to the slower recovery and lower compliance in the patients. Effective management necessitates molecular understanding of the skin microbial niche and developing agents which may replace these excipients which provide a nutrient source with those that would potentiate the killing mechanism.

Fatty acids in the form of phospholipids are important components of the lipid bi-layer of the cell membrane of all cells. But interestingly, all fatty acids and their derivatives are not perceived as the same by *Malasezzia*. Selected FA can insert themselves into the lipid bi-layer of the fungal membranes and physically disturb the membrane, resulting in increased fluidity of the membrane. Such elevations in membrane fluidity can cause a generalized disorganization of the cell membrane that lead to conformational changes in membrane proteins, release of intracellular components, cytoplasmic disorder and eventual cell disintegration in quick succession. Thus, anti-*Malassezia* fatty acids or their derivatives hold great potential not only as environment-friendly antifungal agents but also to synergize with existing antifungal drugs for topical treatment of dandruff and seborrheic dermatitis (Fig. 12.7).

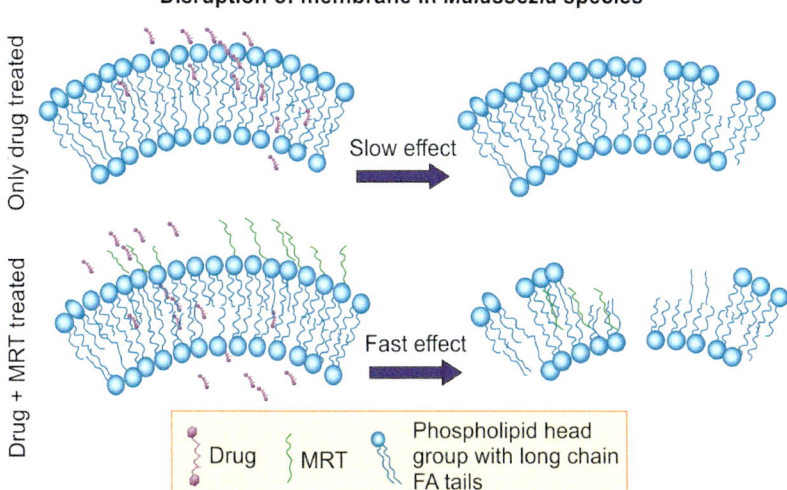

Disruption of membrane in *Malassezia* species

Fig. 12.7: Low concentration of MRT^TM can cause time and dose dependent disruption and discernible increase of membrane fluidity which is not achieved by the antifungal drug alone

Systemic Therapy

Systemic therapy is generally not recommended for treatment of seborrheic dermatitis. A recent systematic review of published data of oral treatments (itraconazole, fluconazole, ketoconazole, pramiconazole, terbinafine, prednisone, isotretinoin and homeopathic mineral therapy) for seborrheic dermatitis concluded that the quality of the evidence was generally low. Considerable variability was noted in the clinical efficacy outcomes between the studies making it difficult to draw direct comparisons or perform statistical analysis between the reported treatments.

It was concluded that ketoconazole therapy was associated with more relapses compared to other treatments. **Terbinafine** is preferred for systemic treatment of seborrheic dermatitis, if the need so arises. In some cases, topical and oral combination therapy has been recommended. **Terbinafine** has been prescribed at 250 mg/day either as a continuous (4–6 weeks) or as an intermittent regimen (12 days per month) for 3 months.

Oral itraconzaole has an affinity for highly keratinized areas of the body and it persists in the skin for long durations. **Itraconazole** has been used in the dose of 200 mg/day for the first week of the month followed by pulse maintenance therapy as 200 mg every two weeks or on the first two days every month. The maintenance treatment has been continued for variable periods ranging from 2 to 11 months.

Fluconazole has been used daily (50 mg/day for 2 weeks) or weekly (200–300 mg) for 2–4 weeks.

Ketoconazole dosing regimen is 200 mg daily for 4 weeks.

Isotretinoin has been used in refractory cases, in varying dosing ranging from 0.1 to 0.5 mg/kg/day and dosing intervals from once daily to alternate day or 3 days a week. Isotretinoin, even in small doses, given for 6 months has been shown to reduce sebaceous gland size by 51% and sebum production by 64% (Giessler et al, 2003). The benefit in seborrheic dermatitis may be due to this effect only or may also be related to its recently detailed anti-inflammatory properties.

CONCLUSION

Seborrheic dermatitis is a common, chronic, recurrent condition causing erythematous scaly patches, typically affecting multiple body sites where sebum production is high, including the face, scalp, chest, back and shoulders. Although there are differing viewpoints regarding the cause of SD, it appears to be related to the presence of *Malassezia* species on sebum-rich areas of the body. The diagnosis is primarily clinical, but seborrheic dermatitis must be distinguished from other skin disorders presenting with similar symptoms.

The goals of therapy are to reduce disease symptoms and prevent recurrences. Antifungal and anti-inflammatory agents comprise the mainstay of therapy and generally affords prompt relief. Alternating use of antifungal agents and anti-inflammatory agents or use of a combination product, may both be effective. Effective management of SD requires clearing of symptoms with antifungal and anti-inflammatory treatment and re-establishing general scalp and skin health to help maintain remission. Comprehensive studies investigating the intra- and inter-associations among dandruff-causing intrinsic and extrinsic agents including host demographics like gender and age, sebum alterations and microorganisms in the affected regions may help identify new targets and allow to carve-out improved treatment regimens with reduced side effects and better management of seborrheic dermatitis.

Acknowledgments

We thank **Dr Chia-Chun ANG** MBBS (Singapore), MRCP (UK), and Dr **Wai-Kwong Cheong** MBBS (Singapore), MRCP (UK), FRCP (Edinburgh), FAMS (Dermatology) for images 12.2, 12.3, 12.4 and **Dr Kabir Sardana** for Figs 12.1, 12.5, 12.6 and 12.7.

Bibliography

1. Comert A, Bekiroglu N, G€urb€uz O, Ergun T. Efficacy of oral fluconazole in the treatment of seborrheic dermatitis: a placebo-controlled study. Am J Clin Dermatol 2007; 8: 235–38.

2. Cassano N, Amoruso A, Loconsole F, Vena GA. Oral terbinafine for the treatment of seborrheic dermatitis in adults. Int J Dermatol 2002; 41: 821–22.

3. Das J, Majumdar M, Chakraborty YU, et al. Oral itraconazole for the treatment of severe seborrhoeic dermatitis. Indian J Dermatol 2011;56:515–16.

4. Faergemann J. Management of seborrheic dermatitis and pityriasis versicolor. Am J Clin Dermatol 2000 Mar–Apr;1(2):75–80.

5. Gary W. Clark, Sara M. Pope, Khalid A. Jaboori. Diagnosis and Treatment of Seborrheic Dermatitis. Am Fam Physician 2015 Feb 1;91(3):185–90.

6. Geissler SE, Michelsen S, Plewig G. Very low dose isotretinoin is effective in controlling seborrhea. J Dtsch Dermatol Ges 2003;1:952–58.

7. Gupta AK, Batra R, Bluhm R, Boekhout T, Dawson TL. Skin disease associated with *Malassezia* species. J Am Acad Dermatol 2004 Nov; 51(5): 785–98.

8. Gupta AK, Madzia SE, Batra R. Etiology and management of Seborrheic dermatitis. Dermatology 2004 ;208(2):89–93.

9. Hammer KA, Carson CF, Riley TV, Nielsen JB. A review of the toxicity of *Melaleuca alternifolia* (tea tree) oil. Food Chem Toxicol 2006 May;44(5): 616–25.

10. Harding CR. The stratum corneum: structure and function in health and disease. Dermatol. Ther 2004 ;17 Suppl 1:6–15.

11. James Q. Adult Seborrheic Dermatitis: A Status Report on Practical Topical Management. Clin Aesthet Dermatol 2011 May;4(5):32–8.

12. Kim T-W, Mun J-H, Wa S-WJ, Song M, Kim H-S, Ko H-C, et al. Proactive treatment of adult facial seborrheic dermatitis with 0.1% tacrolimus ointment: randomized, double-blind, vehicle controlled, multi-center trial. Acta Derm Venereol 2013;93:557–61.

13. Luis J. Borda, Tongyu C. Wikramanayake. Seborrheic Dermatitis and Dandruff: A Comprehensive Review. J. Clin Investig Dermatol 2015 Dec;3(2).

14. Mesquita Kde C, Igreja AC, Costa IM. Seborrheic dermatitis: Is there room for systemic corticosteroids? An Bras Dermatol 2012; 87: 507.

15. Nelson AM, Zhao W, Gilliland KL, et al. Isotretinoin temporally regulates distinct sets of genes in patient skin. J Invest Dermatol 2009; 129: 1038–42.

16. Sampaio AL, Mameri AC, Vargas TJ, Ramos-e-Silva M, Nunes AP, et al. Seborrheic dermatitis. An Bras Dermatol 2011 Nov–Dec;86(6):1061–71.

17. Scaparro E, Quadri G, Virno G, et al. Evaluation of the efficacy and tolerability of oral terbinafine (Daskil) in patients with seborrhoeic dermatitis. A multicentre, randomized, investigator-blinded, placebo-controlled trial. Br J Dermatol 2001; 144: 854–57.

18. Schwartz JR, Cardin CW, Dawson TL. "Seborrheic dermatitis and dandruff" Textbook of Cosmetic dermatology, 2010.

19. Schwartz RA, Janusz CA, Janniger CK.Seborrheic dermatitis: an overview. Am Fam Physician 2006 Jul 1;74(1):125–30.

20. Shemer A, Kaplan B, Nathansohn N, et al. Treatment of moderate to severe facial seborrheic dermatitis with itraconazole: an open non-comparative study. Isr Med Assoc J 2008; 10: 417–18.

21. Tajima M, Sugita T, Nishikawa A, Tsuboi R. Molecular analysis of Malassezia microflora in seborrheic dermatitis patients: Comparison with other diseases and healthy subjects. J Invest Dermatol. 2008.

22. Thomas B, and Noah S, Seborrheic Dermatitis P&T, 2010.

23. Vena GA, Micali G, Santoianni P et al. Oral terbinafine in the treatment of multi-site seborrheic dermatitis: a multicenter, double-blind placebo-controlled study. Int J Immunopathol Pharmacol 2005;18:745–53.

24. Wright MC, Hevert F, Rozman T. "In vitro comparison of anti-fungal effects of a coal tar gel and a ketoconazole gel on Malassezia furfur: Mycoses 1993 May–Jun;36(5–6):207–10.

25. Zisova LG. Fluconazole and its place in the treatment of seborrheic dermatitis—new therapeutic possibilities. Folia Med (Plovdiv) 2006; 48: 39–45.

26. Zisova LG. Treatment of Malassezia species associated seborrheic blepharitis with fluconazole. Folia Med (Plovdiv) 2009; 51: 57–59.

27. Zrinka B. Mokos, Martina K, Aleksandra B. Seborrheic Dermatitis: An Update. Acta Dermatovenereol Croat, 2012.

13

Miscellaneous and Psychogenic Scalp Disorders

Ananta Khurana, Kabir Sardana

INTRODUCTION

Omar Khayyam said that "A hair divides what is false and true". This deep philosophical thought belies the importance of hair for those who feel its crucial for their persona, but it maybe an unnecessary attachment, though given a choice, its rare to find a person who can rise above its loss.

This chapter reviews those disorders of the hair that demonstrate the complex interplay between physiology, psychology and social sequelae. Various types of factitial hair loss, most notably trichotillomania, are discussed with a mention of red scalp syndrome.

RED SCALP DISEASE

Red scalp disease was originally reported by Thestrup-Pedersen and Hjorth in 1987 and subsequently commented on by Moschella in 1994, who described the difficult problem of 'diffuse red scalp disease which can also be itchy and burning, is nonresponsive to any therapy including potent topical steroids or antiseborrheic therapy'. There is only scarce literature available on this topic so far. But the disease is probably underdiagnosed.

Though this condition has an obscure etiology, Dr Ralph Trueb has considered 3 entities to be a part of this disorder and it would be a good idea for now to consider it this way.

These subsets include, *Malassezia allergy, Rosacea-like dermatosis* **of the** *scalp and scalp burnout.*

Clinical Features

Red scalp disease affects both genders and is primarily seen in adult patients. The patient presents with the prominent complaints of itching, stinging and burning over the scalp. On examination, erythema, telangiectasias and follicular papules and pustules are seen (Fig. 13.1).

1. A subset of patients with head and neck dermatitis may have a reaction to resident *Malassezia* flora and this can be due to a admixture of humoral- and cell-mediated immunity. Though the colonization rate may not vary, patients with head and neck dermatitis have a positive skin prick test result and higher *Malassezia*—specific IgE compared to healthy control subjects. *Malassezia* allergy may be suspected in patients with atopic disease with

   a. eczema involving the head and neck region,
   b. exacerbations during adolescence or early adulthood,
   c. lesions recalcitrant to conventional therapy.

2. There have been reports of cases of red scalp disease with clinical and histopathological findings consistent with rosacea and response to oral tetracycline therapy. The finding of scalp telangiectasia was strongly correlated with the presence of trichodynia. But it must be emphasized that this may also be a consequence of photodamage. This entity has been described as a *rosacea-like dermatosis* of the scalp. The morphology has a admixture of erythema, telangiectasia, follicular papules, and pustules.

Demodex infestation (Fig. 13.2) of the scalp has been documented and notwithstanding its commensal nature, active therapy has lead to relief of symptoms.

Pathogenesis

The pathogenesis of this disorder is obscure. The histological changes reported include presence of telangiectasias and perifollicular mixed-cellular inflammation with granuloma formation in the papules. An increased expression of the neuropeptide substance P has been reported in the vicinity of the follicles, suggesting a connection with cutaneous vascular reactivity (Oberholzer et al, 2009). A report of 2 cases with histology suggestive of rosacea and response to tetracycline treatment, supports a possible link between the two diseases. In a series, 18 patients presented by Grimalt, scalp redness was associated with hair loss due to androgenetic alopecia in the majority of cases, leading to speculations over the role of chronic UV exposure of the balding scalp.

Differential Diagnosis

Exclusion of the commoner causes of the scalp symptoms must be considered first. Important conditions to be excluded include contact dermatitis (irritative and allergic), seborrheic dermatitis, actinic keratosis, psoriasis, lichen planopilaris, lupus erythematosus and dermatomyositis.

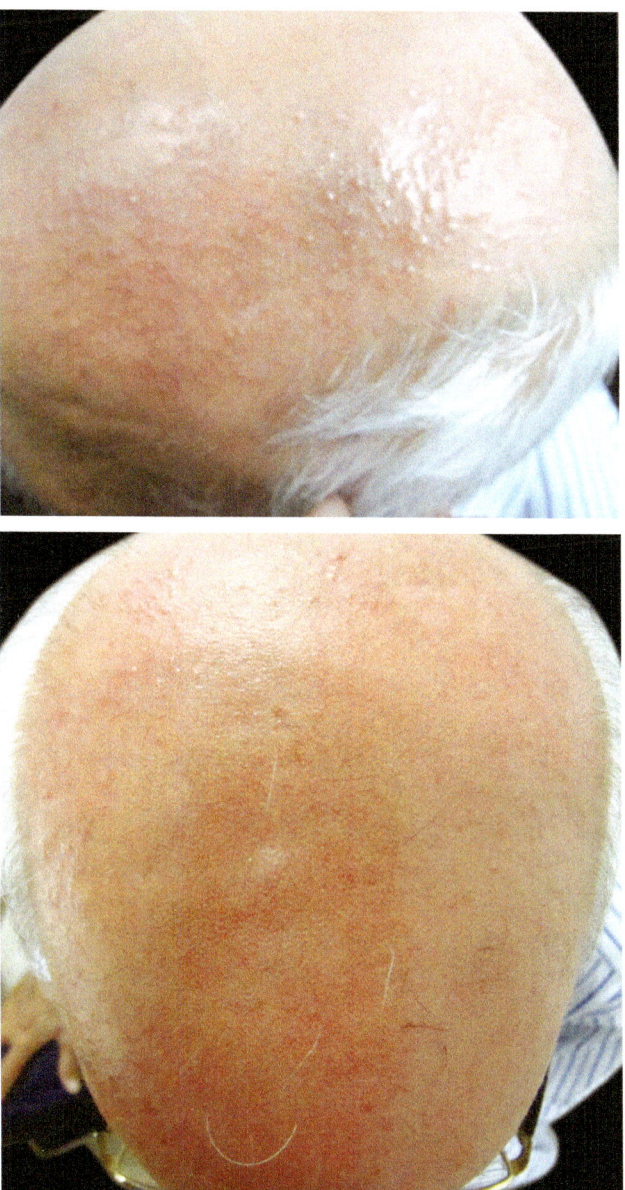

Fig. 13.1: A male patient with persistent itching and burning of the scalp which shows multiple red papules and telangiectasias with a background of erythema. The patient was treated with minocycline and topical metronidazole gel

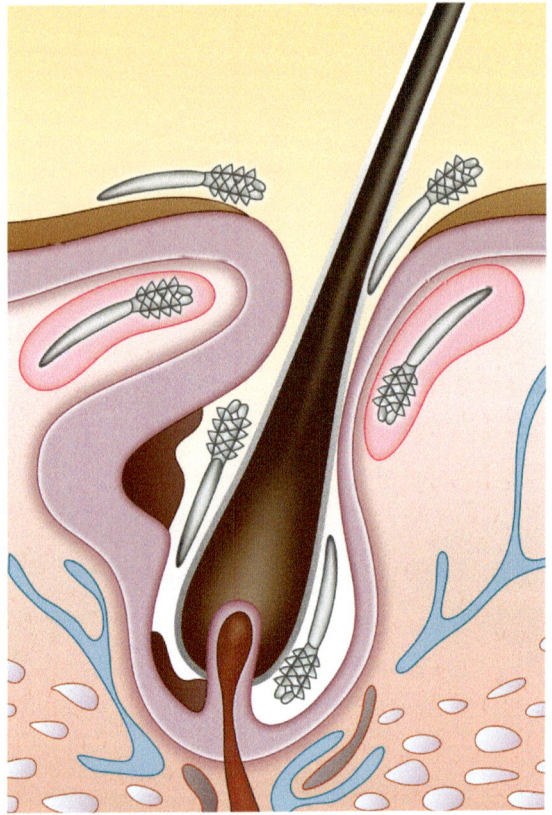

Fig. 13.2: A depiction of demodex infestation of the hair follicle

Treatment

Treatment options are limited but general measures are useful.

The *basic principles* involve protection of the scalp from further noxious environmental, medical, or cosmetic exposures and acting toward appeasement and restoration of the skin. A mild shampoo must be selected, avoiding ingredients with irritation potential or containing frequent contact allergens. Persons with greasy hair (seborrhea) should shampoo their hair often, sometimes even daily, whereas persons with dry hair (sebostasis) should shampoo less often.

Ralph Trueb has recommended the use of herbal additives particularly North American Virginian witch-hazel (*Hamamelis virginiana*). Other components include, chamomile (*Matricaria chamomilla*), heartseed (*Cardiospermum halicacabum*) and peony (*Paeonia lactiflora*). These are specially useful as most minoxidil preparations are alcoholic and irritate the skin.

In cases of *Malassezia allergy*, 1- to 2-month course of daily oral itraconazole followed by long-term weekly treatment in combination with regular use of ketoconazole shampoo is useful.

In *rosacea-like dermatitis*, oral tetracycline has shown benefit. Oral metronidazole (250 mg b.i.d. for 30 days), 5% topical permethrin cream b.i.d., and 0.02% miconazole shampoo may help in *demodex infestations*.

Photoprotection should be advised. Low-dose isotretinoin may be considered. Potent steroids are best avoided.

TRICHODYNIA

Trichodynia refers to complaints such as pain, burning, stinging, and pruritus of the scalp in patients with diffuse alopecia and was described by Sulzberger et al in 1960, though references to it can be found in early dermatology literature as well.

The cause of trichodynia is not yet fully understood, though many are proposed. Changes in the production and activity of substance P (SP) in the skin or increased inflammatory cell activity may play a role (Ericcson et al, Tmasson et al). An interaction between SP and mast cells via NK-1 receptor might be a pathway through which stress may induce abnormalities of hair cycle and the same may apply to trichodynia as well. Another explanation may be an underlying psychiatric disorder in the affected person. Anxiety and depression are possible cause (though reports are conflicting). Some authors consider trichodynia to be equivalent to glossodynia and vulvodynia. Rebora et al found trichodynia in 76 of 222 female patients complaining of hair loss (34.2%) and speculated that trichodynia and hair loss may be associated with peribulbar inflammation. Baldary et al suggested trichodynia is almost exclusive to patients with active telogen effluvium and that it may be a marker of activity of an inflammatory peripilar process.

The predominance of women is almost universally reported across all studies. Women sometimes mention the occurrence of trichodynia whenever they wear a ponytail. But the symptom is often not reported spontaneously by the patient. The type and intensity of trichodynia varies, but the burning type is probably most frequent. Delfrin et al suggested that the intensity of symptoms may be related to the severity of shedding, though other authors have refuted this. The symptom is generally reported to be diffusely present all over the scalp.

Treatment of trichodynia has rarely been discussed in literature. Role of anti-inflammatory agents does not have much evidence backing so far. Anti-depressives have been used by authors who believe in the psychiatric origin of the symptom (Hoss et al). Inhibitors of SP are now available (e.g. cannabinoids, NK-1 receptor inhibitors) and could be tried in the near future (Rebora, 2016).

TRAUMATIC ALOPECIA

Traumatic alopecia is classified with respect to the type of trauma, localization and pattern within the scalp. According to the type of trauma, it can be a cosmetic traumatic alopecia, accidental traumatic alopecia and trichotillomania (TTM). The localization may be marginal or nonmarginal. Marginal may further be frontomarginal or ophiasiform and nonmarginal may be linear or patchy. Traction alopecia and central centrifugal cicatricial alopecias are discussed in Chapter 10. TTM is discussed in detail below. It is noteworthy that the risk of developing traction alopecia increases with age (related to longer history of related hair practices) and the presence of androgenetic alopecia (related to decreased resistance of hair to traction). In India, it may be seen in certain religious communities (Fig. 13.3).

Traumatic alopecia may occur as a part of the battered baby syndrome and physical assault in adults. Alopecia is reported to develop along the line of incision in facelift procedures. Occipital scalp alopecia in infants, alopecia following a scalp hematoma and after prolonged compression as during general anesthesia of long duration

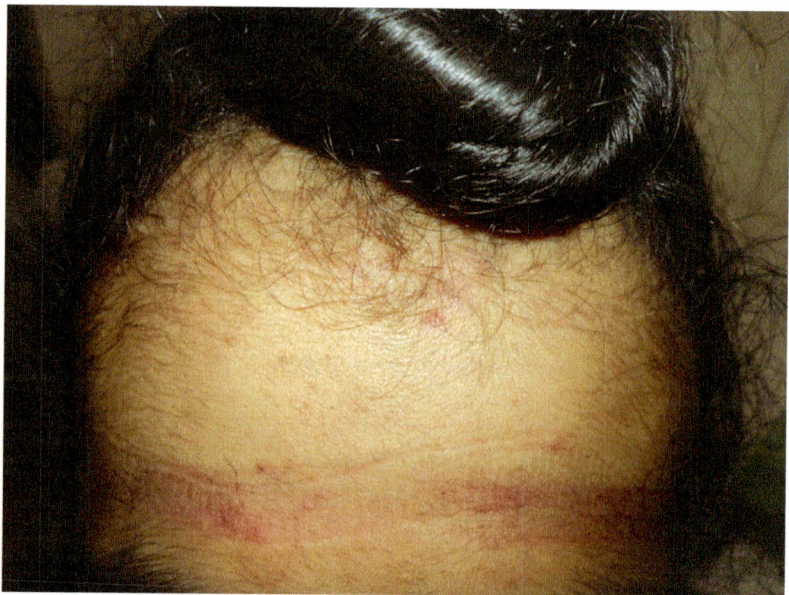

Fig. 13.3: Traction alopecia in a Sikh boy due to tight braiding of hair

are probably related to prolonged ischemia of the hair follicles. Traumatic alopecia is reported to occur following use of orthodontic devices with extensions over the scalp. It may develop under tight headgear and compression by the arms of spectacles or from accidental trauma. It may also develop following radiation and chemical burns.

The treatment and prognosis depends upon the extent of damage to the hair follicles. Modifying hair styling practices helps correct cosmetic traumatic alopecia. Occipital scalp alopecia in infants is temporary and improves with age. Pressure from headgear and devices is another modifiable cause.

PSYCHOGENIC DISORDERS AFFECTING THE SCALP

Dermatologists are the first point of contact for patients with psychiatric conditions manifesting as hair/scalp disorders and must keep the various manifestations thereof in mind. While they play an important role in pointing to an underlying disorder, they must also understand their limitations in dealing with such patients and consider appropriate referrals.

Psychocutaneous disorders of the hair and scalp can be largely grouped into the following categories:

1. Psychophysiological disorders (Box 13.1), in which scalp disorder is exacerbated by emotional factors (e.g. hyperhidrosis, atopic eczema, psoriasis and seborrheic capitis).

Box 13.1: An overview of the varied trichological manifestations of psychological disorders

---

Manifestations of generalized anxiety disorder:
- Neurotic excoriations of the scalp
- Scalp dysesthesia

Manifestations of depressive disorder:
- Neurotic excoriations of the scalp
- Scalp dysesthesia
- Imaginary hair loss (psychogenic pseudoeffluvium)

Manifestations of delusional disorder:
- Delusions of parasitosis
- Imaginary hair loss (psychogenic pseudoeffluvium)

Manifestations of obsessive–compulsive disorder:
- Trichotillomania
- Neurotic excoriations of the scalp
- Factitial dermatitis of the scalp

2. Primary psychiatric disorders, in which there is no real skin condition, and the symptoms are either self-induced (e.g. trichotillomania, factitial dermatitis) or delusional (e.g. psychogenic pseudoeffluvium).

3. Cutaneous sensory disorders, in which the patient has various abnormal sensations of the scalp, wth no primary dermatologic or medical condition responsible for the sensations.

4. Secondary psychiatric disorders in which patients develop emotional problems as a result of hair loss.

The dermatological presentations of primary psychiatric disorders are quite classical, but the underlying psychopathology varies, thus a classification is detailed in Box 13.1 that can help ascertain the underlying psychopathological condition. We believe that most patients would prefer being treated by dermatologists than psychiatrists and believe us, it is a lot more simpler that mesotherapy, PRP and hair transplantation.

Neurotic Excoriations of the Scalp

The term refers to self inflicted excoriations of the scalp in the absence of any specific underlying etiology. The disease may present at any age, but the most severe cases generally present in the third to fifth decade. The excoriations may be limited to the scalp or affect other approachable areas simultaneously (Fig. 13.4). The excoriations may

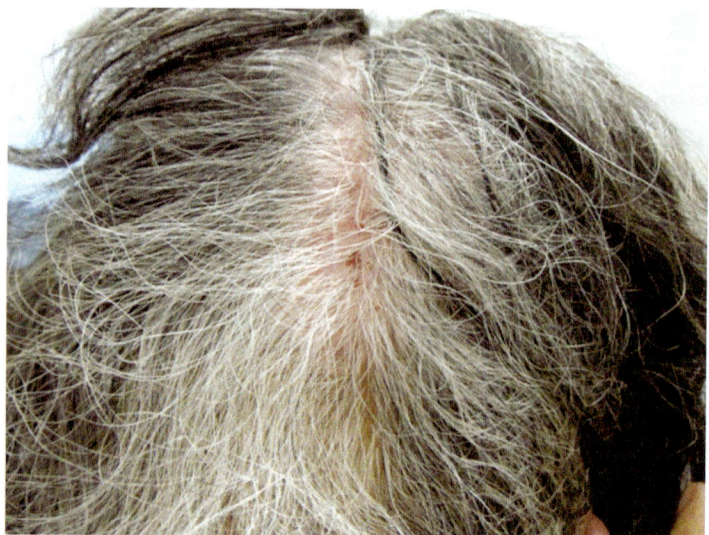

Fig. 13.4: Compulsive scratch marks in an elderly patient with a sleep disorder. He had associated xerosis of the body

be initiated by minor cutaneous irregularities like an irritated hair follicle/insect bite or in case of skin—an acne papule (acne excoriee) or a keratin plug. There is a decreased threshold for itch with tendency to habitual or neurotic scratching. The scratching may start as the hand comes across an irregularity on the surface or it may occur in an organized and ritualistic manner on its own. The patient may scratch with fingers or may use an auxillary instrument, such as the point of a knife. Tissue damage triggers further itching and the cycle continues.

Mild and transient cases may be in response to stress, such as of an examination, especially in younger patients (thinker's itch), mainly in someone with obsessive compulsive personality traits. Psychiatric evaluation is required for the more severe and sustained cases, which may be related to a generalized anxiety disorder, depression or obsessive compulsive disorder.

The lesions are nonspecific and range from minor excoriations to deep scooped out skin defects to hyperpigmented nodules and finally hypopigmented atrophic scars. Regional lymph nodes may be enlarged when secondary bacterial infection develops.

The diagnosis should be made only after careful exclusion of all etiologies of scalp pruritus, neurological disorders and other psychiatric disorders such as cocaine intoxication, delusions of parasitosis and factitial dermatitis. Importantly, the presence of a psychopathology must be ascertained through both clinical observations and patient questioning.

Treatment

The treatment is essentially psychiatric. Dermatological treatment is related to appropriate treatment of scalp lesions as may be required according to the presentation. These include non-irritative shampoos, topical antibiotics or steroid antibiotic combinations. Treatment of pruritus is essential. Options include topical antipruritics, including doxepin 5% cream or a menthol or phenol containing lotion with an emollient base. Oral antihistamines such as doxepin or hydroxyzine should be prescribed alongside. Cool compresses may also be used to provide hydration, accelerate crust removal and sooth the skin. Oral antibiotics are needed in case of secondary infection.

The first-line psychiatric treatment for neurotic excoriations is selective serotonin re-uptake inhibitors **(SSRIs)** as they can reduce depressive and compulsive symptoms. *Anxiolytics* such as benzodiazepines can be used for short-term treatment when an acute social stressor or comorbid anxiety is involved.

Alprazolam differs from the older benzodiazepines such as diazepam and chlordiazepoxide because its half-life is short and predictable. Another advantage is that it has an antidepressant effect, whereas most other benzodiazepines generally have a depressant effect. Because of the possible risk of addiction with long-term use, the most prudent way of using alprazolam would be to restrict its use to 2–3 weeks. *Doxepin* is another useful molecule with an antidepressant and anxiolytic effect.

Additional therapeutic options involve nonpharmacological treatment approaches including cognitive therapy, behavior modification, eclectic approach and psychodynamic psychotherapy, which have demonstrated inconsistency in effectiveness. However, before these methods can be considered, the patient should be willing to accept the psychiatric nature of the condition and be able to identify triggers leading to excoriation.

Factitial Dermatitis of the Scalp

Factitial dermatitis of the scalp is a disorder of self-injurious behavior, and generally presents with lesions over the skin in addition. A patient with this condition produces cutaneous lesions in order to fulfill an unconscious psychological need. The psychological need is typically one of being taken care of by assuming the sick role. This is different from malingering as these patients do it for psychological reasons and not for monetary or other discrete objectives. Patients typically deny their role in the process and seek care from different physicians. There is commonly a history of childhood trauma and deprivation. The patients are more commonly females (3:1 to 20:1 in different series), and the onset is mostly in adolescence and early childhood. They are unable to establish close interpersonal relationships and generally have severe personality disorders. A large number of patients has been reported to work, or have a close family member working in the heath care field. These patients follow through with the medical procedures and are at risk from the complications of procedures and for drug addictions. In the severe form (Munchhausen syndrome), a series of successive hospitalizations becomes a lifelong pattern.

The pathogenesis may be related to traumatic events, especially abuse and deprivations in childhood, and lack of support from relatives/friends in adulthood. Majority suffer from borderline personality disorder. Because of emotional deficits in childhood and frequent history of physical/sexual abuse, these patients do not develop a stable body image with clearly defined physical and emotional boundaries. The factitial lesions provide them excitement and stimulation, easing the sense of emptiness and isolation, and skin sensation defines boundaries and helps establish personal and sexual identity, whereas the sick role gratifies dependency needs.

Patients present with a vague "hollow" history and are seemingly unaffected, while the relatives are anxious and often angry at medical "incompetence" in diagnosing the condition. The lesions are as varied as the different methods employed to create them. On the scalp, these are generally ulcerations or areas of cutting off hair (trichotemnomania). The lesions are bizarre in shape and distribution, and usually appear on normal skin.

Many dermatologic, neurologic and mental disorders may have similar symptoms and need to be ruled out. Important differentials are necrotizing herpes zoster, temporal arteritis, angiosarcoma, neurotrophic ulcerations of the scalp, bullous disorders, pyoderma gangrenosum, other types of vasculitis and neurotic excoriations of the scalp.

Treatment

Psychiatric treatment includes a combination of pharmacological therapies and behavioral therapy. Most essential and difficult is to secure an enduring and stable patient–physician relationship. Physician needs to have a "non-confrontational" approach, understanding that the factitious manifestations are the patients' "cry for help". A dialectical behavioral therapy involving a structured behavioral therapeutic program for borderline personality disorder patients is recommended (Heller et al).

Psychotropic medications can be directed toward depression and anxiety, often experienced by these patients. Selective serotonin reuptake inhibitors **(SSRIs)** such as fluoxetine, sertraline, paroxetine and fluvoxamine, in possibly high doses, are typically first-line treatment for compulsive, self-injurious behavior (Koblenzer, 2000). *Anxiolytics* such as buspirone and benzodiazepines can be prescribed if anxiety is a dominant feature. *Atypical antipsychotics* such as pimozide, olanzapine or risperidone can be helpful in treating the self-injurious behavior, and may be used alone or in combination with a SSRI. Dermatological treatment is symptomatic and directed towards achieving healing of the induced lesions.

Trichotillomania/Trichotillosis (Also see Chapter 10)

Trichotillomania (TTM) was first described in 1889 by Hallopeau. The name is derived from the Greek words thrix (hair), tillein (pull out) and mania (madness). The term 'mania' although is best avoided and trichotillosis may be a more appropriate name for the disorder. It is a psychodermatological disorder characterized by an uncontrollable urge to pull one's own hair, leading to hair loss and functional impairment.

Community prevalence studies suggest that TTM is a common disorder with point prevalence estimate of 0.5 to 2% (though prevalence up to 13% has been reported in other studies, not following the DSM criteria) (King et al, 1995; Duke et al, 2010). As TTM is characterized by repetitive behaviors limited to hair pulling, it is considered as an obsessive compulsive disease (OCD) spectrum disorder. According to this approach, TTM was moved from the group of "impulse control disorders not elsewhere classified" in the previous version of the American Psychiatric Association Classification DSM-IV to the group of disorders of obsessive compulsive spectrum in recent DSM-V (2013), although in International Classification of Diseases 10th Revision (WHO-ICD-10), classification it still belongs to an impulse control disorders.

The disease possibly has a bimodal distribution with patients usually presenting between the ages of 10 and 13 years (quite consistent across studies) where the disorder is considered mild, on the lines of a habit tic (epilation tic) and the more chronic and severe cases who present as adults but who started hair pulling activities in adolescence or early adult life. In adults, TTM appears to have a large female preponderance (4:1). In childhood, the sex distribution has been found to be equal.

Diagnostic and Statistical Manual of Mental Disorders (DSM-5; 2013) criteria for diagnosing TTM are:

1. Recurrent pulling out of one's hair, resulting in hair loss
2. Repeated attempts to decrease or stop hair pulling
3. The hair pulling causes clinically significant distress or impairment in social, occupational, or other important areas of functioning
4. The hair pulling or hair loss is not attributable to another medical condition (e.g. a dermatological condition)
5. The hair pulling is not better explained by the symptoms of another mental disorder (e.g. attempts to improve a perceived defect or flaw in appearance in body dysmorphic disorder).

Clinical Features

Patients may pull hair from the scalp only or also from the eyebrows, eyelashes, pubic region and the trunk. Pediatric patients commonly pull only from the scalp. A variable number of patients also engage in trichophagia, which may lead to further complications. TTM may also be accompanied by nail biting or nail picking. Psychiatric comorbidities include anxiety disorders, mood disorders, substance use disorders and eating disorders in adults.

The classical clinical presentation is of an irregular patch (or patches) of incomplete hair loss, on approachable areas of the scalp (Fig. 13.5). The hair in the patch is of unequal lengths. Hair may be broken mid-shaft or may be present as black dots or stubbles on the scalp (Fig. 13.6). Hair is not easily pulled out on examination and the hair pull test is negative.

Diagnosis

Trichoscopy (Fig. 13.6) is an essential tool in diagnosing difficult cases, where the presentation mimics alopecia areata or tinea capitis (trichoscopic features are detailed in Chapter 10). A biopsy can also be confirmatory in doubtful cases. It has a characteristic pathology with an increased number of hair follicles in catagen phase. Some follicles show follicular plugging with pigment casts. Trichomalacia is a histopathological sign of trauma to the hair shaft. In this condition, the hair shaft within the follicle is small and wavy or spiral-shaped (Figs 13.7 and 13.8).

Treatment

Individuals with TTM rarely seek psychological or psychiatric treatment for their condition. Patients avoid seeking treatment due to social embarrassment or due to a belief that their condition is just a "bad habit" or that it is untreatable. They often refuse to admit to the habit. Without treatment, response rates in adults are low (approximately 14%) (Woods et al, 2006). When diagnosed early and appropriately treated, however, up to 50% of individuals may experience symptom reduction at least for the short term (O Connor et al, 2003).

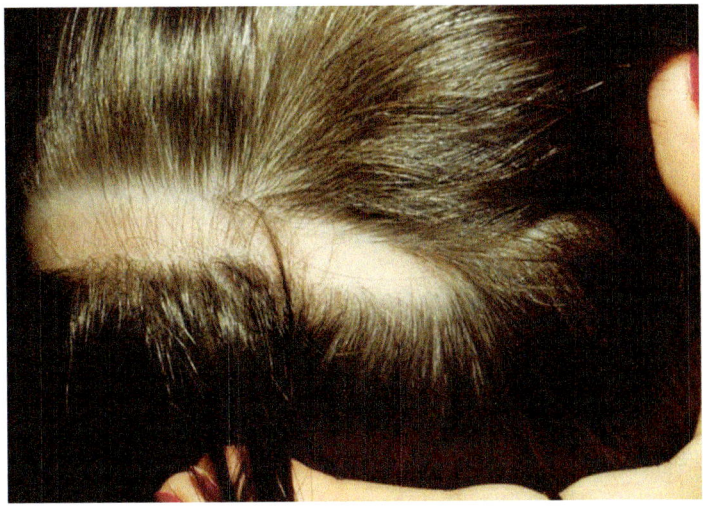

Fig. 13.5: A bizarre shaped area of hair loss in a child

Therapy for TTM lacks scientific evidence and is largely based on case reports. Behavior therapy, in the form of habit reversal therapy is the cornerstone of management. In terms of medication, there are currently no drugs that are universally accepted as first-line treatments. The usual treatment options for OCD are generally ineffective in TTM.

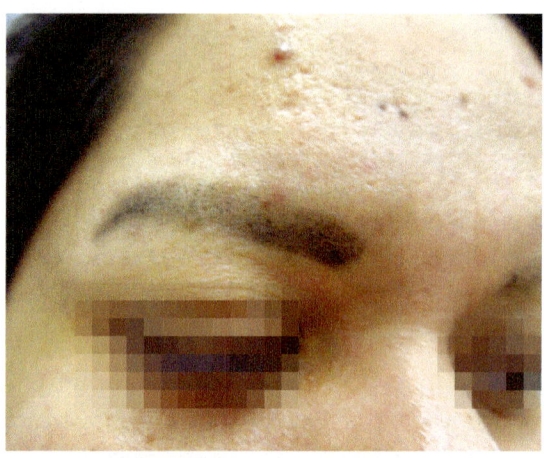

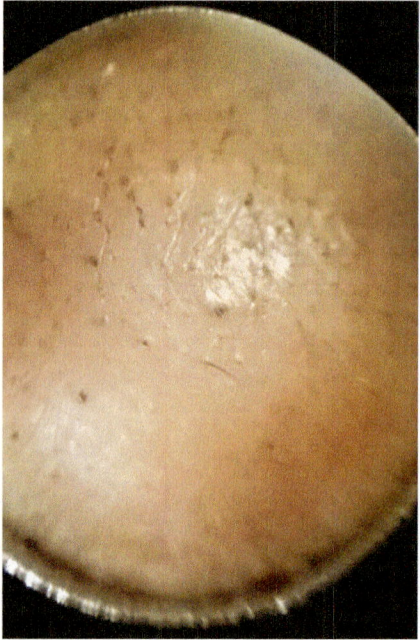

Fig. 13.6: This young lady had been compulsively pulling out her eyebrows, while preparing for her civil service exam. Trichoscopy using a mobile attachment revealed variably broken hair

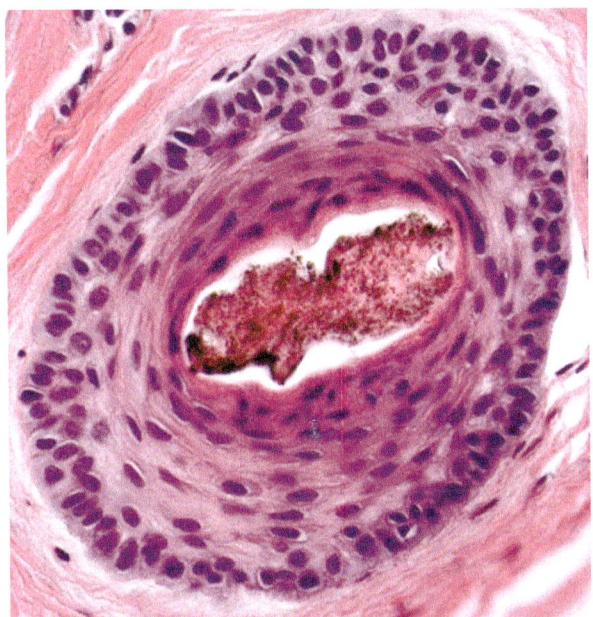

Fig. 13.7: Trichomalacia is evident in this specimen from a patient with trichotillomania. The hair shaft is distorted in shape, irregularly pigmented and incompletely cornified (Dr EA Knopp)

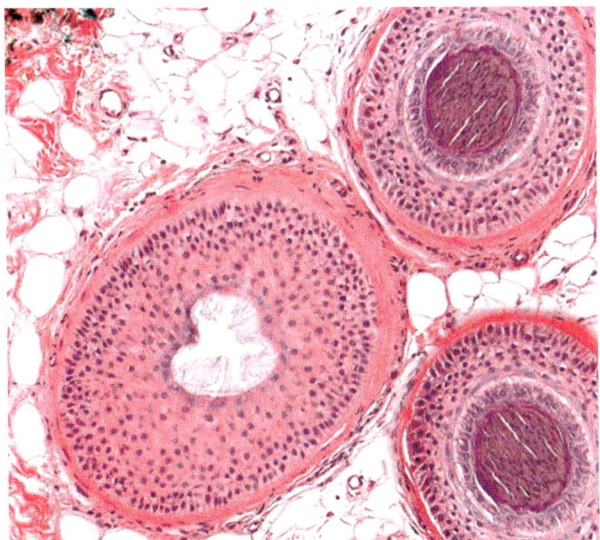

Fig. 13.8: Trichotillomania. A follicle with missing shafts and collapse of the inner root sheath; adjacent (upper and lower right) are unaffected follicles (*Courtesy:* EA Knopp)

A recent Cochrane review concluded that although clomipramine has demonstrated some benefit for trichotillomania, there is no strong evidence of a treatment effect for the selective serotonin reuptake inhibitors (SSRIs). Tricyclic antidepressants, Li salts and antipsychotics have been used with variable success.

But in practice SSRIs remain the most commonly prescribed drugs. These include: Fluoxetine, sertraline, paroxetine, fluvoxamine, escitalopram and clomipramine, prescribed alone or as a combined therapy with atypical antipsychotics such as pimozide, olanzapine or risperidone. At least 4 weeks are necessary for antidepressant effects from these agents, and time to response for TTM is approximately the same. Patients should be advised of this delayed onset of response when medications are prescribed to avoid early discontinuation of treatment (Table 13.1).

Recently, **N-acetylcysteine** has been proposed as an effective alternative treatment since the drug restores the extracellular glutamate concentration in the nucleus accumbens (low levels of extracellular glutamate concentration have been held responsible for the pathogenesis of compulsive behaviors, including the TTM). In a randomized, double-blind clinical trial, N-acetylcysteine at 1200 mg BD was effective and safe (Rodrigues-Barata et al, 2012). Side effects with NAC are generally mild and usually only involve some bloated feelings and flatulence.

The **antipsychotic**, olanzapine, has also been studied in one small (n = 23) double-blind, placebo-controlled trial (Van Ameringen et al, 2010). After 12 weeks using a mean dose of 10.8 mg/day, olanzapine significantly reduced symptoms of trichotillomania.

An open-label study of dronabinol, a **cannabinoid agonist**, demonstrated marked reductions in trichotillomania symptoms during a 12-week trial using a mean dose of 11.6 mg/day (Grant et al, 2011). Dronabinol, a generally well tolerated medication at these low doses with only slight sedation, may be a promising option if similar benefit is demonstrated in controlled trials.

Trichotemnomania

Trichotemnomania (Greek *thrix*—hair, *temnein*—to cut) is hair loss due to cutting or shaving of hair in the setting of obsessive–compulsive disorder. Trichotemnomania is usually a loss of scalp hair, but can also occur in other locations, such as the eyebrows, axilla or pubis. Most reports so far are of European origin. Patients give a vague history of sudden hair loss but appear unperturbed. The diagnostic clue is

Table 13.1: An overview of salient features of SSRIs

Generic name	Usual daily starting dose (mg)	Usual daily dose range (mg)	Relative histamine with H1 receptor-blocking potency	Relative anticholinergic potency	Relative alpha-adrenergic receptor-blocking potency
Selective serotonin reuptake inhibitors					
Fluoxetine	10–20	10–60	Low/absent	Low/absent	Low/absent
Sertraline	25–50	50–200	Low/absent	Low/absent	Low/absent
Paroxetine	10–20	20–60	Low/absent	Very mild	Low/absent
Fluvoxamine	25–50	100–200	Low/absent	Low/absent	Low/absent
Citalopram	10–20	20–60	Low/absent	Low/absent	Low/absent
Escitalopram	10	10–20	Low/absent	Low/absent	Low/absent
Heterocyclic agents					
Clomipramine	25–50	100–225	Moderate	High	Moderate
Doxepin	25–50	100–200	High	High	Moderate/high

Fluoxetine (Fludac); Sertaline (Serta); Paroxetine (Pari CR); Citalopram (Citapam); Escitalopram (Nexito); Clomipramine (Clonil); Doxepin (Spectra).

the presence of follicular openings filled with hair shafts within a healthy-looking scalp. Also, the hair at the difficult to reach areas may still be present. There are no signs of inflammation or scarring. The hairs present are of similar length, suggesting being cut with scissors or shaved. As in TTM, the patients refuse to admit to their habit. Trichoscopy shows no evidence of alopecia areata and histology shows entirely normal structures (c.f. TTM). Regrowing alopecia areata generally shows hair of reduced thickness and pigment and can be differentiated thus. The treatment is essentially psychiatric.

Trichoteiromania (Teiro'-Greek Meaning 'I Rub')

This is another rare obsessive–compulsive habit wherein hair loss occurs due to repeated rubbing. The hallmark of trichoteiromania is short hairs with split, brush-like ends (like weathered hair), giving the impression of white tips. Patients who repetitively rub their scalp secondary to underlying skin or hair pathology usually demonstrate irregular and patchy hair loss and weathering. This differs from trichoteiromania where the hairs in the involved part are all uniformly and equally affected, and the scalp shows no underlying pathology. The underlying mental disorder varies among the patients, though scalp dysaesthesia, not explained through any specific dermatological disorder, is a common denominator. It has no diagnostic histopathological features and has a normal trichogram.

Trichodaganomania

This is another type of hair loss with associated psychiatric comorbidity, characterized by the compulsive habit of biting one's own hair. However, due to its intrinsic mechanism, the hair loss is not located on the head.

Delusions of Parasitosis (Ekbom's Syndrome)

Delusions of parasitosis is a rare psychiatric disorder that is characterized by a solitary delusion, that of a parasitic infestation. By definition, the delusion is firmly believed and cannot be shaken by rationalization. Delusions of parasitosis belongs in a group of disorders called monosymptomatic hypochondriacal psychosis. The delusional disorder is truly isolated to the one concern, unlike schizophrenia, which involves multiple functional deficits such as hallucinations, lack of social skills, and flat affect in addition to the delusional symptoms.

Clinical Features

Patients will commonly complain of a sensation of perceived parasites crawling upon or burrowing into the skin. One constant finding, though, is the lack of primary lesions. The patient has entirely normal skin findings or only secondary lesions as a result of scratching or picking. Individuals suffering from this condition may injure themselves in attempts to be rid of the "parasites".

The diagnosis is one of exclusion and requires a detailed investigation into (i) a possible real infestation, (ii) potential causes of pruritus, and (iii) organic causes of adult onset psychiatric symptoms.

Management

Patients typically are highly resistant to accepting a psychiatric diagnosis as the reason for their symptoms. Antipsychotics are the typical pharmacological treatment of choice. The agents have been divided into two major classes: Typical and atypical. The primary difference between the two classes is the ratio of serotonin blockade compared to dopaminergic blockade. An overview of the doses and side effects is given in Tables 13.2 and 13.3. A baseline ECG before starting antipsychotic medications and periodically thereafter is advised.

Table 13.2: An overview of antipsychotics					
Generic (trade) name	Dose	Sedation	Anticholinergic effect	Extrapyramidal effect	Hypotension
Typical agents					
Haloperidol (Serenace)	1–20	Low	Low	High	Low
Pimozide (Orap)	1–10				
Atypical agents					
Olanzapine (Oleanz)	2.5–15	Moderate	Low	Low	Low
Quietiapine (Qutipin)	25–300	High	—		High
Aripiprazole (Arpizol)	5–30	Low	—		Low

Metabolic effects: Olanzapine: Weight gain.

Table 13.3: Recommended monitoring for patients on atypical antipsychotics

	Baseline	4 weeks	8 weeks	12 weeks	Quarterly	Annually	Every 5 years
Personal/ family history of hyper- lipidemia	X					X	
Weight (BMI)	X	X	X	X	X	X	
Waist circum- ference	X			X		X	
Blood pressure	X			X		X	
Fasting plasma glucose	X			X		X	
Fasting lipid profile	X			X			X

Acknowledgment

Dr EA Knopp, Connecticut, USA & Dr Kabir Sardana for select images in the chapter.

Bibliography

1. American Psychiatric Association. Diagnostic and statistical manual of mental disorders (5th edn). Arlington, VA: American Psychiatric Publishing, 2013.
2. Baldari M, Montinari M, Guarrera M, Rebora A. Trichodynia is a distinguishing symptom of telogen effluvium. J Eur Acad Dermatol Venereol 2009;23:733–4.
3. Bernhard JD: Itch: Mechanisms and Management of Pruritus. New York, McGraw-Hill, 1994;p.51.
4. Blume-Peytavi U, Tosti A, Whiting DA, Trueb R (eds). Hair growth and disorders. 2008, Srpinger Publishers. Germany.
5. Buchanan JA, Zakrzewska JM. Burning mouth syndrome. Clin Evid (Online) 2010;19:1301.
6. Christenson GA. Trichotillomania—from prevalence to comorbidity. Psychiatric Times 1995;12(9):44–8.
7. Cohen LJ, Stein DJ, Simeon D, Spadaccini E, Rosen J, Aronowitz B, Hollander E. Clinical profile, comorbidity, and treatment history in 123 hair pullers: a survey study. Journal of Clinical Psychiatry. 1995;56(7):319–26.

8. Defrin R, Lurie R. Indications for peripheral and central sensitization in patients with chronic scalp pain (trichodynia). Clin J Pain 2013;29: 417–24.

9. Dougherty DD, Loh R, Jenike MA, Keuthen NJ. Single modality versus dual modality treatment for trichotillomania: Sertraline, behavioral therapy, or both. J Clin Psychiatry 2006;67:1086–92.

10. Duarte Pinto ACV, de Brito FF, et al. Trichotillomania: a case report with clinical and dermatoscopic differential diagnosis with alopecia areata. An Bras Dermatol 2017;92(1):118–20.

11. Duke DC, Keeley ML, Geffken GR, Storch EA. Trichotillomania: A current review. Clin Psychol Rev 2010 Mar; 30(2):181–93.

12. Durusoy C, Ozenli Y, Adiguzel A, Budakoglu IY, Tugal O, Arikan S, et al. The role of psychological factors and serum zinc, folate and vitamin B_{12} levels in the aetiology of trichodynia: A case-control study. Clin Exp Dermatol 2009;34:789–92.

13. Ericson M, Gabrielson A, Worel S, Lee WS, Hordinsky MK. Substance P (SP) in innervated and non-innervated blood vessels in the skin of patients with symptomatic scalp. Exp Dermatol 1999;8:344–5.

14. Freyschmidt-Paul P, Hoffmann R, Happle R. Trichoteiromania. Eur J Dermatol 2001;11:369–71.

15. Gallouj S, Rabhi S, Baybay H, Soughi M, Meziane M, Rammouz I, Mikou O, Bono W, Mernissi FZ. Trichotemnomania associated to trichotillomania: a case report with emphasis on the diagnostic value of dermoscopy. Dermatol Venereol 2011 Feb;138(2):140–1.

16. Grant JE, Chamberlain SR. Trichotillomania. Am J Psychiatry. 2016 September 01;173(9):868–74.

17. Grant JE, Odlaug BL, Chamberlain SR, Kim SW. Dronabinol, a cannabinoid agonist, reduces hair pulling in trichotillomania: a pilot study. Psychopharmacology (Berl) 2011 Dec; 218(3):493–502.

18. Grzesiak M1, Reich A, Szepietowski JC, Hadry T, Pacan P. Trichotillomania among young adults: Prevalence and Comorbidity. Acta Derm Venereol 2017 Apr 6;97(4):509–12.

19. Happle R. Trichotemnomania: obsessive-compulsive habit of cutting or shaving the hair. J Am Acad Dermatol 2005 Jan;52(1):157–9.

20. Heller MM, Koo JM. Neurotic excoriations, acne excoriee, and factitial dermatitis. In: Heller MM, Koo JY, editors. Contemporary Diagnosis and Management in Psychodermatology. 1st edn. Newton: Handbooks in Health Care Co; 2011: pp. 37–44.

21. Hoss D, Segal S. Scalp dysesthesia. Arch Dermatol 1998;134:327–330.

22. Jafferany M, Feng J, Hornung RL. Trichodaganomania: the compulsive habit of biting one's own hair. J Am Acad Dermatol 2009;60:689–91.

23. Jermain DM, Crismon ML. Pharmacotherapy of obsessive–compulsive Disorder Pharmacotherapy 1990;10:175–98.

24. King RA, Zohar AH, Ratzoni G, Binder M, Kron S, Dycian A, Cohen DJ, Pauls DL, Apter A. An epidemiological study of trichotillomania in Israeli adolescents. J am Acad Child Adolesc Psychiatry 1995;34:1212–15.

25. Kivanç-Altunay I, Sava C, Gökdemir G, Kölü A, Ayaydin EB. The presence of trichodynia in patients with telogen effluvium and androgenetic alopecia. Int J Dermatol 2003;42:691–3.

26. Koblenzer CS. Dermatitis artefacta. Clinical features and approaches to treatment. Am J Clin Dermatol 2000;1:47–55.

27. Koblenzer CS. Pharmacology of psychotropic drugs useful in dermatologic practice. Int J Dermatol 1993;32:162–8.

28. Koblenzer CS. Psychiatric syndromes of interest to dermatologists. Int J Dermatol 1993;32:82–8.

29. Koblenzer CS. Psychocutaneous Disease. Orlando, Fl: Grune and Stratton; 1987.

30. Koo JY, Smith LL. Obsessive–compulsive disorders in the pediatric dermatology practice. Pediatr Dermatol 1991;8:107–13.

31. Moore PA, Guggenheimer J, Orchard T. Burning mouth syndrome and peripheral neuropathy in patients with type 1 diabetes mellitus. J Diabetes Complications 2007;21:397–402.

32. Oberholzer PA, Nobbe S, Kolm I, Kerl K, Kamarachev J, Tr€ueb RM. Red scalp disease—a rosacea-like dermatosis of the scalp. Successful therapy with oral tetracycline. Dermatology 2009;219:179–81.

33. O'Connor K, Brisebois H, Brault M, Robillard S, Loiselle J. Behavioral activity associated with onset in chronic tic and habit disorder. Behav Res Ther. 2003;41(2):241–49.

34. Orgaz-Molina J, Husein-Elahmed H, Soriano-Hernández MI, Arias-Santiago S. Trichotemnomania: hair loss mediated by a compulsive habit not admitted by patients. Acta Derm Venereol 2012 Mar;92(2):183–4.

35. Rebora A, Semino MT, Guarrera M. Trichodynia. Dermatology 1996;192: 292–3. 18. Tomasson K, Kent D, Coryell W. Somatization and conversion disorders: Comorbidity and demographics at presentation. Acta Psychiatr Scand. 1991;84:288–93.

36. Rebora A. Trichodynia: a review of the literature.Int J Dermatol 2016 Apr;55(4):382–4.

37. Reich S, Tru¨eb RM. Trichoteiromanie. J Dtsch Dermatol Ges 2003;1:22–8.

38. Rief W, Hiller W, Geissner E, Fichter MM. A two-year follow-up study of patients with somatoform disorders. Psychosomatics 1995;36:376–86.

39. Rodrigues-Barata AR, Tosti A, Rodríguez-Pichardo A, Camacho-Martínez F. N-acetylcysteine in the treatment of trichotillomania. Int J Trichology 2012;4:176–8.

40. Rothbart R, Amos T, Siegfried N, Ipser JC, Fineberg N, Chamberlain SR, Stein DJ. Pharmacotherapy for trichotillomania. Cochrane Database Syst Rev 2013 Nov 8;11:CD007662.

41. Rothbaum BO, Shaw L, Morris R, Ninan PT. Prevalence of trichotillomania in a college freshman population. J Clin Psychiatry 1993;54:72–3.

42. Szepietowski JC, Salomon J, Pacan P, Hrehorów E, Zalewska A. Frequency and treatment of trichotillomania in Poland. Acta Derm Venereol 2009; 89(3):267–70.

43. Thestrup-Pedersen K, Hjorth N. Red scalp: a previously undescribed disease of the scalp. Ugeskr Laeger 1987;149:2141–42.

44. Tirado MIM. Tratamientocognitivo-conductualenunaadolescente con trichotillomania. Revista de PsicologíaClínica con Niños y Adolescentes 2015;2:9–17.

45. Trüeb RM. Idiopathic chronic telegon effluvium in the woman. Hautarzt 2000;51:899–905.

46. Trüeb RM. Telogen effluvium and trichodynia. Dermatology 1998;196: 374–5.

47. Trüeb, Ralph M. The Difficult Hair Loss Patient Guide to Successful Management of Alopecia and Related Conditions. Swinger International Publishing, Switzerland, 2015.

48. Van Ameringen M, Mancini C, Patterson B, Bennett M, Oakman J. A randomized, double-blind, placebo-controlled trial of olanzapine in the treatment of trichotillomania. J Clin Psychiatry 2010;71(10):1336–43.

49. Willimann B, Trüeb RM. Hair pain (trichodynia): Frequency and relationship to hair loss and patient gender. Dermatology 2002;205:374–7.

50. Wollina U. Three orphans one should know: red scalp, red ear and red scrotum syndrome. J Eur Acad Dermatol Venereol 2016 Nov;30(11):e169–e70.

51. Wong JW, Nguyen TV, Koo JY. Primary Psychiatric Conditions: Dermatitis Artefacta, Trichotillomania and Neurotic Excoriations. Indian J Dermatol 2013 Jan–Feb;58(1):44–48.

52. Woods DW, Flessner CA, Franklin ME, Keuthen NJ, Goodwin RD, Stein DJ, Walther MR, TLC-Scientific Advisory Board. The Trichotillomania Impact Project (TIP): exploring phenomenology, functional impairment, and treatment utilization. J Clin Psychiatry 2006;67:1877–88.

53. World Health Organization. The ICD-10: classification of mental and behavioural disorders: clinical description and diagnostic guidelines. Geneva: WHO, 1992.

54. Zaidens SH. Self-inflicted dermatoses and their psychodynamics. J Nerv Ment Dis 1951;113:395–404.

14

Newer and Investigational Drugs for Androgenetic Alopecia

Kabir Sardana, Ananta Khurana

Androgenetic alopecia (AGA) is the major type of alopecia affecting 60–70% of the population and is reliably believed to be caused by the overproduction of 5α-dihydrotestosterone (5α-DHT), a potent androgen, within the hair follicle, specifically the dermal papilla (DP) cells that are the main regulators of hair growth and are the only site of 5α-DHT action (Tobin DJ). Minoxidil and finasteride are the only two FDA-approved drugs used for the treatment of AGA. Minoxidil, a vasodilator and potassium channel opener, is known to prolong the anagen phase and possibly converts vellus hair to terminal hair. The effects are consequent to the upregulation of VEGF and FGF-7 within the dermal papilla (DP) cells and due to the growth-promoting activity on the hair epithelial cells (Iino M). Other mechanisms proposed include stimulation of potassium channel and prostaglandin endoperoxide synthase-1, which increases levels of prostaglandin E_2 (PGE_2).

However, **minoxidil** is only effective in **30–35%** of the patients treated and the treatment must be continued for lifetime. **Finasteride**, a synthetic azosteroid, is a 5α-reductase (5αR) type 2 inhibitor which reduces the level of 5α-DHT in serum by 68% but is effective in only **48%** of patients. Further, the role of both these approved drugs in conversion of vellus to terminal hair has been challenged by way of unit area trichogram based evaluations, which show no decrease in absolute vellus hair count (in contrast with vellus hair percentage which reduces) following successful treatment with minoxidil/minoxidil + finasteride (Rushton et al, 2016). Thus, there is a pressing need for more effective and long-lasting treatments for androgenetic alopecia affecting men and women.

Mediators of Hair Growth

There are various mediators that play a role in the transition through different phases of the hair growth cycle (Fig. 14.1). But for AGA, androgens play a role in both sexes (Cotsarelis et al).

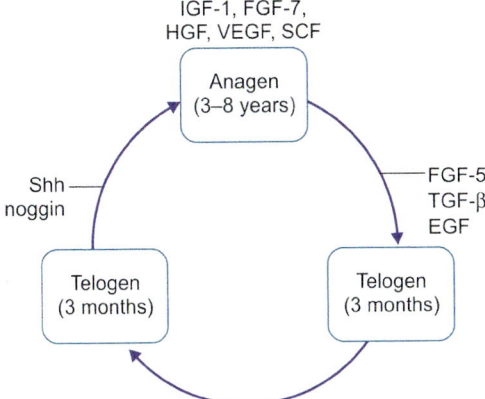

Fig. 14.1: Mediators of the hair growth cycle (Shh: Sonic Hedgehog, IGF-1: Insulin like growth factor 1, FGF-7: Fibroblast growth factor-7, HGF: Hepatocyte growth factor, VEGF: Vascular endothelial growth factor, SCF: Stem cell factor, TGF: Transfroming growth factor, EGF: Epidermal growth factor)

The mechanism of androgen action within DP cell is depicted in Fig. 14.2. Testosterone (T) and 5α-DHT are the two major types of androgens that cause AGA. Both T and 5α-DHT can bind to the AR, a member of steroid–thyroid hormone nuclear receptor superfamily, to form a receptor-ligand complex. The complex is then translocated to the nucleus where it acts as a transcriptional factor, regulating the

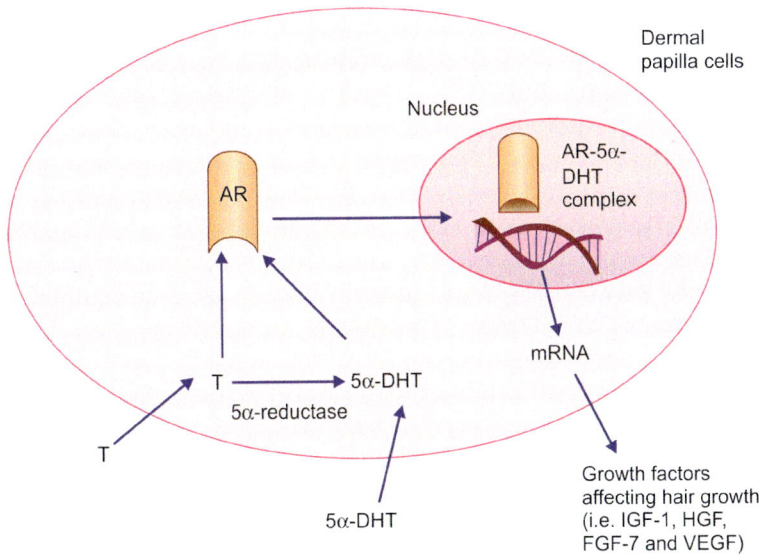

Fig. 14.2: Mechanism of androgens action within dermal papilla cell

expression of androgen-sensitive genes. The androgen sensitive genes are the growth factor genes produced by DP cells during the hair cycle (Itami S). However, 5α-DHT has five times higher binding affinity to AR and 10-fold higher potency than T in inducing androgen-sensitive genes and is known to be overproduced during AGA (Azzouni F).

Therapeutic Targets for Novel Drugs

Thus, in essence the therapeutic targets are primarily the androgenetic pathways, via inhibition of the following:

a. The 5α-R enzyme
b. The interaction of 5α-DHT and AR
c. Translocation of 5α-DHT-AR complex

A combination of these three activities would lead to a promising treatment in the near future.

But the most crucial target, potentially permanent, is the so-called "God site" of hair growth, that is

d. Activating, growth factors and stem cells of the hair

A summary of the novel targets of therapies that will be discussed in Box 14.1.

5α-Reductase Inhibitors

Three isoforms of 5α-R have been found. These are 5α-R type 1 (5α-R1), type 2 (5α-R2) and type 3 (5α-R3). 5α-R1 shows a broad pH range of 6.5–8 with lower affinity to T (kM > 1 μM), whereas 5α-R2 shows a narrow acidic pH of 5.5 and has a higher affinity to T (kM < 10 nM). 5α-R3 has a narrow pH range of 6.5–6.9, while there is no information on the affinity to T (Azzaouni).

Sites: Within the human body, 5α-R1 has been found in the sebaceous glands, chest and back skin, liver, adrenal glands and kidney tissues (Chen W), whereas 5α-R2 has been found in the *beard*, chest skin, liver, seminal vesicles, prostate gland, testis and epididymis, foreskin and scrotum (Chen W). 5α-R3 is known to have a ubiquitous property within the body but is overexpressed in the prostate during cancer.

Box 14.1: Overview of novel targets of drugs for AGA

i. 5α-reductase inhibitors
ii. Androgen receptor (AR) blocking agents
iii. Growth factor—producing factors related to hair growth
iv. Stem cell research
v. Miscellaneous agents

Within the hair follicle, 5α-R1 is present in the DP cells, epidermal and follicular keratinocytes (KZs), whereas 5α-R2 is present in the inner layer of the ORS, IRS, interfollicular KZs and might be present in the DP cells (Bayne E). Although the distribution of the two forms is relatively clear, it has been proven through RT-PCR that the DP cells, which are the main site of hair growth regulation, express 5α-R1 (Bayne E). But research works on active anti-AGA compounds have still been conducted on both the 5α-R1 and 5α-R2 isoforms. This might be due to the clinical findings that finasteride, which is a 5α-R2 inhibitor, can exert hair growth-promoting activity.

The 5α-reducatse inhibitors are of two types, **steroidal** and **nonsteroidal**. Most of the so-called "biological agents" are non-steroidal and the clinicians must understand that they are not clinically equivalent to the steroidal inhibitors. Also, the method of assessing equivalence is important as *ex vivo* or *in vitro* data does *not* correlate with *in vivo* results.

The steroidal inhibitors are listed in Table 14.1. Among the three 4 azasteroids, 4-MA exhibited the highest 5α-R1 and 5α-R2 inhibitory activity with IC 50 (half maximal inhibitory concentration) of 1.7 nM and 1.9 nM, respectively (Agarwal S), while dutasteride exhibited the highest 5α-R3 inhibitory activity with an IC 50 of 0.33 nM (Yamana K). In addition, epristeride, an androstene carboxylic acid, also exhibits 5α-R2 inhibitory activity. Those compounds detailed below (natural nonsteroidal inhibitors) have been extracted mostly from medicinal plants and/or active compounds isolated from plant extracts, as summarized in Table 14.2.

Is Dutasteride Better than Finasteride?

An elegantly immaculate study that has been completed [NCT01231607] answers this question. Herein various doses of dutasteride were compared with finasteride and the winner is undeniably dutasteride (Table 14.3). But this is strictly an off-label use.

Table 14.1: Steroidal 5α-R inhibitors		
Class	*Drug*	*5α-R type*
4-Azasteroid	Finasteride	R2/R3
	Dutasteride	R1/R2/R3
	4-MA	R1/R2
6-Azasteroid	GIIS7669X	R1/R2
10-Azasteroid	AS97004	R1
Androstene carboxylic acid	Epristeride	R2

Table 14.2: Natural nonsteroidal 5α-R inhibitors. Please note that the inhibition of the receptors are largely studied in nonhuman cell lines and are not bio-equivalent

Drug	5α-R1	5α-R2
Alizarin	Yes	
Avicequinone C	Yes	
Bromopyrogallol red	Yes	Yes
Caffeic acid phenethyl ester, biochanin A, kaempferol	Yes	
Epigallocatechin-3-gallate	Yes	Yes
Gossypol, nordihydroguaiaretic acid, octyl gallate	Yes	Yes
Linoleic, monolinoleic acids	Yes	Yes
Oleic, linoleic, palmitic acids	Yes	Yes
Osthenol, bisabolangelone	Yes	
Soyasaponin, kaikasaponin III	Yes	Yes
Terpenoids, aliphatic alcohols	Yes	
Triolin	Yes	

Topical or Intradermal Delivery of 5α-reductase Inhibitors

One 6-month double-blind study on 45 patients showed that 1% finasteride gel (40% water and 60% ethanol in hydroxyl-propyl-methyl-cellulose) is as effective as 1 mg oral finasteride (Hajheydari Z et al, 2009).

Another study compared the efficacy and safety of the application of 3% minoxidil lotion (MNX) versus combined 3% minoxidil and 0.1% finasteride lotion (MFX) in 40 men with AGA over a period of 24 weeks. The results showed no statistically significant change in hair count between the two groups; however, global photographic assessment exhibited substantial improvement in the MFX compared with the MNX group. Possible new vehicles to improve finasteride delivery include liquid crystalline nanoparticles (Madheswaran et al, 2013) and hydroxypropyl-chitosan (Caserini et al, 2012) may be an effective option. In India, the DCGI had approved a combination of minoxidil and finasteride based on its evaluation of data, though the same is not in public domain, but the combination is widely used and is believed to be superior to minoxidil alone.

Dutasteride: Data on efficacy of topical dutasteride are anecdotal. A recent placebo-controlled study of 126 female patients evaluated the efficacy of locally injected dutasteride in female AGA. Treatment was delivered with mesotherapy by intradermal injections in the vertex, of 2 ml of a solution containing 0.5 mg of dutasteride, 20 mg of biotin,

Table 14.3: Overview of results of NCT01231607 study

	Placebo	Dutasteride 0.02 mg	Dutasteride 0.1 mg	Dutasteride 0.5 mg	Finasteride 1 mg
Participants analyzed [Units: Participants]	148	155	158	150	141
Change from baseline (BL) in target area hair count (HC) within a 2.54 centimeter (cm) (1 inch) diameter circle at the vertex at week 24, as assessed by macrophotographic technique (MT) [Units: Hair count] Least squares mean (standard error)	4.9 (7.89)	17.1 (7.74)	63.0 (7.67)	89.6 (7.87)	56 5 (8.12)

Dutasteride 0.02 mg vs. Finasteride 1 mg (<0.001); Dutasteride 0.5 mg vs. Finasteride 1 mg (0.002); Dutasteride 0.02 mg vs. Finasteride 1 mg (<0.001)

200 mg of pyridoxine and 500 mg of D-panthenol. Injections were repeated weekly for 8 weeks, then every 2 weeks for 4 weeks and a last application at 16 weeks. Photographic improvement occurred in 62.8% of patients treated, after the 18th week ($p < 0.05$). Shedding diminished ($p < 0.05$) and the hair diameter increased ($p < 0.05$). The side effects most commonly reported were headaches, itching and tolerable pain at the site of injections (Moftah et al, 2012).

However, we forewarn that mesotherapy is probably not the best way of delivery of 5α-reductase inhibitors as there are reports of severe adverse effects such as scarring and nonscarring alopecias, scalp abscess and subcutaneous fat necrosis after scalp mesotherapy (Kadry et al, 2008).

Androgen Receptor (AR) Inhibitors

AR is a member of steroid–thyroid hormone nuclear receptor superfamily that functions as ligand-activated transcription factor. T and/or 5α-DHT activate AR, resulting in the upregulation or down-regulation of androgen-sensitive genes within the DP cells, leading to hair loss. Therefore, another possible way to reduce the effect of androgens causing AGA type of hair loss is to inhibit the interaction between the androgens and its receptor. AR inhibitory compounds are either **AR antagonists** commonly known as AR blockers or *inhibitors* of androgen-induced **AR translocation** to the nucleus. These compounds are divided into steroidal and nonsteroidal inhibitors, based on their molecular structures, and are summarized in Table 14.4. All the compounds are AR antagonists *except* from emodin and diallyl trisulfide, while a few compounds also act as translocation inhibitors. Though unapproved, common drugs used off-label for AGA include spironolactone, CPA and estrogens, usually in females, are also AR inhibitors.

Topical Antiandrogens

There is one phase II clinical trial that aims to determine the efficacy of oral spironolactone compared with topical minoxidil in the treatment of female pattern hair loss. The study has been completed but the results are still awaited (NCT00175617). **Cortexolone 17α-propionate** is a new steroidal antiandrogen that has been shown to have a strong topical antiandrogenic activity without systemic side effects (Trifu et al, 2011).

A multicenter, RCT has been completed wherein cortexolone 17α-propionate (CB-03-01) 5% solution was compared with minoxidil 5% solution, and vehicle solution. Though this study has been completed, its results are awaited and will be of great use in AGA (NCT02279823).

Table 14.4: AR inhibitory compounds	
Steroidal compounds	17-Deacetylnorgestimate 4-Azasteroid (4-MA) Chlormadinone acetate Corticosterone Cyproterone thiopivalate Cyproterone acetate Norethindrone Norethynodrel Norgestimate Norgestrel **Spironolactone**
Nonsteroidal compounds	3-[4-Cyano-3 (trifluoromethyl) phenyl]-5, 5-dimethyl-2, 4-(4, 4-Dimethyl-2, 5-dioxo-3- (4-hydroxybutyl) 1-4-(Alkylthio)-benzonitrile [*RU 58841*] 4-(Arylthio)-4-Aryl-2-trifluoromethyl benzonitrile and 4-dioxo-1-imidazolidine acetonitrile [*RU 58462*] 4-OH-Tamoxifen Bicalutamide Diphenyl ethers **Flutamide** Hydroxyflutamide (4-imidazolidinyl)-2-(trifluoromethyl)-benzonitrile Nafoxidine Nilutamide Tamoxifen
Naturally available compounds	Ganoderol B-ethanolic fruiting body extract of *Ganoderma lucidus* β-Zearalenol Guggulsterone Equol Indole-3-carbinol Pterocarpan Lupeol Atraric acid and N-buytlbenzene sulfonamide Dichloromethane bark extract of *Pygeum Africanum* (TI) Decursin, Decursinol and Decursinolangelate *Angelica gigas* (TI) Nonylphenol and Bisphenol A (TI) Emodin–*Rheum palmatum* (TI) Diallyl trisulfide–*Allium sativum* (TI)

TI: Translocation inhibitor; compounds in bold are used clinically

Growth Factor Modulation

IGF-1, FGF-7, HGF and VEGF are growth factors produced by the DP cells and are responsible for maintaining the hair follicle in the anagen phase of the hair cycle. These growth factors are responsible for the proliferation and differentiation of the hair matrix cells (HMs) into the outer root sheath (ORS), inner root sheath (IRS) and hair shaft (HS). However, the exact pathway of each growth factor related to hair growth has not been studied (Tsuboi R). Therefore, a potential target would be to upregulate these growth factors within the DP cells, which would lengthen the anagen phase, countering AGA type of hair loss.

Only two extracts, namely the ethanolic extract of the root of *Asiasari radix* and the methanolic root extract of *Sophora flavescens*, have been identified so far to increase the expression of VEGF, IGF-1 and FGF-7, respectively, within the DP cells (Roh SS).

Compounds with Multiple Activities

Till date, only the ethanolic root extract of *A. radix* and methanolic root extract of *S. flavescens* possess both 5α-R inhibitory activity and growth factor inducing capability in absence of androgens (Roh SS). In addition, ganoderol B obtained from the ethanolic extract of fruiting body of *G. lucidus* exhibits both 5α-R inhibitory and antiandrogenic activities (Bovee TF).

Stem Cell Activation

AGA is a nonscarring type of alopecia and is potentially reversible, as the hair follicle stem cells are preserved. Various stem cells, cytokines and growth factors regulate the process of hair growth (Fig. 14.3). The use of hair follicle stem cells (HFSCs) located in the bulge area is promising for the treatment of nonscarring alopecia (Mokos ZB). The bulge area is an immune privileged zone mostly because of down-regulation of MHC-I molecules and upregulation of immunosuppressant molecules, protecting HFSCs from aggressive autoimmune attacks. HFSCs can differentiate into cells of a *hair follicle, sebaceous gland or interfollicular epidermis*, depending on the surrounding chemical environment (Choi YS). Moreover, the hair cycle can be affected by alterations of the pathways involved in the activation and suppression of HFSCs.

One of the main pathways currently being studied is the **Wnt/β-catenin pathway**. The activation of this pathway induces the differentiation of bulge stem cells into hair follicles. Activation of Wnt signaling is essential for hair follicle development, hair cycling, hair growth and wound healing. Wnt, especially **Wnt10b**, has been shown

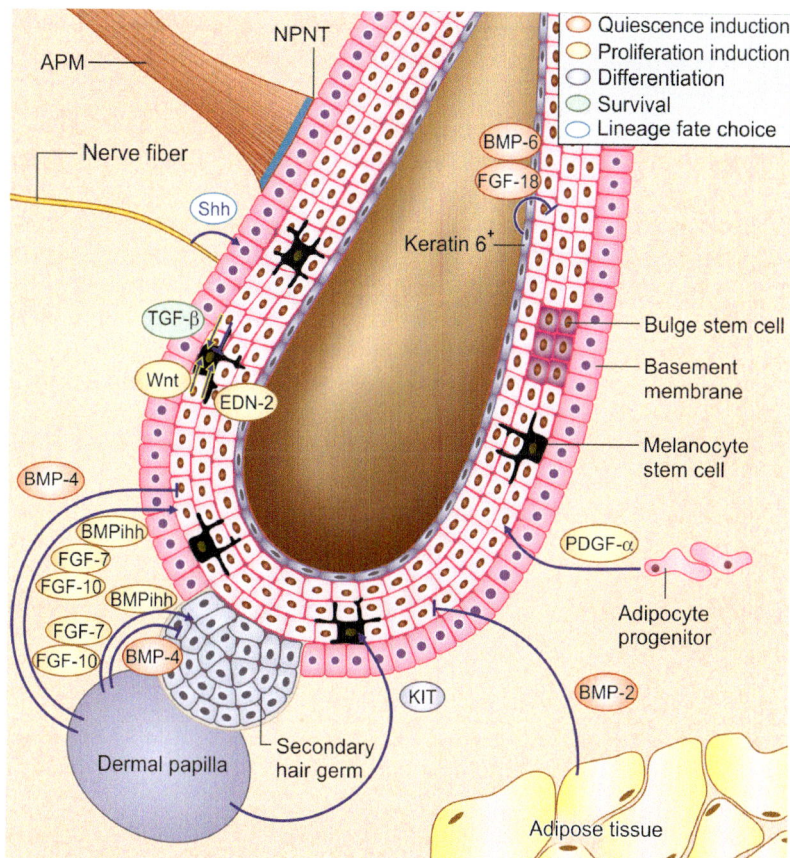

Fig. 14.3: Diagrammatic overview of various mediators of hair growth quiescence, proliferation and differentiation

to be the *first trigger* that stimulates the dermal papilla to induce hair growth, through hair follicle induction, initiation of hair follicle formation and prolongation of anagen (Shimuzu H). A recent study has described a Wnt7a-containing conditioned medium (Wnt-CM), from the supernatant of cultured human umbilical cord-multipotent stem cells (UC-MSCs) overexpressing Wnt7a, in order to examine the effects of this CM on cutaneous healing. This preparation could accelerate wound closure and induce regeneration of hair follicles. Jo et al demonstrated that topical application of **valproic acid**, which inhibits GSK3b, promotes hair formation in a mice model and on human hair follicle *in vitro*, by increasing β-catenin (Jo SJ, 2013). Recently, in a randomized, double-blind, placebo-controlled trial, men with moderate AGA were treated with a spray containing 8.3%

valproic acid or placebo for 24 weeks resulting in significant increase in total hair count in the experimental group (Jo SJ, 2014).

a. **Hair follicle gene reawakening:** Follica Inc. is presently evaluating a way to regenerate hair follicles by reawakening genes from embryonic development. During wound healing, cells become susceptible to signals that induce hair follicle development in embryonic life. These signals are Wnt dependent, as shown by Ito et al in mice after full-thickness wounds. Although factors that may trigger and regulate follicle neogenesis in humans are unknown, the goal of Follica Inc., research is to identify the molecules that are critical in hair follicle regeneration, and then deliver them to the scalp after creating wounds using lasers or other techniques. One of the substances that may be critical in hair regeneration is **lithium**, since it has been established that it increases the **Wnt** canonical signaling pathway through stabilization of β-catenin. Thus, lithium seems to restore the hair differentiation.

b. **Hair stimulating complex:** Hair stimulating complex (HSC) is a bioengineered human cell-derived formulation containing **Wnt7a** protein, **epidermal growth factors** and **follistatin** (Zimber MP et al, 2011). The culture of newborn cells in a simulated embryonic environment with very low oxygen and low gravity conditions produces naturally secreted growth factors, proteins and other synergistic bioproducts, which are then harvested to produce this formula. The intradermal application of 0.1 cc of HSC was found to increase hair shaft thickness ($p = 0.04$), hair density ($p = 0.025$) and number of total terminal hair ($p = 0.003$) compared with placebo at 12 weeks. Most importantly, these results were maintained after 1 year of treatment without any significant side effects reported in the HSC-treated sites.

c. **Adipose-derived stem cells have also been studied:** The primary roles of mesenchymal stem cells (MSCs) are to maintain the stem cell niche, facilitate recovery after injury, and ensure healthy aging and the homeostasis of organ and tissues. MSCs have recently emerged as a new therapeutic option for hair loss. Since adipose-derived stem cells (ADSCs) are the most accessible sources of MSCs, ADSC-based hair regeneration is currently under investigation. Besides replacing degenerated cells in affected organs, ADSCs exhibit their beneficial effects through the paracrine actions of various cytokines and growth factors. However, their survival and regeneration potential are induced by hypoxia, and alternative methods of induction have been looked for. Therefore, preconditioning adipose stem cells with ultraviolet B (UVB) to stimulate the hair growth promoting effects was studied (Jeong YM). It was found that only low-dose UVB (< 20 mJ/cm^2) was able to increase cell survival, migration, angiogenic differentiation and paracrine effects. By performing this technique prior to cell transplantation, it was observed that mice had increased hair follicle formation and hair weight. UVB preconditioning promotes these effects by generating reactive oxygen species and upregulating NADPH oxidase.

Several laboratory experiments and animal studies have shown that ADSC-related proteins can stimulate hair growth.

d. **Stem, dermal, epidermal and hair follicle cells:** Japanese scientists had showed the possibility of regenerating functional bioengineered hair follicles through the rearrangement of various follicular stem cells. Stem cells and dermal papillae were combined in the laboratory to create a follicular germ. This germ, once implanted in the scalp, grew into a viable hair follicle that was able to repeat the hair cycle, connect properly with surrounding skin tissues and achieve piloerection (Toyoshima KE, 2012). The same group has now described a detailed protocol for the regeneration of functional hair follicles and their stem cell niches by the rearrangement of embryonic or adult hair follicle-derived epithelial and mesenchymal cells.

Currently, **Aderans** and **RepliCel** are carrying out phase II trials to evaluate the possibility of restoring miniaturized follicles or to create new hair follicles by injecting autologous dermal and/or epidermal cells. Trichogenic cells from the hair matrix, the dermal papilla or the outer root sheath are isolated from a biopsy taken from patient's scalp. These cells are then expanded in culture and injected into the balding areas of the scalp (Adams JU).

RepliCel (previously Tricho Science Innovations) already has preliminary results of their phase I/IIa clinical trial, in which they included 19 patients who were injected with autologous dermal sheath cup cells to determine the safety and efficacy on hair growth at 6 months post-injection. RepliCel's product was found not only to be safe for human use, but also to increase the number of vellus hair by 24.9%, increase the number of terminal hair by 14.9%, increase the total hair density by 19.2% and to increase the overall hair thickness per area by 15.4%. Currently, RepliCel is working on initiation a phase IIb clinical trial to optimize regimen including different concentrations of cells and different treatment schedules, including single and repeat injections.

Miscellaneous Agents

a. **Prostaglandins analogs and antagonists:** A serendipitous finding of trichomegalia of the eyelashes in patients using latanoprost (a prostaglandin F_2 (PGF_2) analog) for glaucoma (Johnstone et al, 1997) lead to the use of bimatoprost, for increasing eyelash length, thickness and darkness, an apparent sign of "beautiful eyes" desirous in some patients (Smith et al, 2012). As minoxidil's mode of action is mediated by increase in PGE_2 levels, this is another potential target of action. It is pertinent to note that, the study of Blume-Peytavi et al, used latanoprost 0.1%, in patients with AGA, which is higher than the eye drop concentration, which is 0.005%.

Garza et al (2012) made a breakthrough in the pathogenesis of AGA where prostaglandin D_2 (PGD_2) and its synthetase (PGD_2S) were found to be highly expressed in the scalp of balding men and increased levels of PGD_2 were linked with miniaturization of hair follicles in mice. Together these findings suggest that a balance between PGE_2 and PGD_2 controls hair growth and that a deregulation in the prostaglandin pathway may be responsible for hair loss in AGA. Therefore, supplemental PGE_2 could be therapeutic since increasing its levels in bald scalp could overcome the inhibitory effects of PGD_2. Also inhibiting PGD_2 signaling through agents like indole acetic acids (e.g. OC000459), ramatroban, phenyl acetic acids or tetrahydroquinolines could be beneficial.

b. **Platelet-rich plasma:** Platelet-rich plasma (PRP) is an autologous preparation of plasma with $> 1,000,000/\mu l$ platelets that are capable of secreting growth factors and cytokines, which stimulate dermal fibroblasts and stem cells. An overview is given below, though we do not believe that the results justify the possibly "passing hype" over this procedure.

One study by Uebel et al (2006) demonstrated that pre-treatment of follicular units with PRP before transplantation, improved hair density and growth. This salubrious effect is believed to be due to stimulation of bulge stem cells by growth factors released from the platelets. Another study showed that PRP induces proliferation of dermal papilla cells, prolongs anagen, delays progression into catagen, increases the survival of hair follicles and stimulates hair growth in mice. A recent study in 26 humans with thin hair established that injections of 3 ml of PRP every 2 weeks for a total of 5 injections increased number of hair and the diameter of the hair shaft when compared with placebo ($p < 0.01$).

Two, potentially result oriented, trials were initiated by an Indian lab, Kasiak Research. One study was a phase I/II multicenter, open-label, randomized pilot study to determine the safety and efficacy of human platelet lysate (HPL) in patients with AGA undergoing hair transplantation. The other clinical trial was a phase I/II multicenter, open-label, randomized pilot study that aims to compare the effect of three injections of autologous HPL with the standard treatment for AGA (2% minoxidil and/or finasteride). These two trials initiated in 2012, were listed on clincial trials. gov, but the completion date has passed and the status has not been verified in more than two years. We can presume that results were not satisfactory, thus in a proper intervention trial PRP may not work.

Though most of us using PRP are averse to discuss its side effects, psoriasiform scalp dermatitis 2–6 weeks after being treated with PRP can be disconcerting to the patients.

c. **Human placental extract:** The use of placental extract in promoting hair loss pre dates the use of PRP and has not been practiced simply as there is a little commercial gain in this versus the widely popular PRP. Many clinicians have used the placentral extract preparation in India (Placentrex™) as an off-label indication to promote hair growth. The science behind this exists and is based on the finding that HPE (human placental extract) leads to an increase β-catenin levels and inhibits GSK 3β (Ser9) by phosphorylation thus promoting the hair-inductive capacity of hDPCs (Kwon TR). In communication with minoxidil it prolonged anagen phase. A recent study by Seo HS found that it significantly increased the expression of FGF-7, which plays pivotal roles to maintain anagen phase both protein and mRNA levels. It seems that this may be a simpler and cheaper option than PRP specially as the injectible variant of this HPE is available in India. We hope the clinical experience can be translated into clinical studies, which may supplement the molecular basis of HPE.

d. **Nitric oxide:** A trial was initiated on topical nitric oxide (NO) gel based on its role in promoting hair follicle formation through stem cell development, hair regeneration, hair shaft elongation and increased growth rate in rats and mice. But the study did not find any favourable findings (NCT01347957).

e. **Roxithromycin:** Roxithromycin (RXM), a macrolide antibiotic, has two ancillary actions, including inhibiting apoptosis of keratinocytes by inhibiting the production of oxygen reactive species and suppressing the androgen receptor in human dermal fibroblasts.

Ito et al developed a randomized, double-blind, placebo-controlled study to determine the efficacy of topical application of RXM on hair growth. The study group included 13 men with AGA who had to daily apply 3–5 ml of a 0.5% RXM solution for 6 months, and a control group of 11 men who had to apply the same amount of a vehicle-only solution for the same amount of time established. After 6 months, global photographic assessment showed that 58% of patients in the study group presented with favorable results, while no patient in the control group showed hair regrowth ($p < 0.01$). Histological examination of treated areas showed that the global increase in hair density was mainly due to increase in hair shaft thickness rather than an increase in the number of hair follicles.

f. **Vitamin D_3:** Vitamin D_3 (VD_3) works via its interaction with the VDR which is expressed in hair follicle keratinocytes during late anagen and catagen, which suggests that VD_3 may play a role in the haircycle (Reichrath et al, 1994). VD_3 has also been shown to modulate Wnt10b gene expression (Aoi et al, 2012).

Vegesna et al developed a study in which nude mice were either given VD_3 analogs or a placebo. The mice in the VD_3 analog group developed hair, while the control group did not. Furthermore, formation of new, fully formed hair follicles was confirmed by histological examination in the VD_3 analog group, while the placebo group presented no hair follicles or only distorted hair follicles. It was also observed that the mice treated with VD_3 analogs showed a higher maximum hair growth than the controls.

Whether this is a tool with *in vivo* application, is plagued by the universally low values exhibited by laboratories which may not have a clinical correlate.

g. **KROX20: From hair pigmentation to hair growth:** A recent study by Le LQ identified that the transcription factor KROX20 marks a cell lineage differentiating towards the hair shaft and that stem cell factor (SCF) in these hair shaft progenitor cells acts as a critical intrinsic rheostat of hair pigmentation by managing mature melanocytes in the upper HF matrix. Ablation of Scf in KROX20 lineage cells consequently leads to a complete absence of hair pigmentation, showing an indispensable non-cell autonomous SCF contribution to melanocytes. KROX20 lineage cells are the main source of SCF, which stimulates follicular mature melanocytes to produce hair pigment. As an extension, the completion of hair regeneration is dependent on the presence of HF KROX20 lineage cells as the cells give rise directly to hair shafts (Fig. 14.4). This may be a potential treatment agent in the near future.

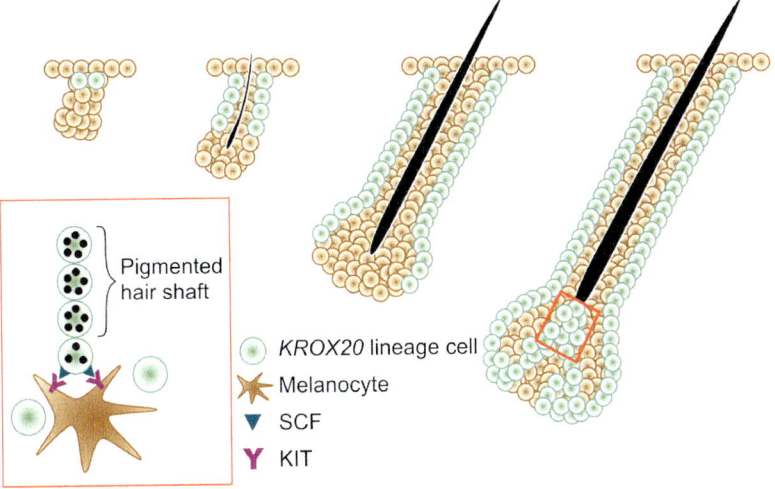

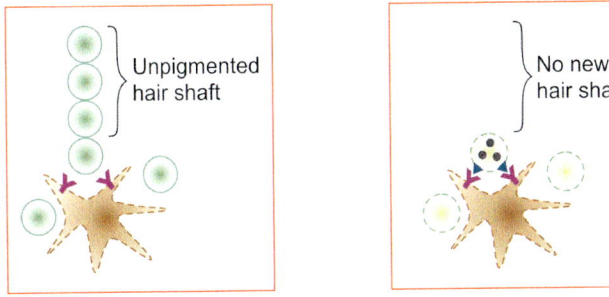

Fig. 14.4: The role of KROX20 in hair shaft development: Lineage tracing of KROX20 lineage cells revealed a dynamic expansion toward the direction of hair-producing cells during HF morphogenesis in the upper HF matrix. Hair progenitor cells sustain differentiated melanocytes through non-cell autonomous SCF/KIT signaling. Depletion of SCF in hair progenitor cells results in loss of hair pigmentation. Depletion of KROX20 lineage cells, the cells that differentiate into hair-producing cells, results in impaired hair regeneration (redrawn with kind permission of Dr Lu Q. Le)

Future of Hair Restoration: Medical Agents beyond Surgery— Target 2020

Though hair restoration by surgical means is the "in thing", we believe that its days are possibly numbered. The frenetic pace of trials on novel methods of achieving hair growth, portends a future where possibly stem cells can be injected with gratifying results. Probably another 5 years from now, such an agent will be in the FDA approved list with potentially revolutionary changes in the way we treat AGA. A list of such future projects is detailed below.

1. **Shiseido/RepliCel:** RepliCel's hair growth treatment, RCH-01, involves culturing a person's own hair follicle cells and then re-injecting them back into their scalp. This entails taking a small punch biopsy from the scalp and then dissecting our hair follicles from which the stem cells are cultured in a growth medium. The cells are replicated into the millions and then injected back into the person's scalp.

   RepliCel has been involved in a lot of activity over the past years to further develop their RCH-01 treatment into a worldwide success. For starters, RepliCel created a partnership with Shiseido, which is the fourth largest cosmetic company in the world. Also Japan's new legislation which is designed to help expedite the trial process for stem cell technologies makes Japan an ideal place to launch a new cellular-based technology and get it to market quickly. To be clear, Shiseido and RepliCel are separate companies. RepliCel has licensed Shiseido the rights to bring RCH-01 to the world through an expedited regulatory path in Japan.

   Points of interest: Shiseido is currently trialing RepliCel's RCH-01 in Japan for market approval by the end of 2018. RepliCel is also planning on launching its own RCH-01 phase II trial, hopefully sometime in 2017, for the regulatory approval pathway in North America.

2. **Histogen:** Histogen's hair stimulating complex (HSC) is a cell conditioned media that is derived from neonatal cells grown under embryonic-like conditions. It is an injectable serum that is used to stimulate the growth of new hair follicles as well as existing ones in a person's scalp. This treatment was first announced around 2008 and a lot of people are eager for it to be released in the market. The treatment has been trialed on both men and women and is said to be effective at regrowing hair throughout the scalp.

   Points of interest: This is a treatment that has a very high appeal due to its ease of application. Theoretically, you could walk in, receive injections, and walk out. No need to harvest your own cells and come back to get them re-injected such as with other cellular-based treatments.

   Status: Phase III trial, for approval in Mexico, awaiting to be initiated. Histogen is also presently looking to launch a trial for approval in Japan and China. Potentially on the market in Mexico in 2018.

3. **Brotzu lotion:** The "Brotzu lotion" is a product discovered by a vascular surgeon in Italy Dr Giovanni Brotzu. His chance

discovery was based on a drug trial for vascular insufficiency wherein the patients regrew hair on legs. The formula was then modified to use di-homo-γ-linolenic acid (DGLA) instead of PGE1, because DGLA would not be classified as a drug and would require much less clinical trials to be approved for hair growth. The known ingredients of this lotion include DGLA, carnitine, S-equol, and cationic liposomes. The pharmaceutical company Fidia Pharma has acquired the rights to manufacture the Brotzu formula and is apparently performing a clinical study with the lotion for use in people with AGA. The study is still ongoing and Fidia pharmaceuticals has said that the treatment should be available by the end of 2018.

Points of interest: Fidia Pharma purchased the rights to develop this hair growth lotion after viewing its preliminary data. The USP of this product is that it is classified as a cosmetic and could be acquired over-the-counter.

Status: Clinical efficacy trial is ongoing and Fidia Pharma has said the lotion should be released by the end of 2018.

4. **RiverTown Therapeutics Inc.:** RT1640 is composed of **minoxidil, cyclosporine-A**, and a novel drug RT175. This compound has been developed by the founder of RiverTown Therapeutics Inc., David Weinstein MD, PhD. In a phase I trial, 100% of the people who used the treatment had satisfactory hair growth and, reportedly, several people had complete hair regeneration. The three agents in RT1640 act on distinct pathways of AGA and synergize to promote the growth and maintenance of hair follicles. RT1640 also reanimates the melanocytic progenitor cells which give hair its color, hence, RT1640 is said to restore pigment to regenerated hair as well.

Points of interest: The dual results of regrowing hair and restoration of pigment to the hair makes this a potentially useful drug.

Status: Currently raising funds for a phase Ib/IIa study in 2017.

5. **Tsuji-Riken/organ technologies:** Dr Takashi Tsuji runs one of the most advanced stem cell labs in the world at the Riken Institute in Japan. Thankfully, he took up the task of using stem cells to grow hair in his R&D and subsequently got some major partners to help further his work. In mid-2016, it was announced that Riken would be establishing a joint venture with the electronics company Kyocera and the regenerative medicine company. Organ Technologies to bring Dr Tsuji's hair regeneration treatment to the market. The treatment involves extracting a small number of hair follicles from a person's donor scalp area and then isolating two specific types of cells from the follicle—papilla cells and

epidermal cells from the bulge region. These cells are then cultured, expanded, and combined to create a hair follicle "germ" or "follicular primordium." Once the hair follicle germs are ready, they are transported to a facility where they can be implanted back into a person's scalp to grow hair.

Points of interest: Tsuji has been doing hair follicle research for several years now. Organ technologies will develop this treatment in Japan which currently has the fastest track to market approval in the world for cellular therapies. Kyocera has announced that they aim for this treatment to be on the market in 2020.

Status: Currently undergoing research and development with a goal of market release in 2020.

6. **Follica:** Known for being one of the quietest companies on the horizon of hair growth treatments. Follica is also one of the most anticipated. Follica was founded in 2007 and its science is based on creating tiny wounds in the scalp to create hair follicle generation. The name of Follica's treatment has been revealed to be an acronym: **RAIN.** The RAIN treatment is a two-part process which consists of (1) a micro-wounding therapy combined with applied compounds which takes place in the clinic, (2) followed by a treatment package to be used at home consisting of a topical formula and an application device.

Points of interest: Follica's co-founder Dr George Cotsarelis is one of the household names in the hair follicle research world and has an array of hair growth related patents belt. About 10 years deep in development, Follica is planning to initiate a pivotal trial in early 2017, which, pending results, could lead to Follica's hair growth therapy being approved for the market in 2018.

Status: Aiming at FDA clearance in 2017 for a commercial release in 2018.

7. **Follicum:** Follicum is a Swedish biotechnology company that is developing human peptides for the use of stimulating hair growth and inhibiting hair growth. The lead candidate peptide of Follicum is called FOL-005. Specifically, it is called FOL-S-005 when being used to stimulate hair growth. FOL-S-005 is aimed to be commercialized as a topical solution according to Follicum's website. A phase IIa trial of FOL-005 will be completing in January 2017. Follicum has previously mentioned that they expect to observe hair inhibition from this safety trial, so we will have to wait and see what kind of data is acquired through this study.

Points of interest: The hair growth effect of this peptide was discovered accidentally in mice in 2004. This means they have had 11 years to conduct R&D on this discovery. Follicum has been working with renowned hair researcher Ralf Paus since 2012 to further their R&D. They have initiated human trials which began in early 2016 and have secured two major manufacturing partners for their peptide technology.

Follicum has shown that their compound works faster than minoxidil 5% which is a compelling thought as most newer products never compare with minoxidil.

Status: Phase IIa trial to conclude in January 2017, those results to follow in early 2017.

8. **Samumed:** SM04554 is a small-molecule topical solution that activates the **Wnt** pathway to grow hair. In March 2016, Samumed presented their highly anticipated phase II results at the American Academy of Dermatology. The phase II results got a mixed response from the online world of hair growth enthusiasts, but the bottom line is that the treatment grew hair in the trial. Approximately, a 10% overall increase in hair density was observed in the best responding group who used SM04554. Before that study came to completion, Samumed initiated a second phase II study with a scalp biopsy analysis to better understand how their molecule gets the hair to grow. The initial phase II trial lead to the conclusion that this drug does not contain a "dose response" in patients who use it. This means that adding more of the drug to a patient's anatomy does not lead to more results. Finding the "just right" dosage and application is important for this drug to work its best.

Points of interest: Samumed began by breezing their way through clinical trials and completed an important phase II within about two years time from their initial startup. Now the company is looking into ways to optimize its drug to grow hair without a dose response and get to a phase III trial.

Status: Have recently completed the biopsy analysis phase II trial. Samumed has announced a third phase II trial will happen sometime in 2017 before moving into a phase III trial.

9. **Allergan (from Kythera): Setipiprant** is an oral medication. Specifically, it is a prostaglandin D_2 receptor (PGD_2R) antagonist. Setipiprant was originally developed for medical applications aside from hair growth and has undergone clinical trials for other indications. Setipiprant is now undergoing a phase IIa clinical trial in which finasteride is one of the control vehicles. The study is to be completed in September 2017.

Points of interest: Setipiprant has already undergone a phase III trial in the US. This should save it some time in its FDA trial process. As a medication taken by mouth it is easy to administer and comply with.

Status: Undergoing phase IIa clinial trial with a completion date of September 2017.

10. **Dr Angela Christiano and Dr Colin Jahoda (Aclaris and Rapunzel):** Two of the most prominent names when it comes to hair follicle research. Dr Jahoda's latest public work has been focused on 3D dermal papilla culturing, while Dr Christiano has been popping up frequently in news headlines for her research on JAK inhibitors and hair growth. Dr Christiano has even recently sold her JAK inhibitor portfolio to Aclaris therapeutics who is carrying out trials for JAK inhibtor's use in treating AGA and alopecia areata. Even better, these two researchers are reportedly teaming up on Christiano's new startup "Rapunzel" to develop a treatment using cultured hair follicle cells to regenerate hair.

Points of interest: Dr Jahoda implanted his own hair cells into his wife's arm and found that his cells grew hair on her arm all the way back in 1999. In other words, the man is experienced in cellular hair growth research. Also, Jahoda and Christiano have both been issued a new patent related to 3D hair follicle culturing in January 2017.

Status: Rapunzel could enter headlines as early as 2nd Q 2017.

Acknowledgments

We acknowledge the permission given for re drawing the image (Fig. 14.4) from the seminal work by Dr Lu Q. Le, MD, PhD, Associate Professor, Department of Dermatology, Simmons Comprehensive Cancer Center, Hamon Center for Regenerative Medicine and Science University of Texas, Southwestern Medical School, USA.

Bibliography

1. Adams JU. Raising hairs. Nat Biotechnol 2011;29(6):474–6.
2. Aggarwal S, Thareja S, Verma A, et al. An overview on 5α-reductase inhibitors. Steroids 2010;75(2):109–53.
3. Aoi N, Inoue K, Chikanishi T, et al. 1, 25-dihydroxyvitamin D_3 modulates the hair-inductive capacity of dermal papilla cells: therapeutic potential for hair regeneration. Stem Cells Transl Med 2012;1(8):615–26.
4. Asakawa K, Toyoshima KE, Tsuji T. Functional Hair Follicle Regeneration by the Rearrangement of Stem Cells. Methods Mol Biol. 2017;1597: 117–34.
5. Azzouni F, Godoy A, Li Y, Mohler J. The 5α-reductase isozyme family: a review of basic biology and their role in human diseases. Adv Urol 2011;2012.

6. Bayne E, Flanagan J, Einstein M, et al. Immunohistochemical localization of types I and II 5α-reductase in human scalp. Br J Dermatol 1999;141:481–91.

7. Bovee TF, Schoonen WG, Hamers AR, et al. Screening of synthetic and plant-derived compounds for (anti) estrogenic and (anti) androgenic activities. Anal Bioanal Chem 2008;390(4):1111–19.

8. Caserini M, Radicioni M, Annoni O, Palmieri R. Pharmacokinetics and pharmacodynamics of finasteride topical solution after single and repeated dose in subjects with androgenetic alopecia. 42nd Annual ESDR Meeting; 18–22 September 2012; Venice.

9. Chen W, Orfanos C. The 5α-recluctase system and its inhibitors. Dermatology 1996;193(3):177–84.

10. Choi YS, Zhang Y, Xu M, et al. Distinct functions for Wnt/β-catenin in hair follicle stem cell proliferation and survival and interfollicular epidermal homeostasis. Cell Stem Cell 2013;13(6):720–33.

11. Cotsarelis G, Millar SE. Towards a molecular understanding of hair loss and its treatment. Trends Mol Med 2001;7(7):293–301.

12. Digiuni M, Manni G, Vetrugno M, et al. An evaluation of Therapeutic Noninferiority of 0.005% lanatoprost ophthalmic solution and Xalatan in patients with glaucoma or ocular hypertension. J Glaucoma 2012.

13. Dong L, Hao H, Liu J, Ti D, Tong C, Hou Q, et al. A Conditioned Medium of Umbilical Cord Mesenchymal Stem Cells Overexpressing Wnt7a Promotes Wound Repair and Regeneration of Hair Follicles in Mice. Stem Cells Int, 2017.

14. Eppley BL, Pietzak WS, Blanton M. Platelet-rich plasma: a review of biology and applications in plastic surgery. Plast Reconstr Surg 2006;118(6):147e–59e.

15. Garza LA, Liu Y, Yang Z, et al. Prostaglandin D_2 inhibits hair growth and is elevated in bald scalp of men with androgenetic alopecia. Sci Transl Med 2012;4(126):126ra34.

16. Hajheydari Z, Akbari J, Saeedi M, Shokoohi L. Comparing the therapeutic effects of finasteride gel and tablet in treatment of the androgenetic alopecia. Indian J Dermatol Venereol Leprol 2009;75(1):47–51.

17. Hugh Rushton D, Norris MJ, Van Neste D. Hair regrowth in male and female pattern hair loss does not involve the conversion of vellus hair to terminal hair. Exp Dermatol 2016 Jun;25(6):482–4.

18. Iino M, Ehama R, Nakazawa Y, et al. Adenosine stimulates fibroblast growth factor-7 gene expression via adenosine A2b receptor signaling in dermal papilla cells. J Invest Dermatol 2007;127(6):1318–25.

19. Inui S, Nakajima T, Fukuzato Y, et al. Potential anti-androgenic activity of roxithromycin in skin. J Dermatol Sci 2001;27(2):147–51.

20. Itami S, Inui S. Role of androgen in mesenchymal epithelial interactions in human hair follicle. J Investig Dermatol Symp Proc 2005;10(3):209–11.

21. Jeong YM, Sung YK, Kim WK, et al. Ultraviolet B preconditioning enhances the hair growth-promoting effects of adipose-derived stem cells via

generation of reactive oxygen species. Stem Cells Dev 2013;22(1):158–68.

22. Jo SJ, Choi SJ, Yoon SY, et al. Valproic acid promotes human hair growth in *in vitro* culture model. J Dermatol Sci 2013;72(1):16–24.

23. Jo SJ, Shin H, Park YW, et al. Topical valproic acid increases the hair count in male patients with androgenetic alopecia:a randomized, comparative, clinical feasibility study using phototrichogram analysis. J Dermatol 2014;41(4):285–91.

24. Johnstone MA. Hypertrichosis and increased pigmentation of eyelashes and adjacent hair in the region of the ipsilateral eyelids of patients treated with unilateral topical latanoprost. Am J Ophthalmol 1997;124(4):544–7.

25. Kadry R, Hamadah I, Al-Issa A, et al. Multiple scalp abscess with subcutaneous fat necrosis and scarring alopecia as a complication of scalp mesotherapy. J Drugs Dermatol 2008;7(1):72–3.

26. Kwon TR, Oh CT, Park HM, Han HJ, Ji HJ, Kim BJ. Potential synergistic effects of human placental extract and minoxidil on hair growth-promoting activity in C57BL/6J mice. Clin Exp Dermatol 2015 Aug;40(6):672–81.

27. Lee SH, Yoon J, Shin SH, Zahoor M, Kim HJ, Park PJ, et al. Valproic acid induces hair regeneration in murine model and activates alkaline phosphatase activity in human dermal papilla cells. PLoS One. 2012;7(4):e34152.

28. Li ZJ, Choi HI, Choi DK, et al. Autologous platelet-rich plasma: a potential therapeutic tool for promoting hair growth. Dermatol Surg 2012;38(7 Pt 1):1040–6.

29. Liao CP, Booker RC, Morrison SJ, Le LQ. Identification of hair shaft progenitors that create a niche for hair pigmentation. Genes Dev 2017 Apr 15;31(8):744–756.

30. Madheswaran T, Baskaran R, Thapa RK, et al. Design and *in vitro* evaluation of finasteride-loaded liquid crystalline nanoparticles for topical delivery. AAPS Pharm Sci Tech 2013;14(1):45–52.

31. Meyer KC, Klatte JE, Dinh HV, et al. Evidence that the bulge region is a site of relative immune privilege in human hair follicles. Br J Dermatol 2008;159(5):1077–85.

32. Moftah N, Moftah N, Abd-Elaziz G, et al. Mesotherapy using dutasteride-containing preparation in treatment of female pattern hair loss: photographic, morphometric and ultrastructural evaluation. J Eur Acad Dermatol Venereol 2012;published online 6 April 2012.

33. Mokos ZB, Mosler EL. Advances in a rapidly emerging field of hair follicle stem cell research. Coll Antropol 2014;38(1):373–8.

34. Randall VA. Androgens and human hair growth. Clin Endocrinol (Oxf) 1994;40(4):439–57.

35. Reichrath J, Schilli M, Kerber A, et al. Hair follicle expression of 1, 25-dihydroxyvitamin D_3 receptors during the murine hair cycle. Br J Dermatol 1994;131(4):477–82.

36. Roh SS, Kim CD, Lee MH, et al. The hair growth promoting effect of *Sophora flavescens* extract and its molecular regulation. J Dermatol Sci 2002;30(1):43–9.

37. Seo HS, Lee DJ, Chung JH, Lee CH, Kim HR, Kim JE, Kim BJ, Jung MH, Ha KT,Jeong HS. Hominis placenta facilitates hair re-growth by upregulating cellular proliferation and expression of fibroblast growth factor-7. BMC Complement Altern Med 2016 Jul 7;16:187.

38. Shimizu H, Morgan BA. Wnt signaling through the β-catenin pathway is sufficient to maintain, but not restore, anagen-phase characteristics of dermal papilla cells. J Investig Dermatol 2004;122(2):239–45.

39. Shin H, Won CH, Chung WK, Park up-to-date Clinical Trials of Hair Regeneration using Conditioned Media of Adipose-derived Stem Cells in Male and Female Pattern Hair Loss BS. Curr Stem Cell Res Ther. 2017 May 4.

40. Smith S, Fagien S, Whitcup SM, et al. Eyelash growth in subjects treated with bimatoprost: a multicenter, randomized, double-masked, vehicle-controlled, parallel-group study. J Am Acad Dermatol 2012;66(5):801–6.

41. Tobin DJ. The biogenesis and growth of human hair. In: Tobin DJ, editor. Hair in toxicology—an important bio-monitor. RSC Publishing, Cambridge; 2005.

42. Toyoshima KE, Asakawa K, Ishibashi N, et al. Fully functional hair follicle regeneration through the rearrangement of stem cells and their niches. Nat Commun 2012;3:784.

43. Trifu V, Tiplica GS, Naumescu E, et al. Cortexolone 17α-propionate 1% cream, a new potent antiandrogen for topical treatment of acne vulgaris. A pilot randomized, double-blind comparative study vs placebo and tretinoin 0.05% cream. Br J Dermatol 2011;165(1):177–83.

44. Tsuboi R. Growth factors and hair growth. J Invest Dermatol 1997;4(2):103–8.

45. Uebel CO, da Silva JB, Cantarelli D, Martins P. The role of platelet plasma growth factors in male pattern baldness surgery. Plast Reconstr Surg 2006;118(6):1458–66.

46. Vegesna V, O'Kelly J, Uskokovic M, et al. Vitamin D_3 analogs stimulate hair growth in nude mice. Endocrinology 2002;143(11):4389–96.

47. Yamana K, Labrie F. Human type III 5α-reductase is expressed in peripheral tissues at higher levels than types I and II and its activity is potently inhibited by finasteride and dutasteride. Horm Mol Biol Clin Invest 2010;2(3):293–9.

48. Zimber MP, Ziering C, Zeigler F, et al. Hair regrowth following a Wnt and follistatin containing treatment: safety and efficacy in a first-in-man phase I clinical trial. J Drugs Dermatol 2011;10(11):1308–12.

15

Role of Nutrition and Off-Label Treatments for Hair Loss

Ananta Khurana

INTRODUCTION

The medical therapy of hair loss is a multi-million dollar industry and is based on the psychological consequences of hair loss and the rampant OTC advertised products, most of which have a little evidence to back their claims. The self-limiting nature of acute telogen effluvium and the variation of seasons that affect the hair loss, is one of the reasons that some so-called "successful" therapies might work.

A European consensus group (Blumeyer A et al) that examined the various therapies for the treatment of androgenetic alopecia in a systematic literature review found that, of the plethora of products, there was excellent evidence levels for the therapeutic use of topical minoxidil and of oral finasteride with low evidence levels for hormonal treatments (in women), even though most of the products listed in Table 15.1 are frequently prescribed by practitioners.

But conversely, it must be accepted that there is a well established list of essential nutrients (Table 15.2) required for hair integrity, and in India, because of varying levels of nutritional intake, a deficiency might manifest as hair loss. Vegetarian diet and concomitant iron deficiency can be a major factor in hair loss in a proportion of patients. Therefore, good medical practice involves integrating personal clinical expertise with the best available clinical evidence. There are compounded preparations that possibly exhibit a profound effect in patients, even though not covered in scientific databases.

NUTRITIONAL AGENTS

Though there is some evidence to show that some nutritional supplements may have a role in alopecia, but the moot point is whether increasing the content of an already adequate diet with specific amino acids, vitamins, and/or trace elements can promote hair growth.

Table 15.1: A list of miscellaneous treatments proposed for treatment of hair loss

Promotion of hair regrowth	Aloe vera
	Amino acids
	Bergamot
	Caffeine
	Chinese herbals
	Cyclosporine
	Electromagnetic/electrostatic field
	Ginkgo biloba
	Ginseng
	Hibiscus
	Iron supplements in the absence of deficiency
	Low-level laser
	Marine extract and silicea component
	Melatonin
	Millet seed (silicic acid, amino acids, vitamins, minerals)
	Proanthocyanidins
	Retinoids
	Sorphora
	Vitamins (biotin, niacin derivates)
Improved perifollicular vascularization	Aminexil
	Glycerol oxyesters and silicium
	Mesotherapy
	Minerals
	Niacin derivatives
	Prostaglandins (viprostol, latanoprost)
DHT inhibitory activity	*Cimicifuga racemosa*
	Green tea
	Polysorbate 60
	Saw palmetto
	β-sitosterol
Anti-inflammatory activity	Ketoconazole
	Zinc pyrithione
	Corticosteroids
Improved hair nutrition	Vitamins (biotin, niacin derivates)
	Trace elements (zinc, copper)
Others	Botulinum toxin

Table 15.2: Micronutrients relevant to the hair and recommended daily allowances

Vitamins

B vitamins
- Biotin (vitamin H): 30 µg
- Niacin (vitamin B$_3$): 20 mg
- Folic acid: 300 µg
- Riboflavin (vitamin B$_2$): 1.7 mg
- Pantothenic acid (vitamin B$_5$): 5 mg
- Pyridoxine (vitamin B$_6$): 1.5 mg
- Cyanocobalamin (vitamin B$_{12}$): 3 µg

Other vitamins
- Vitamin A/β-carotene: 6 mg
- α-tocopherol (vitamin E): 10 IU

Trace metals

Iron: Depending on age and sex (in men: 8–10 mg)
Zinc: 15 mg
Selenium: 50 mg

It is pertinent to note that in urban India, paradoxically, the consumption of junk food may predispose to nutritional imbalances as opposed to rural areas where this is not a issue. Thus, the consequent malnutrition may cause hair loss. A vegetarian diet, followed by a large chunk of our population, also predisposes to specific nutrient deficiencies and consequences thereof.

Iron

Iron deficiency (ID)/iron deficiency anemia (IDA) is the most common nutritional deficiency around the world. The interest in its association with hair disorders has generated many papers over past several decades. But conclusive evidence for the role of iron deficiency causing hair loss is still lacking.

While the mechanism of action by which iron affects hair growth is not known, hair follicle matrix cells are some of the most rapidly dividing cells in the body, and ID may contribute to hair loss via its role as a cofactor for ribonucleotide reductase, the rate-limiting enzyme for DNA synthesis. In addition, multiple genes have been identified in the human hair follicle, some of which may be regulated by iron. In a mouse model, reversal of iron deficiency in Tmprss 6 mutated mice, following iron administration, lead to a reversal of the associated hair loss as well.

Table 15.3 summarizes the studies done on iron deficiency on different causes of hair loss so far. However, it is difficult to derive

Table 15.3: Summary of studies on iron deficiency in hair loss			
Chronic telogen effluvium			
Authors/year of publication	*Patients and controls included*	*Parameters measured and compared/ intervention done*	*Result*
Rushton, 2002	12 female patients	7/12 treated with 72 mg iron and 1.5 g L-lysine for 6 months; 5/12 given placebo	31% reduction in hair fall in treated group vs 9% increase in placebo group Ferritin levels increased from 41.3 to 68.9 µg/ml in treated group (insignificant rise in controls)
Rushton, 2002	22 females, no controls	All given 72 mg iron plus 1.5 g L-lysine for 6 months	Mean ferritin increased from 33 to 89 µg/L Telogen % reduced from 19.5 to 11.3%
Rushton, 2003	20 females, no controls	Serum ferritin measured	65% had levels <40 µg/L; 95% had levels <70 µg/L
Kantor, 2003	Total 196 patients; 30 of CTE, 11 healthy controls	Serum ferritin	Values of patients not lower than controls; hemoglobin levels also did not differ
Sinclair, 2002	Total 194 patients; 12 had ferritin <20 µg/ml; 3 classified as CTE in view of normal histology	Oral iron given for 3–6 months till ferritin increased to >20 µg/ml	No improvement in hair fall
Olsen, 2010	96 women with CTE, 76 healthy controls	Serum ferritin	When ferritin <15 µg/L taken as cut-off: ID in 12.1% of pre-menopausal CTE patients and 29.8%

(Contd.)

Table 15.3: Summary of studies on iron deficiency in hair loss (*Contd.*)

Chronic telogen effluvium

Authors/year of publication	Patients and controls included	Parameters measured and compared/ intervention done	Result
			pre-menopausal controls; and in 10.5% post-menopausal CTE patients vs 6.9% post-menopausal controls. With cut-off of ferritin >40 µg/L: ID seen in 63.8% of pre-menopausal women vs 72.3% of pre-menopausal controls and 36.8% post-menopausal CTE women vs 20.7% post-menopausal controls. No statistically signifi-cant difference between any group
Rasheed et al, 2013	42 patients included, 40 controls	Serum ferritin	Levels in TE (14.7 ± 22.1 µg/L) were significantly lower than in controls (43.5 ± 20.4 µg/L)
Androgenetic alopecia			
Rushton et al, 1990	100 women included, 20 controls	50/100 underwent investigations	36 of these (72%) had serum ferritin below the lowest value seen in control subjects
Rushton and Ramsay, 1992	40 pre-menopausal females with androgenetic alopecia	20 patients (10 with ferritin <40 µg/L and 10 with ferritin	Increase in total hair density (hair/ cm²) and meaningful hair

(Contd.)

Table 15.3: Summary of studies on iron deficiency in hair loss (*Contd.*)

Androgenetic alopecia

Authors/year of publication	Patients and controls included	Parameters measured and compared/ intervention done	Result
		>40 µg/L) treated with cyproterone acetate—ethyl estradiol in reverse sequential regime for 12 months 20 untreated (again with equal distribution of ferritin <40 µg/L and >40 µg/L levels)	density (non-vellus hair/cm²) only in treated patients with serum ferritin above 40 µg/L, but not in those with ferritin below 40 µg/L. In the control group a significant mean decrease in total hair density and meaningful hair density after 12 months
Aydingoz et al, 1999	43 female patients with androgenetic alopecia, 46 healthy controls	Serum ferritin compared	No difference between the two groups
Sinclair, 2002 (same as above)	117/194 AGA with ferritin >20 µg/L 7 patients with AGA had serum ferritin <20 µg/L (Hb normal)	All treated with spironolactone *plus* iron given in addition to those with ferritin <20 µg/L, for 3–6 months	4/7 low ferritin patients improved with treatment Results were similar to the response rates seen in the other 108 patients who received oral antiandrogens only. Thus, concluded no role of ID in AGA
Olsen, 2010 (same as above)	285 FPHL, 76 controls	Serum ferritin compared	When ferritin <15 µg/L taken as cut-off: ID in 12.4% of pre-menopausal FPHL women and

(Contd.)

Table 15.3: Summary of studies on iron deficiency in hair loss (*Contd.*)

Androgenetic alopecia

Authors/year of publication	Patients and controls included	Parameters measured and compared/ intervention done	Result
			29.8% pre-menopausal controls, and in 1.7% post-menopausal FPHL patients vs 6.9% post-menopausal controls. Cut-off ferritin >40 µg/L: ID 58.8% pre-menopausal FPHL patients and 72.3% pre-menopausal controls and in 26.1% post-menopausal patients vs 20.7% of post-menopausal controls. No statistically significant difference between any group
Rasheed et al, 2013	38 patients included, 40 controls	Serum ferritin	Levels in FPHL (23.9 ± 38.5 µg/L) were significantly lower than in controls (43.5 ± 20.4 µg/L)

Alopecia areata

White, 1994	9 males and 21 female patients, no controls	Assessed for IDA/ID, did not mention criteria	71% female patients had ID and 14% had IDA. No male patient had ID/IDA

(*Contd.*)

Table 15.3: Summary of studies on iron deficiency in hair loss (*Contd.*)			
Alopecia areata			
Authors/year of publication	Patients and controls included	Parameters measured and compared/ intervention done	Result
Boffa et al, 1995	32 patients (21 females and 11 males), No controls	Serum ferritin and Hb measured. ID defined as ferritin <15 µg/L, IDA as Hb <12 in females and <13 in males	No increase in incidence of ID in alopecia areata patients
Esfandiarpour et al, 2008	23 female and 29 male patients, 63 controls	Serum iron, ferritin and TIBC measured	No difference in parameters between patients and controls

conclusive answers from these owing to different criteria used to label iron deficiency, absence of controls in some and variability in criteria used to include controls in others.

Serum ferritin is an indicator of iron stores in the body and the most commonly used criteria to define an iron deficient state, the only disadvantage being that it is unreliable in the presence of infection/inflammation. The cut-offs used to define ID have been variable. WHO recommends the cut-off of <15 ng/ml in adults and <12 ng/ml in children, below which iron stores are considered to be depleted. However, others have commented that levels lower than 30 ng/ml are sensitive (92%) and specific (98%) for identifying absolute ID, correlating with the absence of iron stores in the bone marrow. Further increase in sensitivity (98%) is achieved by raising the cut-off to 40 ng/ml. Rushton et al recommend using the ferritin cut-off of 70 ng/ml (along with ESR <10 mm/hr) for patients complaining of increased hair fall.

Other markers have also been used but are less reliable. Iron deficiency results in a reduction in serum iron levels, an elevation in transferrin (total iron-binding capacity [TIBC]) levels, and hence a net reduction in transferrin saturation (i.e. SI/TIBC). However, the diurnal variation both in serum iron and transferrin saturation is considerable. In addition, there is a marked overlap in these indices between normal and iron-deficient subjects. Serum soluble transferrin receptor has been used in epidemiological studies but lacks standardization to be employed in clinical practice. Serum hepcidin is a novel biomarker, which may be used in near future.

Thus, the literature available so far has not been able to give a definite answer as to whether ID without anemia needs to be treated in patients with hair fall (particularly FPHL and CTE/CDTHL). Further, excess of iron is toxic to the body and unnecessary treatment must be avoided. However, ID associated with anemia is an important cause of telogen effluvium and hence measurement of Hb, RBC indices and serum ferritin makes perfect sense in all patients with chronic telogen loss. On the same lines, it is essential to treat ID associated with anemia, as hair fall is just one of the myriad manifestations of IDA.

Typically, for iron replacement therapy, up to 200 mg of elemental iron per day is given, usually as three or four iron tablets (each containing 50–65 mg elemental iron) given over the course of the day. Ideally, oral iron preparations should be taken on an empty stomach, since food may inhibit iron absorption. A dose of 200 mg of elemental iron per day results in the absorption of up to 50 mg of iron. This supports a red cell production level of two to three times normal in an individual with a normally functioning marrow and appropriate erythropoietin stimulus. The reticulocyte count should rise in 1 week and hemoglobin should start rising by the second week of therapy. However, as the hemoglobin level rises, erythropoietin stimulation decreases, and the amount of iron absorbed is reduced. The goal of therapy in individuals with iron deficiency anemia is not only to repair the anemia but also to provide stores of at least 0.5–1 g of iron. Sustained treatment for a period of 6–12 months after correction of the anemia will be necessary to achieve this. Gastrointestinal distress is the most prominent adverse effect with oral iron therapy and is seen in 15–20% of patients. Abdominal pain, nausea, vomiting, or constipation may occur, leading to noncompliance. Of late, there have been studies supporting lower doses/less frequent administration of iron to achieve desired response. A trial comparing 15, 50, and 150 mg oral elemental iron showed that there was no difference in ferritin rise with any dose and showed less gastrointestinal toxicity with the smallest dose. This is because enterocyte iron absorption appears to be saturable, and one dose of iron can "block" absorption of further iron doses for the rest of the day. Another study highlighted that giving 60 mg ferrous sulphate on alternate days maximized fractional iron absorption, increased efficacy and reduced GI side effects. However, iron toxicity can occur with excessive use resulting in gastrointestinal bleeding, abdominal pain and metabolic acidosis in the acute phase and hemochromatosis over prolonged duration.

Biotin

Biotin, or vitamin H, serves as a cofactor for carboxylation enzymes. Biotin deficiency is rare, as intestinal bacteria produce biotin more than the body's daily requirements. Moreover, biotin is consumed from a wide range of food sources in the diet. Deficiency is seen in cases of congenital or acquired biotinidase or carboxylase deficiency, antibiotic use disrupting the gastrointestinal flora, and antiepileptic use (especially valproate). Interestingly, reversal of alopecia induced by valproate has been reported with 10 mg/day of oral biotin. The requirement of biotin is increased in pregnancy and lactation. Smoking may further accelerate biotin catabolism in women. Alcoholics have been found to have greater incidence of biotin deficiency than the general population. Further, relatively low levels of biotin have been reported in patients on parenteral nutrition, those who have had a partial gastrectomy or other causes of achlorhydria, patients on isotretinoin for acne treatment, elderly individuals, and athletes. Deficiency of biotin can also occur with excessive ingestion of raw egg whites due to binding by avidin. Symptoms of deficiency include eczematous skin rash (seborrheic dermatitis like picture), alopecia, conjunctivitis and neurological features like depression, lethargy, hallucination, and numbness and tingling of the extremities.

Biotin treatment has shown efficacy in treating brittle fingernails and onychoschizia. However, no clinical trials have shown role of biotin in treating hair loss of any etiology. Yet, it is the most commonly marketed and prescribed supplement for hair loss. When biotin deficiency is suspected on clinical grounds, the serum biotin level must be determined, and in case of biotin deficiency (<100 ng/L), the cause must be sought (unless obvious from the patient history) and treated. Regardless of the cause, the deficiency can usually be successfully addressed directly with supplementation with oral biotin supplements (which generally have a good bio availability), usually in a dosage of 5 mg/day. Fortunately (in contrast to other nutritional supplements, such as vitamin A, selenium, iron, and zinc), there is no known toxicity of biotin supplementation in an order of magnitude greater than of the nutritional requirements.

Zinc

Zinc is an essential mineral required by many enzymes and transcription factors that regulate gene expression. It plays an important role in the Hedgehog pathway governing hair follicle morphogenesis. It is also an essential component of numerous metalloenzymes important in protein synthesis and cell division. Zinc deficiency may be either inherited (acrodermatitis enteropathica) or acquired (with malabsorption syndromes or gastric bypass surgery). In addition, deficiency can occur with liver or renal dysfunction, malignancy, alcoholism, and drugs (mainly valproate and some anti-hypertensives). Patients may experience diarrhea, immunological effects, abnormalities in taste and smell and delayed wound healing. Cutaneous effects include acral and periorificial dermatitis, while hair changes include TE and brittle hair.

Only a few studies have studied the role of Zinc deficiency in hair loss conditions. Kil et al (2013) measured zinc concentration in 312 patients with alopecia areata, MPHL, FPHL, or TE and showed that all groups had statistically lower zinc concentrations as compared to 30 healthy controls. Karashima et al (2012) reported 5 patients, with telogen effluvium and zinc deficiency, who responded to supplementation with a proprietary zinc preparation Promac®. In another study (Park et al, 2009), in patients with alopecia areata and low serum zinc levels, oral supplementation with 50 mg/day zinc was shown to have therapeutic effects, although this did not reach statistical significance.

There is even sparse information on the effects of zinc supplementation on hair growth in those without documented deficiency. Slonim et al (1992) described a single patient with dry brittle hair and alopecia, without clear deficiency, who experienced improvement following oral zinc therapy.

Excess supplementation can however be toxic causing acute effects including epigastric pain, nausea, vomiting diarrhea, and headache and chronic toxic effects including reduced copper status, interaction with iron, reduced immune function, and decreased concentrations of HDL cholesterol (Table 15.4).

Vitamin E

Vitamin E deficiency results in hemolytic anemias, neurologic findings, and skin dryness. Tocotrienols and tocopherols are members of the vitamin E family and are potent antioxidants. Tocotrienols possess more potent antioxidant property owing to their ability to better distribute within the fatty layers of the cell membranes and hence permit better interaction with lipid radicals.

Vitamin E deficiency is rare, but may occur with fat malabsorption disorders. There is no literature backing the use of vitamin E in hair loss conditions. But it is still widely used with the assumption of improvement in hair growth owing to its antioxidant properties.

Beoy et al (2010) conducted a randomized double blinded controlled trial, wherein 21 patients with alopecia (type not classified further) were given 100 mg of mixed tocotrienols daily and 17 volunteers given

Table 15.4: Nutrient deficiencies associated with drugs/medical diseases

Disease/drug	Associated deficiency
History of blood loss (menstrual in pre-menopausal women, GI in post-menopausal women and men)	Iron
Malabsorption disorders	Multiple vitamin deficiencies
Pregnancy	Iron, folic acid, zinc
Alcoholism	Folic acid, zinc, niacin
Malignancy	Iron, zinc, can depend on type of malignancy
Renal dysfunction	Selenium, zinc
H2 blocker use	Iron
Antiepileptics	Biotin, Zinc
Antihypertensives	Zinc
Prolonged antibiotic use	Biotin
Isoniazid	Niacin
Inadequate sun exposure	Vitamin D
Vegans/vegetarians	Iron, zinc
Excessive ingestion of raw egg whites	Biotin
Malnutrition	Multiple vitamin deficiencies

placebo, for 8 months. The authors reported an increase in number of hair in a pre-determined scalp area in the treated group, after 8 months.

Toxicity with excessive use manifests as increased risk of bleeding, decreased thyroid hormone production and possibly adverse effect on hair growth.

Vitamin D

Vitamin D receptors are found in the outer root sheath keratinocytes during growth phase of the hair cycle. Animal models have shown hair loss in vitamin D deficient states. Vitamin D deficiency has been linked with alopecia areata and treatment with topical vitamin D analogs has been shown to be beneficial in a few studies. Eight women with TE or FPHL were found to have significantly lower values compared with healthy controls (Rasheed et al, 2013).

Thus, sufficient data on vitamin D supplementation is still lacking.

Selenium

Selenium is an essential trace element that has anti-oxidant role and plays a part in hair follicle morphogenesis. Two animal studies have shown sparse hair growth in deficient mice but exact role in humans is not known. It is a part of popular supplements sold in India, but without any evidence backing.

Risk factors for deficiency include living in areas with low selenium soil content, long-term hemodialysis, HIV, and malabsorption disorders. A recent meta-analysis (Jin et al, 2017) commented on possible role of selenium deficiency in alopecia areata. Toxicity can occur with overdose and result in hair loss, GI symptoms, blistering skin lesions and memory difficulties.

Vitamin A

Retinoids, isotretinoin and acitretin, have known association with hair loss. However, the effect of vitamin A on hair is complex, with both low and excess levels causing adverse effects on hair in animal models (Everts et al, 2013). Interestingly, a report mentions resolution of extensive alopecia areata with alitretinoin, given for concomitant hand eczema (Kolesnik et al, 2013). Further, topical application of Bexarotene, another retinoid, has been tried, with variable success, for treating alopecia areata (Talpur et al, 2002).

However, there are no reports on successful use of vitamin A supplementation in hair loss disorders.

And oversupplementation is known to cause hypervitaminosis A leading to hair loss and effects on skin, vision, bones and raised intracranial pressure.

Niacin

Pellagra, due to niacin deficiency, is associated with alopecia in some. However, niacin deficiency is rare and mostly occurs in the setting of alcoholism now. Other causes may be malabsorption disorders and with drugs especially isoniazid. No studies regarding niacin levels in hair loss patients are available so far.

Folic Acid

No difference in folate levels was observed between 91 patients complaining of diffuse hair loss and controls (Durusoy et al, 2009). There is no literature on the effects of folic acid supplementation on hair loss.

Essential Fatty Acids (EFA)

Deficiency of the polyunsaturated essential fatty acids, linoleic acid (an omega-6 fatty acid) and alpha-linolenic acid (an omega-3 fatty acid) can result from prolonged parenteral nutrition and malabsorption disorders such as cystic fibrosis. Hair changes include loss of scalp hair and eyebrows and lightening of hair. Unsaturated fatty acids may also modulate androgen action by inhibition of 5α-reductase, similar to finasteride (Liang et al, 1992). Additionally, arachidonic acid, an omega-6 fatty acid, may promote hair growth by increasing the expression of growth factors in human dermal papilla cells and enhancing follicle proliferation and survival (Munkhbayar et al, 2016).

However, there is no good evidence on the effects of EFA supplementation on hair loss. Cutaneous manifestations of EFA deficiency (scalp dermatitis, alopecia, and depigmentation of hair), in a 19-year-old on intravenous hyperalimentation fluids, were reportedly reversed with continued topical application of safflower oil, which contains 60 to 70% linoleic acid (Sklonik et al, 1977).

Amino Acids and Proteins

Protein malnutrition, such as in kwashiorkor and marasmus, can result in hair thinning, discoloration and hair loss. However, with a normal diet, the effect of protein/amino acid supplementation is not clear.

In the 1960s, the role of the sulfur-containing amino acids L-cystine and L-methionine in the production of wool in sheep was investigated, and it was found that enrichment of a normal diet with L-cystine and L-methionine increased wool production. When considering which dietary supplements could be used for improving hair growth in humans, L-cystine was therefore considered, and starting in the early 1990s, studies on the effect of dietary supplements containing L-cystine in combination with B complex vitamins and medicinal yeast, a rich natural source of amino acids and B complex vitamins, were performed and showed improvements in anagen rates, in hair swelling as a criterion for hair quality, and in the tensile strength of hair fibers.

Further, chemically relaxed hair were shown to have reduced cystine content leading to fragility (Khumalo, 2010). Another amino acid L-lysine may play a role in iron and zinc uptake. Rushton et al have reported successful use of L-lysine with iron as mentioned previously. Other trials have evaluated supplements containing marine proteins in conjunction with multiple other nutrients. However, it is difficult to evaluate the results of these trials, as the composition of these nutritional supplements is not disclosed.

Antioxidants

Components of antioxidant formulations, including Vitamin A, vitamin E, zinc, selenium have been described previously. Oxidative stress has been implicated in the pathogenesis of alopecia areata and in *in vitro* studies on androgenetic alopecia. However, effect of potentially antioxidant molecules in these states has not been researched. In general, it is prudent to keep in mind that high doses of exogenous antioxidants may actually disrupt the balance between oxidation and antioxidation (Bouayed, 2010). *In vitro* studies have shown that while polyphenols have antioxidant properties at low concentrations, they can potentiate ROS generation at higher concentrations. Thus, dietary antioxidants may be safer and reliable, rather than high doses of isolated exogenous antioxidants.

OFF-LABEL TOPICAL AND ORAL HAIR LOSS PRODUCTS

There are a number of molecules, available in combinations, in various products marketed for hair loss. Most **oral** preparations have varying combinations of vitamins, minerals and amino acids, while the **topical 'serums'** contain peptides and herbal products, most of which have minimal or no scientific evidence to their credit. The information regarding some of these has been taken from proprietary sites, as the same is lacking on the medical literature search engines.

1. **Capixyl™:** Capixyl™ is a combination of a biomimetic peptide (acetyl tetrapeptide-3) combined with a red clover extract rich in biochanin A. Although the two ingredients are also used separately in some products, the manufacturers claim that the combination has synergistic effects.

   The following are the claimed biological effects of the 2 ingredients/ Capixyl™:

   a. The combination decreases pro-inflammatory cytokines with a synergistic action compared to the inhibition caused by red clover extract alone.

   b. Biochanin A inhibits 5α-reductase activity, thus reducing miniaturization.

   c. Acetyl tetrapeptide-3 stimulates collagen production for better ECM integrity leading to a "better anchoring".

   d. Capixyl™ induces a visible increase in the anagen hair density and a reduction in the telogen hair density in comparison with placebo.

2. **Procapil™:** Procapil™ is the trademark name for the patented compound biotinyl tripedtide-1.

   It is a combination of a vitaminated matrikine with apigenin and oleanolic acid from olive tree leaves. Matrikines refers to peptides originating from the fragmentation of matrix proteins and presenting biological activities especially tissue repair processes. We could not find any information on the specific matrikine being referred to, with respect to Procapil™.

   Procapil™ allegedly acts by improving scalp microcirculation and counters the follicle aging and follicle atrophy caused by dihydrotestosterone (DHT) by its "DHT-blocking mechanism". It is also claimed to activate a number of genes responsible for tissue repair mechanisms which helps in "keeping hair strong and healthy".

3. **Saw palmetto extract:** Saw palmetto is an extract made from the fruits of a small palm tree (*Serenoa repens*), which is endemic to the South-Eastern USA. It is the primary active ingredient in many hair loss products. It is rich in fatty acids and phytosterols and it is often claimed to be able to block dihydrotestosterone (DHT). There are published studies of saw palmetto both of the oral (Prager N et al) and topical preparations (Wessagowit V et al), but the results are inferior to finasteride (Rossi A et al).

4. **Sapindus trifoliatus (syn reetha):** The shell of the fruit of this plant is a popular component of herbal hair loss remedies and shampoos in India. Dixit et al (1982) reported its antiandrogenic activity in male rodents. There are no studies on its use in hair disorders.

5. **Eclipta alba extract (syn "Bhringraj"; "False Daisy"):** Four studies on rodents have shown hair growth promoting activity of this ayurvedic herb.

   Begum et al (2016) demonstrated that the extract reduced the levels of transforming growth factor-$\beta 1$ (TGF-$\beta 1$) expression during early anagen and anagen-catagen transition and acts as an important exogenous mediator stimulating follicular keratinocyte proliferation.

6. ***Emblica officianalis* extract (syn *Phyllanthus emblica*, amla):** Kumar et al (2012) have reported 5α-reductase inhibition with it, using enzymes from rat liver.

7. **Arnica montana extract:** This is a homeopathic drug, with no studies on hair growth to its credit.

8. **Hibiscus extract (syn gudhal):** Hibiscus leaf extracts have been reported to promote hair growth in a rodent model (Adhirajan et al, 2003). It is a common component of ayurvedic hair cleansers, conditioners and oils.

9. **Other components of the hair loss 'serums' include**
   Amino acids/proteins: Glycine, taurine, cystine, hydrolyzed collagen
   Vitamins: Niacinamide, biotin, ascorbic acid, pantothenate, folate compounds. The inactive components include fragrances, mineral oils, conditioners/humectants/moisturisers (D-panthenol, carboxymethylcellulose, propylene glycol), emulsifying agents (PPG-26 Buteth-26, hydroxyethyl acrylate, sodium acryloyl dimethyl taurate co-polymer) and preservatives (phenoxyethanol, sodium benzoate).

Bibliography

1. Ablon G. A 3-month, randomized, double-blind, placebo-controlled study evaluating the ability of an extra-strength marine protein supplement to promote hair growth and decrease shedding in women with self-perceived thinning hair. Dermatol Res Pract, 2015.

2. Ablon G. A double-blind, placebo-controlled study evaluating the efficacy of an oral supplement in women with self-perceived thinning hair. J Clin Aesthet Dermatol 2012;5(11):28–34.

3. Adhirajan N, Ravi Kumar T, Shanmugasundaram N, Babu M.In vivo and *in vitro* evaluation of hair growth potential of hibiscus rosa sinensis Linn. J Ethnopharmacol 2003 Oct;88(2–3):235–9.

4. Akar A, Arca E, Erbil H, Akay C, Sayal A, Gür AR. Antioxidant enzymes and lipid peroxidation in the scalp of patients with alopecia areata. J Dermatol Sci 2002;29(2):85–90.

5. Aydingoz I, Ferhanoglu B, Guney O. Does tissue iron status have a role in female alopecia? J Eur Acad Dermatol Venereol 1999;13:65–7.

6. Bakry OA, El Farargy SM, El Shafiee MK, Soliman A. Serum vitamin D in patients with alopecia areata. Indian Dermatol Online J 2016 Sep–Oct;7(5):371–77.

7. Begum S, Lee MR, Gu LJ, Hossain J, Sung CK. Exogenous stimulation with *Eclipta alba* promotes hair matrix keratinocyte proliferation and downregulates TGF-β1 expression in nude mice. Int J Mol Med 2015 Feb;35(2):496–502.

8. Begum S, Lee MR, Gu LJ, Hossain MJ, Kim HK, Sung CK. Comparative hair restorer efficacy of medicinal herb on nude (Foxn1nu) mice. Biomed Res Int, 2014.

9. Beoy LA, Woei WJ, Hay YK. Effects of tocotrienol supplementation on hair growth in human volunteers. Trop Life Sci Res 2010 Dec;21(2):91–9.

10. Blumeyer A, et al. Evidence-based (S3) guideline for the treatment of androgenetic alopecia in women and in men. J Dtsch Dermatol Ges 2011;9 Suppl 6:S1–S57.

11. Boffa MJ, Wood P, Griffiths CE. Iron status of patients with alopecia areata. Br J Dermatol 1995;132:662–4.

12. Bouayed J, Bohn T. Exogenous antioxidants—double-edged swords in cellular redox state: Health beneficial effects at physiologic doses versus deleterious effects at high doses. Oxid Med Cell Longev 2010;3(4):228–37.

13. Camaschella C. New insights into iron deficiency and iron deficiency anemia. Blood Rev 2017 Feb 13. pii: S0268-960X(16)30078–9.

14. Datta K, Singh AT, Mukherjee A, Bhat B, Ramesh B, Burman AC. Eclipta alba extract with potential for hair growth promoting activity. J Ethnopharmacol 2009 Jul 30;124(3):450–6.

15. De Marchi U, Biasutto L, Garbisa S, Toninello A, Zoratti M. Quercetin can act either as an inhibitor or an inducer of the mitochondrial permeability

transition pore: a demonstration of the ambivalent redox character of polyphenols. Biochim Biophys Acta 2009;1787(12):1425–32.

16. Deloche C, Bastien P, Chadoutaud S, Galan P, Bertrais S, Hercberg S, et al. Low iron stores: a risk factor for excessive hair loss in non-menopausal women. Eur J Dermatol 2007;17:507–12.

17. Du X, She E, Gelbart T, Truksa J, Lee P, Xia Y, et al. The serine protease TMPRSS6 is required to sense iron deficiency. Science 2008;320:1088–92.

18. Durusoy C, Ozenli Y, Adiguzel A, et al. The role of psychological factors and serum zinc, folate and vitamin B_{12} levels in the aetiology of trichodynia: a case-control study. Clin Exp Dermatol 2009;34(7):789–92.

19. Esfandiarpour I, Farajzadeh S, Abbaszadeh M. Evaluation of serum iron and ferritin levels in alopecia areata. Dermatol Online J 2008;14:21.

20. Everts HB, Silva KA, Montgomery S, et al. Retinoid metabolism is altered in human and mouse cicatricial alopecia. J Invest Dermatol 2013 Feb;133(2):325–33.

21. Finner AM. Nutrition and hair: deficiencies and supplements. Dermatol Clin. 2013;31(1):167–72.

22. Goldberg LJ, Lenzy Y. Nutrition and hair. Clin Dermatol 2010;28 (4):412–19.

23. Greenway FL, Ingram DK, Ravussin E, Hausmann M, Smith SR, Cox L, et al. Loss of taste responds to high dose biotin treatment. J Am Coll Nutr 2011;30:178–81.

24. Guo EL, Katta R. Diet and hair loss: effects of nutrient deficiency and supplement use. Dermatol Pract Concept 2017;7(1):1.

25. Holler PD, Cotsarelis G.Retinoids putting the "a" in alopecia. J Invest Dermatol 2013 Feb;133(2):285–6.

26. Jin W, Zheng H, Shan B, Wu Y. Changes of serum trace elements level in patients with alopecia areata: A meta-analysis. J Dermatol 2017 Feb 2.

27. Kantor J, Kessler LJ, Brooks DG, Cotsarelis G. Decreased serum ferritin is associated with alopecia in women. J Invest Dermatol 2003;121(5):985–88.

28. Kantor J, Kessler LJ, Brooks DG, Cotsarelis G. Decreased serum ferritin is associated with alopecia in women. J Invest Dermatol 2003;121:985–8.

29. Karashima T, Tsuruta D, Hamada T. Oral zinc therapy for zinc deficiency-related telogen effluvium. Dermatol Ther 2012 Mar–Apr;25(2):210–3.

30. Khumalo NP, Stone J, Gumedze F. et al. Relaxers' damage hair: evidence from amino acid analysis. J Am Acad Dermatol 2010 Mar;62(3):402–8.

31. Kil MS, Kim CW, Kim SS. Analysis of serum zinc and copper concentrations in hair loss. Ann Dermatol 2013;25(4):405–9.

32. Kumar N, Rungseevijitprapa W, Narkkhong NA, Suttajit M, Chaiyasut C. 5α-reductase inhibition and **hair** growth promotion of some Thai plants traditionally used for **hair** treatment. J Ethnopharmacol 2012 Feb 15;139(3):765–71.

33. Lengg N, Heidecker B, Seifert B, Trüeb RM. Dietary supplement increases anagen hair rate in women with telogen effluvium: results of a double-blind, placebo-controlled trial. Therapy 2007;4 (1):59–65.

34. Liang T, Liao S. Inhibition of steroid 5α-reductase by specific aliphatic unsaturated fatty acids. Biochem J 1992;285(Pt 2):557–62.

35. Mast AE, Blinder MA, Gronowski AM, Chumley C, Scott MG. Clinical utility of the soluble transferrin receptor and comparison with serum ferritin in several populations. Clin Chem 1998;44:45–51.

36. Mock DM, Baswell DL, Baker H, Holman RT, Sweetman L. Biotin deficiency complicating parenteral alimentation: Diagnosis, metabolic repercussions, and treatment. J Pediatr 1985;106:762–9.

37. Mock DM, Dyken ME. Biotin catabolism is accelerated in adults receiving long-term therapy with anticonvulsants. Neurology 1997;49:1444–7.

38. Munkhbayar S, Jang S, Cho AR, et al. Role of arachidonic acid in promoting hair growth. Ann Dermatol 2016;28(1):55–64.

39. Narang T, Daroach M, Kumaran MS. Efficacy and safety of topical calcipotriol in management of alopecia areata: A pilot study. Dermatol Ther 2017 Jan 30.

40. O'Neil-Cutting MA, Crosby WH. Blocking of iron absorption by a preliminary oral dose of iron. Arch Intern Med 1987;147(3):489–91.

41. Olsen EA, Reed KB, Cacchio PB, Caudill L. Iron deficiency in female pattern hair loss, chronic telogen effluvium, and control groups. J Am Acad Dermatol 2010 Dec;63(6):991–9.

42. Park H, Kim CW, Kim SS, Park CW. The therapeutic effect and the changed serum zinc level after zinc supplementation in alopecia areata patients who had a low serum zinc level. Ann Dermatol 2009;21(2):142–46.

43. Rasheed HI, Mahgoub D, Hegazy R, El-Komy M, Abdel Hay R, Hamid MA, Hamdy E. Serum ferritin and vitamin D in female hair loss: Do they play a role? Skin Pharmacol Physiol 2013;26(2):101–7.

44. Rizer RL, Stephens TJ, Herndon JH, Sperber BR, Murphy J, Ablon GR. A marine protein-based dietary supplement for subclinical hair thinning/loss: results of a multisite, double-blind, placebo-controlled clinical trial. Int J Trichology 2015;7(4):156–66.

45. Rizer RL, Stephens TJ, Herndon JH. A marine based dietary supplement for subclinical hair thinning/loss: results of a multisite, double-blind, placebo-controlled clinical trial. Int J Trichology 2015;7(4):156–66.

46. Roy RK, Thakur M, Dixit VK. Hair growth promoting activity of Eclipta alba in male albino rats. Arch Dermatol Res 2008 Aug;300(7):357–64.

47. Rushton DH, Norris MJ, Dover R, Busuttil N. Causes of hair loss and the developments in hair rejuvenation. Int J Cosmet Sci 2002;24:17–23.

48. Rushton DH, Norris MJ, Dover R, Busuttil N. Causes of hair loss and the developments in hair rejuvenation. Int J Cosmet Sci. 2002 Feb;24(1): 17–23.

49. Rushton DH, Ramsay ID, James KC, Norris MJ, Gilkes JJ. Biochemical and trichological characterization of diffuse alopecia in women. Br J Dermatol 1990;123:187–97.

50. Rushton DH. Nutritional factors and hair loss. Clin Exp Dermatol 2002;27:396–404.

51. Rushton DHI, Ramsay ID. The importance of adequate serum ferritin levels during oral cyproterone acetate and ethinyl oestradiol treatment of diffuse androgen-dependent alopecia in women. Clin Endocrinol (Oxf) 1992 Apr;36(4):421–7.

52. Schrier SL. So you know how to treat iron deficiency anemia. Blood 2015;126:1971.

53. Schulpis KH, Georgala S, Papakonstantinou ED, Michas T, Karikas GA. The effect of isotretinoin on biotinidase activity. Skin Pharmacol Appl Skin Physiol 1999;12:28–33.

54. Schulpis KH, Karikas GA, Tjamouranis J, Regoutas S, Tsakiris S. Low serum biotinidase activity in children with valproic acid monotherapy. Epilepsia. 2001;42:1359–62.

55. Sealey WM, Teague AM, Stratton SL, Mock DM. Smoking accelerates biotin catabolism in women. Am J Clin Nutr 2004;80:932–5.

56. Skolnik P, Eaglstein WH, Ziboh VA. Human essential fatty acid deficiency: treatment by topical application of linoleic acid. Arch Dermatol 1977 Jul;113(7):939–41.

57. Slonim AE, Sadick N, Pugliese M, Meyers-Seifer CH. Clinical response of alopecia, trichorrhexis nodosa, and dry, scaly skin to zinc supplementation. J Pediatr 1992;121(6):890–95.

58. St Pierre SA, Vercellotti GM, Donovan JC, Hordinsky MK. Iron deficiency and diffuse nonscarring scalp alopecia in women: more pieces to the puzzle. J Am Acad Dermatol 2010;63(6):1070–76.

59. Talpur R, Vu J, Bassett R, Stevens V, Duvic M. Phase I/II randomized bilateral half-head comparison of topical bexarotene 1% gel for alopecia areata. J Am Acad Dermatol 2009 Oct;61(4):592.e1–9.

60. Thom E. Efficacy and tolerability of hair gain in individuals with hair loss: a placebo-controlled, double-blind study. J Int Med Res 2001;29(1):2–6.

61. Trost LBI, Bergfeld WF, Calogeras E. The diagnosis and treatment of iron deficiency and its potential relationship to hair loss. J Am Acad Dermatol 2006 May;54(5):824–44.

62. Trüeb RM. Serum Biotin Levels in Women Complaining of Hair Loss. Int J Trichology 2016 Apr–Jun;8(2):73–77.91.

63. Upton JH, Hannen RF, Bahta AW, Farjo N, Farjo B, Philpott MP. Oxidative stress-associated senescence in dermal papilla cells of men with androgenetic alopecia. J Invest Dermatol 2015;135(5):1244–52.

64. WHO. Iron deficiency anaemia, assesment, prevention and Control, a guide for programme managers. Available from: http://www.who.int/nutrition/publications/micronutrients/anaemia_iron_deficiency/WHO_NHD_01.3/en/; 2001.

65. Zhou SJ, Gibson RA, Crowther CA, et al. Should we lower the dose of iron when treating anaemia in pregnancy? A randomized dose-response trial. Eur J Clin Nutr 2009;63(2):183–90.

Basics of Hair Restoration

Rajat Gupta

INTRODUCTION

Hair restoration is one of the most common aesthetic procedures performed in the male population. However, of all the fields of aesthetic surgery, it has suffered probably one of the worst reputations for producing variable and unnatural results and consequently unhappy patients. Part of this is due to the initial years of hair restoration surgeries which included microsurgeries, bald skin excision, flaps, expanders and bigger punch surgeries. The true objective of hair restoration must go beyond these artificial results to a point where the patient who has had hair restoration does not look like he has had any procedure done at all. The final result should be a natural-appearing hairline and natural-appearing density.

The modern discussion of transplantation refers to micrografts or minigrafts, or more specifically in current nomenclature, follicular grafts. Follicular units refer to the naturally occurring clusters of, typically, one to three hairs that emerge from the scalp. A successful hair restoration requires a sense of aesthetics just as demanding as in any other aesthetic procedure. This chapter discusses those factors necessary for a successful aesthetic and natural looking outcomes as well as focusing primarily on the science of current hair transplantation techniques. These aspects are rarely covered in most the chapters written on hair transplant.

The most common type of hair loss in both men and women is referred to as androgenetic alopecia. The mechanism of androgenetic alopecia is inherent in each individual hair follicle as it responds to external stimuli, essentially androgens. The progressive loss of hair is predetermined by genetic characteristics associated with these responsive scalp follicles. In regions of the scalp susceptible to androgenetic alopecia, androgens reduce the growth rate, the hair shaft diameter, and the length of the anagen phase. The mode of action of androgens on the target cells occurs at the bulbar region of the follicle. It appears that androgenetic alopecia is under the control of a single dominant sex-linked autosomal gene. However, this may be influenced by other modifying factors, and there is probably a polygenic component to the expression of male pattern hair loss. In most men with hair loss, the hair follicles in the frontal and crown regions of the scalp appear most likely to be affected by androgenetic alopecia.

Numerous classifications of hair loss have been described on a morphologic basis, which compare the hair-bearing with the non-hair-bearing areas. Norwood, suggested modifications of Hamilton's classification (Fig. 16.1). This classification divide the patterns of baldness into eight main groups.

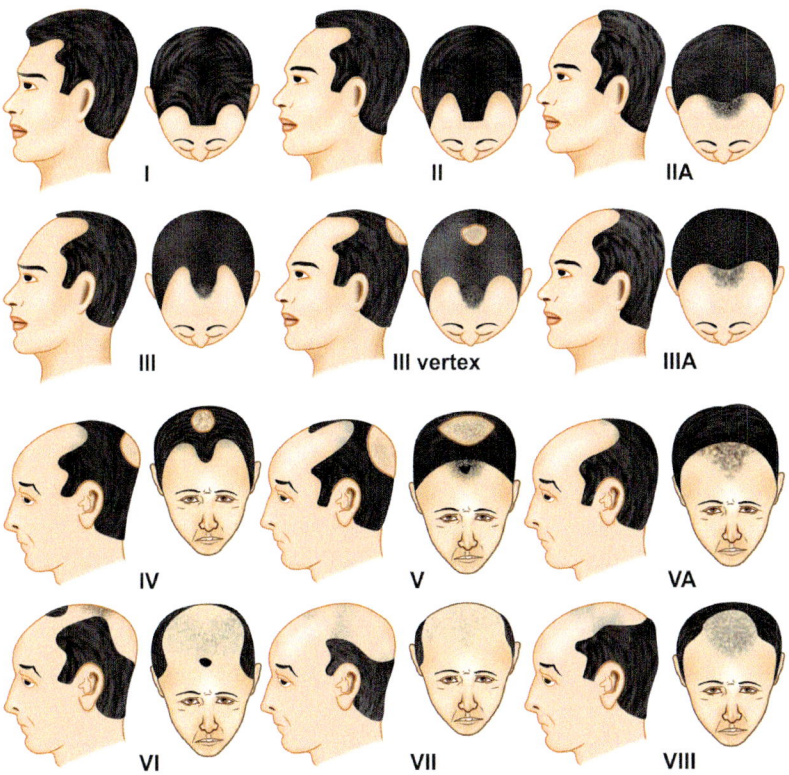

Fig. 16.1: Grade of hair loss (*Courtesy:* Norwood OT). Male pattern baldness: Classification and incidence. South Med J 1975;68:1359–65

Basic Concept and Science

Patients suffering from androgenetic alopecia is due to the hairs being susceptible to DHT. However, in all men even with grade VI or VII baldness there is a zone in scalp at the back of our head which is DHT resistant, hair bearing and shall remain so up to 80–90 years of age. This zone is called *permanent or safe donor area* (Fig. 16.2). The science of hair transplant is to harvest the hair follicles from this permanent zone and subsequently transplant them to the front or bald zone, to achieve a long-lasting result. The transplanted follicles look natural and subsequently grows out as normal hair. Also these hairs can be shampooed, dyed or styled.

In case the transplantation is done of hair follicles harvested away from permanent donor area the result achieved is not long lasting. Using the measurement of donor area as depicted in Fig. 16.2, the number of prominent follicles in it can also be calculated. This varies depending upon the individual characteristics like, density of hairs and grade of hair loss. A survey of 39 of the world's most experienced practitioners of hair restoration surgery with a collective professional experience of nearly 1000 years concluded that a 30-year-old male

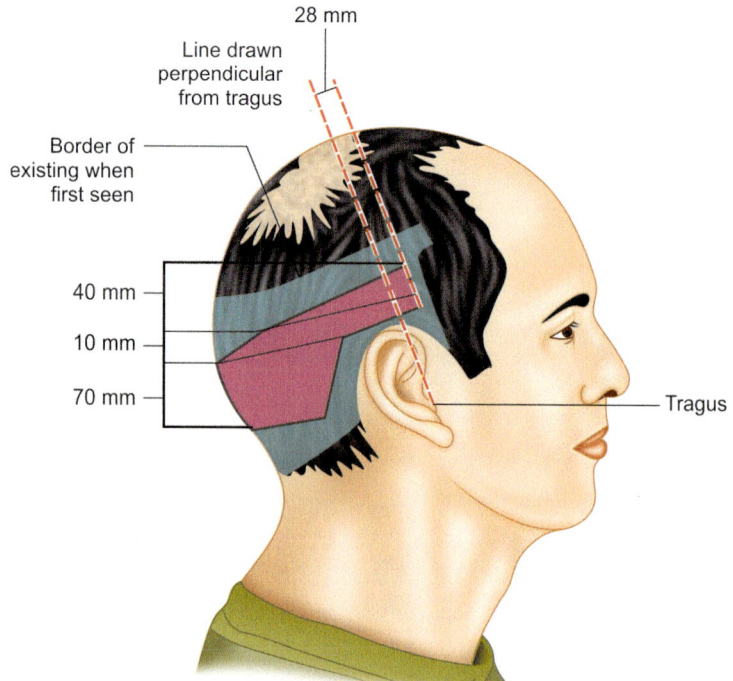

Fig. 16.2: The importance of donor evaluation (*Courtesy:* Unger W)

destined to develop Norwood type V or VI would yield a variable numbers of follicular units (Fig. 16.3), based on the various degrees of donor hair density upon presentation.

Understanding this is very important, before attempting transplant surgery as since we have a finite and fixed amount of permanent follicles, we need to ensure that only the permanent follicles are harvested for the transplant to ensure that the results are permanent. This also ensures that the donor area is used judiciously. Apart from harvesting an adequate number of follicles it is important to appreciate that none should be wasted. Also a decent area of the donor area has to be preserved for subsequent hair transplant if the patient needs it after a few years. The last point is important as we have started getting hair transplant patients in early twenties for covering the frontal area. These patients may have further hair loss from the middle of the scalp as they age and then may require second surgery. If we do not preserve a substantial amount of donor area keeping this point in mind, we may cause more harm than good in the long run.

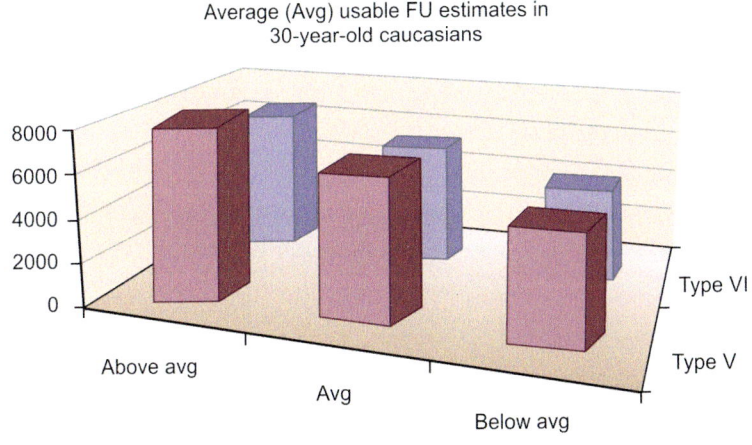

	Above avg density	Avg density	Below avg density
Type V	7904 (3,000–12,000)	6404 (2,000–10,000)	4963 (1,000–9,000)
Type VI	6661 (2,000–10,000)	5393 (1,250–9,000)	4204 (500–8,000)

Numbers represent mean of each category with range in parentheses.

Fig. 16.3: Unger WP et al, estimating the number of lifetime follicular units: A survey and comments of experienced hair transplant surgeons. Dermatol Surg 2013 May;35(50):755–60

Indications for Hair Transplantation or Ideal Patient Selection

When to do hair transplant or when not or when to delay is a question which every hair transplant surgeon should be very clear about. One should avoid doing hair transplant for a patient <20 years of age specially if he/she is having a progressive hair loss. This is important so that we get a fair idea of what will be the expected balding area and perform the transplant accordingly.

Patient should be emotionally stable and understand the limitations of the surgery. We should also rule out any skin or hair disorder and get a thorough dermatological assessment done before proceeding for hair transplant surgery. We should also take into account the patients expectations of the area to be covered, density needed and the donor area. Any mismatch in the above should be a cause for alarm in the surgeons' perception as patients with high expectation will never be satisfied and in the long-term will be a poor advertisement for the hair transplant technique as well.

Methods of Transplant

There are essentially two techniques of hair transplant and both of them differ in how the hair follicles are harvested from the donor area. These are the *follicular unit transplant* (FUT) or strip technique and *follicular unit extraction* (FUE) technique. Another technique the direct hair implant (DHI) is nothing but a variation of FUE. In patients with high grade of hair loss requiring more number of grafts, one can combine the use of both the techniques. Combining the two techniques usually give more number of follicles, better density and hence better results.

Follicular Unit Transplant

In this technique a strip of up to 1.6 × 30 cm (depending upon individual case) is harvested up to the depth of the hair follicle bulb encompassing the subcutaneous fat. As this harvesting remains above the galea the neurovascular bundles are preserved (Fig. 16.4A and B). Then this strip is taken and dissected under magnification into small slivers. Slivers are single thin layer of tissue having hair follicles arranged in a row in a single plane. These slivers are then further dissected into each follicular unit under magnification (Fig. 16.5A to C). Meanwhile the donor site which is a raw area is closed by a special technique of plastic surgery called trichophytic closure (Fig. 16.4C and D). In this technique one edge of cut margin is just de-epithelialized for 1–2 mm followed by a closure which is done kin to skin. Hair follicles from the de-epithelialized area then grow out which makes

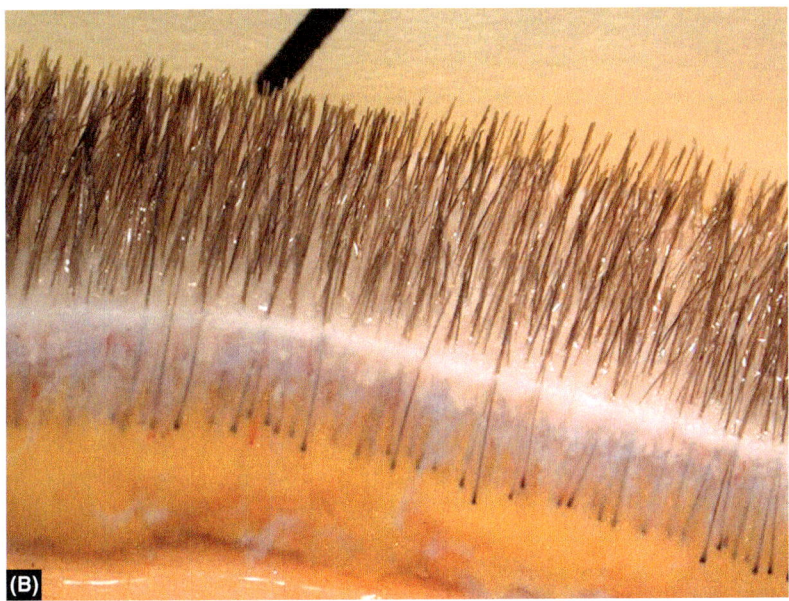

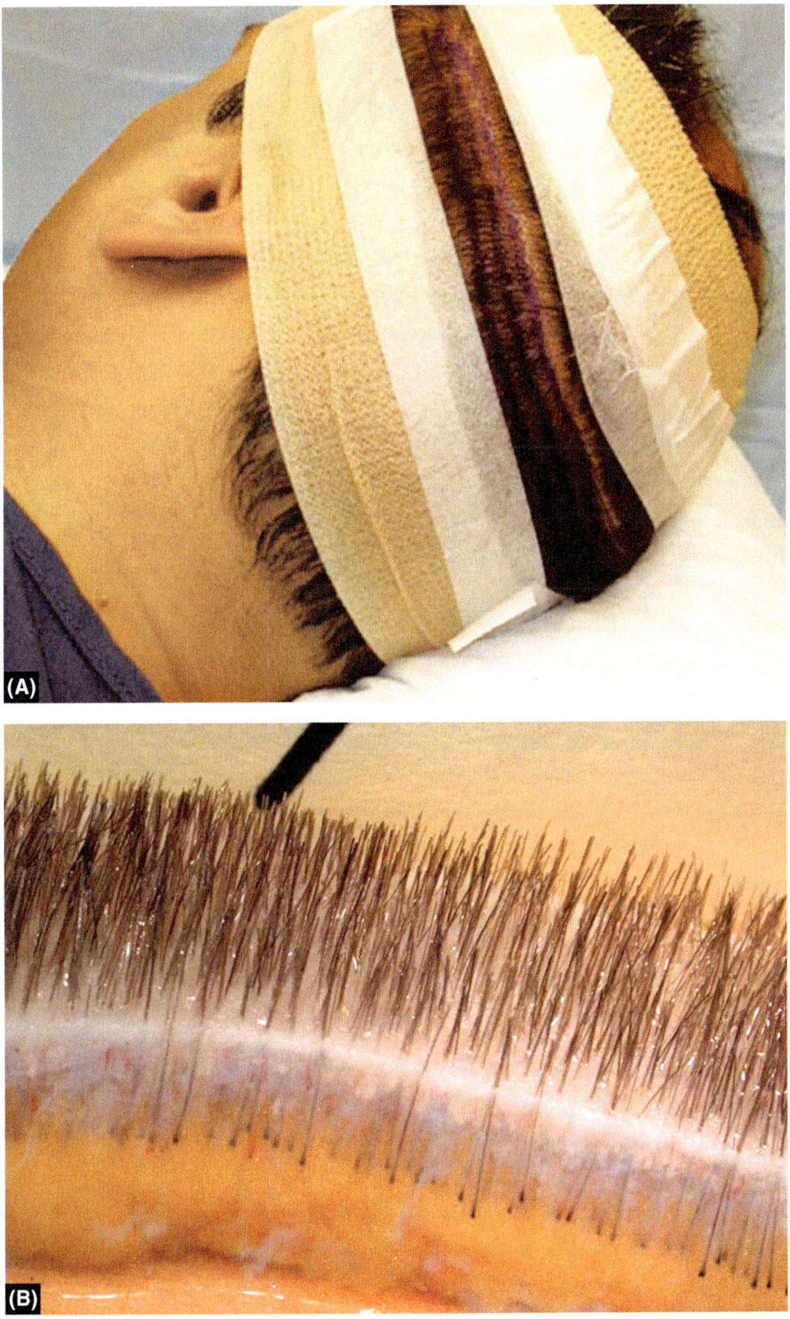

Fig. 16.4A and B: (A) Marking of donor site of strip harvest; (B) Strip after harvest

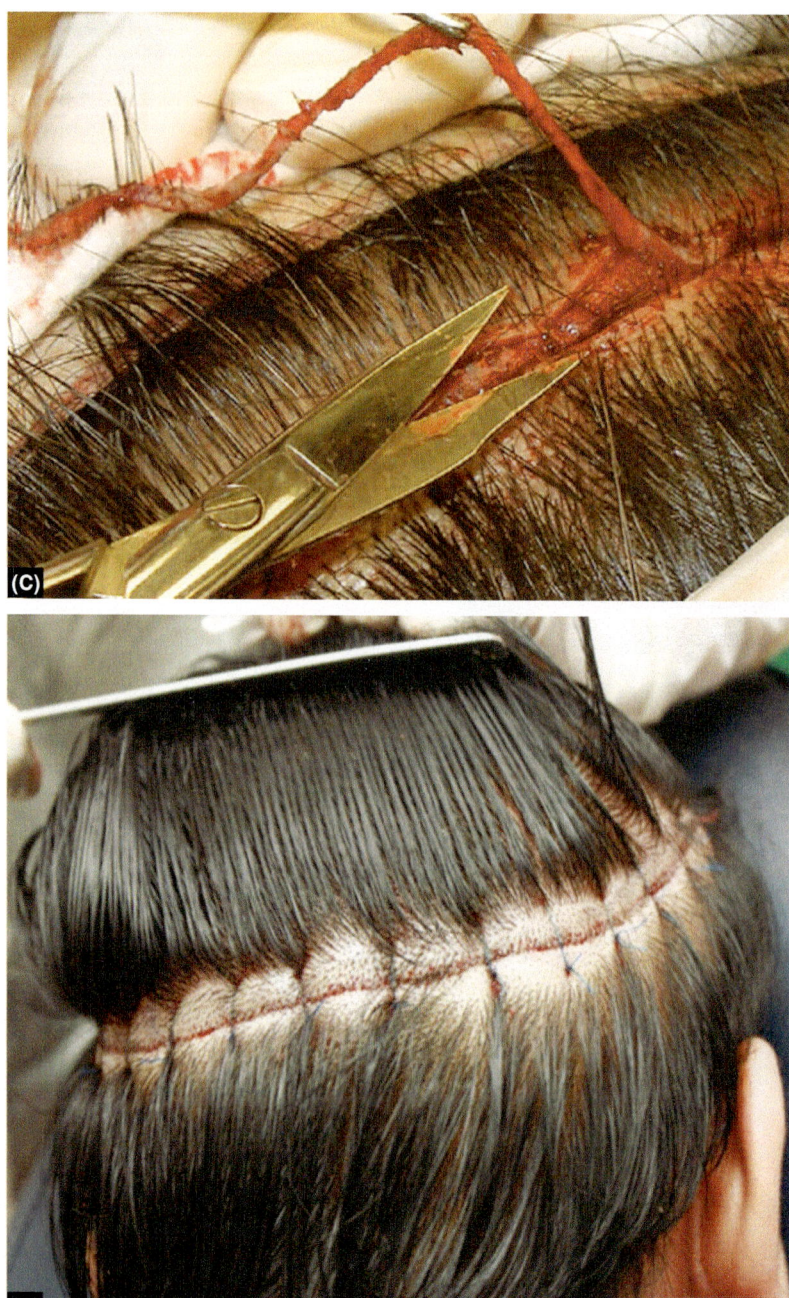

Fig. 16.4C and D: (C) De-epithelialization of cut edge being done; (D) Trichophytic closure

the scar as inconspicuous as possible and is hardly visible (Fig. 16.5D). With the strip technique, it is usually possible to harvest around 2500–3500 follicular units in one sitting.

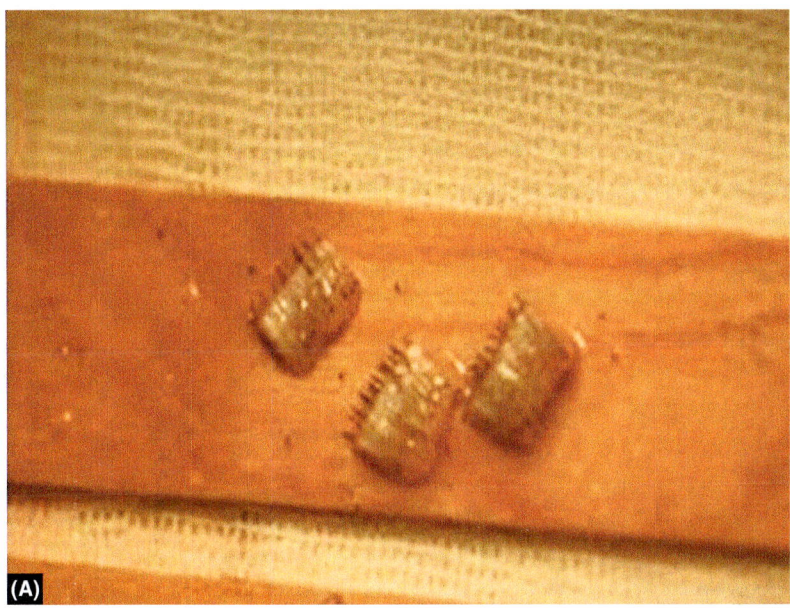

(A)

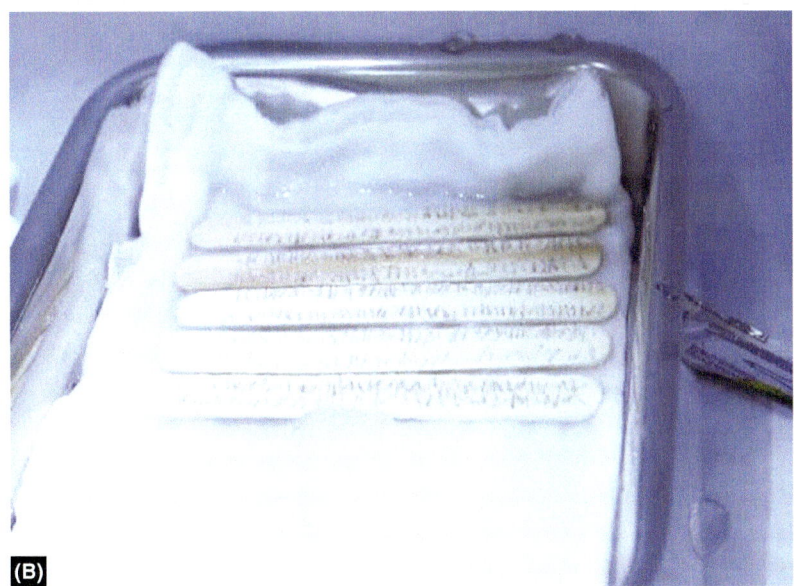

(B)

Fig. 16.5A and B: (A) Slivers dissected out of the strip; (B) Follicular units dissected and kept in cold saline

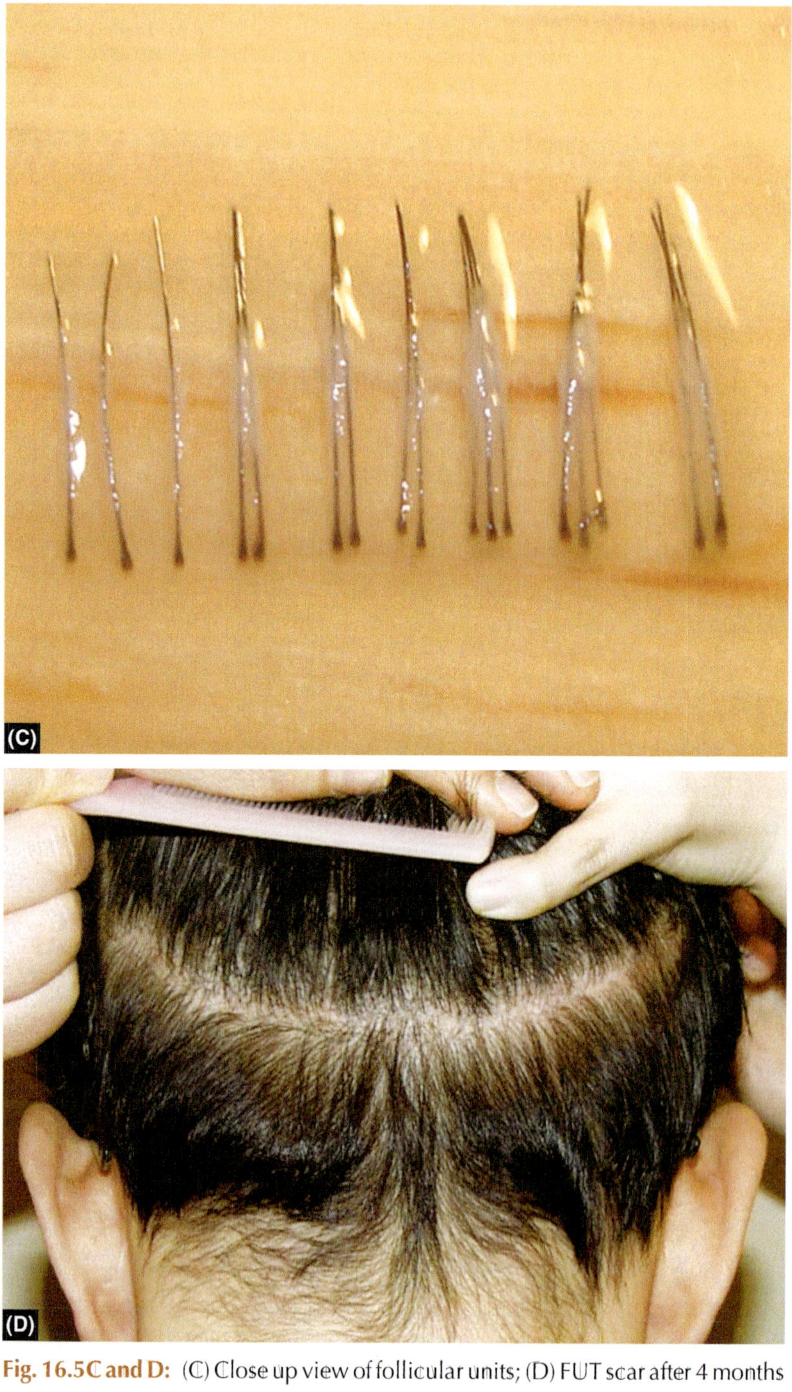

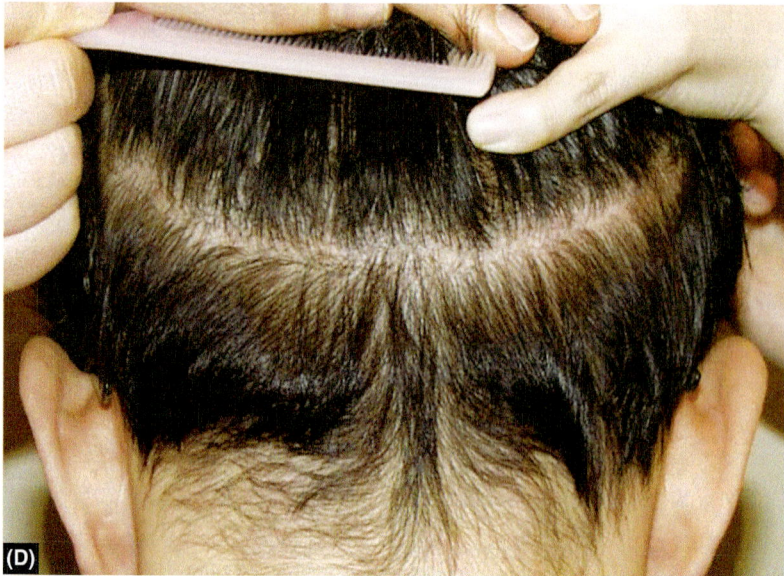

Fig. 16.5C and D: (C) Close up view of follicular units; (D) FUT scar after 4 months

Follicular Unit Extraction

In this technique all the donor hairs are trimmed short. These hair follicles are then cannulated by a small punch usually motorised so that a small punch cut is ensured around the follicle (Fig. 16.6A). This punch is made till the depth of arrector pili muscle which hold the hair follicle in. After the muscle is cut the hair follicle is pulled out carefully with the help of a forceps. During the whole process, it is important to ensure that the direction of the punch and its extraction is the same as the direction of hair follicle inside the scalp. With refinement in techniques and the use of motorised punches, it has been possible to use very minute punches ranging from 0. 7 to 0. 9 mm. These small punches consequentially heal with secondary intention to leave small moth-eaten scars (Fig. 16.6B and C). Although these are also not visible once patient keeps the hair long, advertisements advocating this surgery as "scarless surgery" is morally, ethically and factually incorrect.

With this technique the residual donor density decreases. Thus, it is recommended that one should harvest only one-third of follicles so that the donor site does not look bald. Moreover harvesting may make the scars unsightly as the density will decrease. Since the permanent donor area consists of around 6000 follicular units on an average, it is said that through this technique a surgeon can only harvest up to 2200 follicular units if one strictly restricts to the permanent donor area. Cole, the father of FUE surgery says, "depletion of donor density and overharvesting of hair vulnerable to androgenetic alopecia is a concern with extensive FUE ".

Operative Procedure

Preoperative Period

Preoperative instructions include discontinuation of any herbal medicines that may increase bleeding tendencies, 3 weeks prior to surgery. Patient should also abstain from any drugs which influence platelet activity for at least 1 week prior to surgery. He is also recommended to be off smoking and alcohol intake for at least one week prior to surgery. Patients with relatively tight scalp are instructed how to massage their scalp few weeks before surgery.

Written consent for the procedure and anesthesia and photography must be obtained from the patient on the morning of the surgery.

Hairline Designing

Creating a natural hairline is one of the most important elements of a successful hair transplant. Patients expect and deserve undetectable hairlines. We are better equipped now to create hairlines that meet

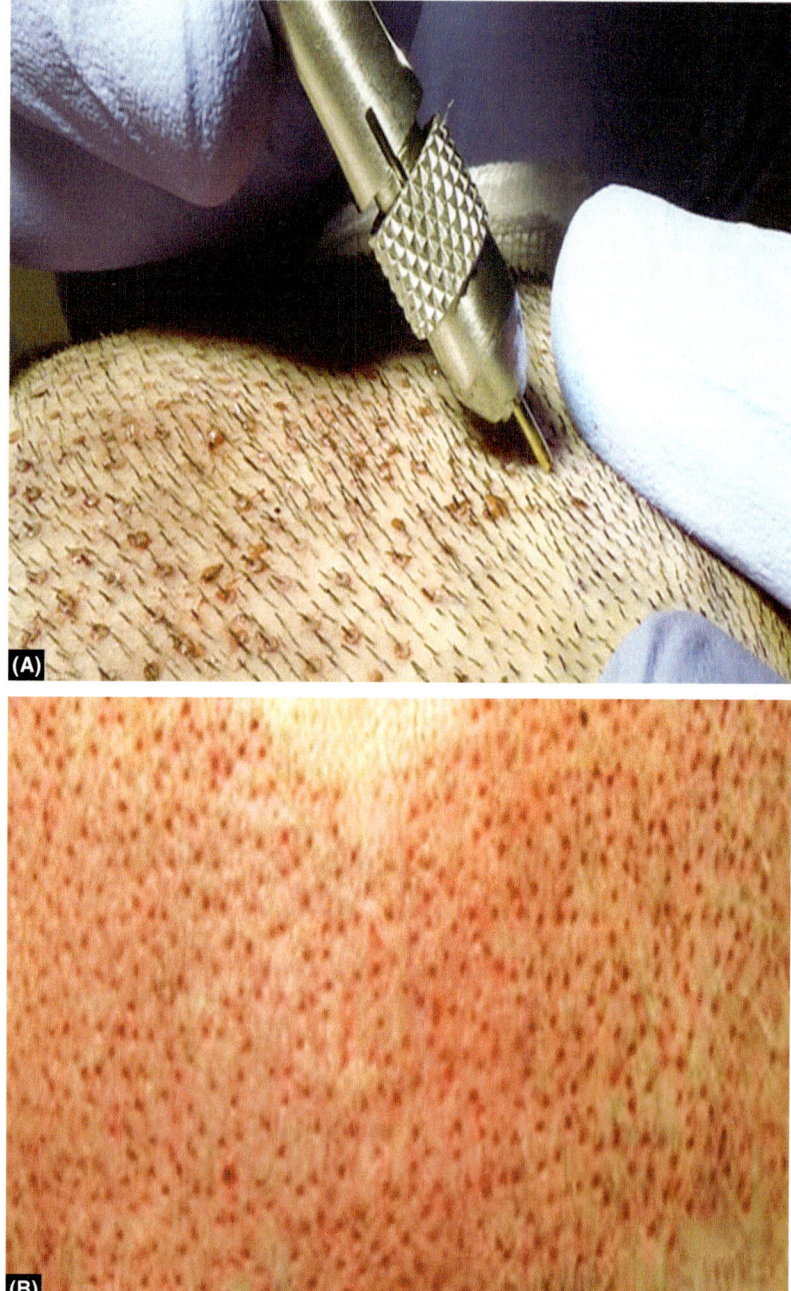

Fig. 16.6A and B: (A) FUE in progress; (B) Wounds left for secondary intention healing

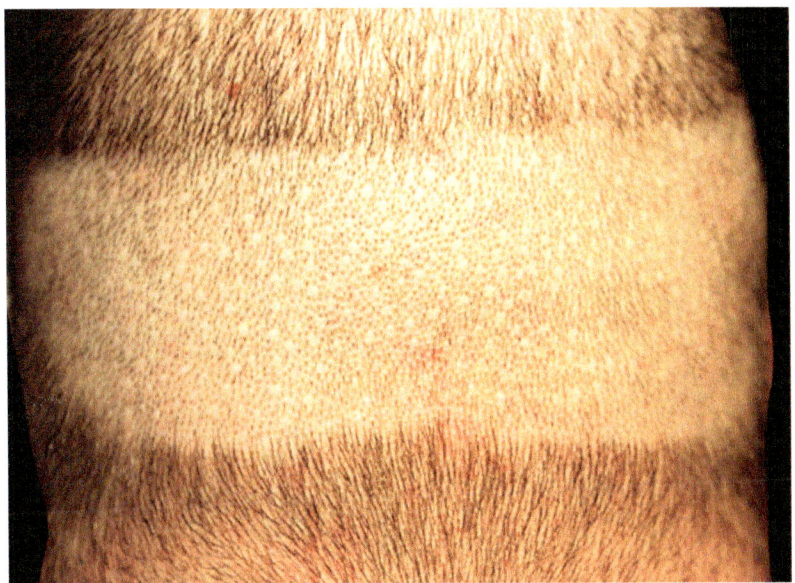

Fig. 16.6C: Moth-eaten scars of FUE visible when hair shaven

this high expectation. This is a result of the exclusive use of follicular unit (FU) grafts in the hairline region. FU grafts have given us a paintbrush with which to create a hairline. Equally important has been a better understanding and recognition of the visual characteristics that make up a normal hairline. Simply using FU grafts without a deliberate attempt to reproduce these characteristics do not guarantee natural-ness. There are 2 major skills needed to "paint" a natural hairline:

1. The ability to locate the appropriate borders of a hairline and adjust these borders based on donor/recipient ratio.
2. The ability to mimic the visual characteristics of a natural hairline at these borders.

Locating Appropriate Borders

A. Mid-frontal point

The mid-frontal point (MFP) is located in the midline and is the most anterior point of the frontal hairline. A number of guidelines can aid in the proper location of the MFP (Fig. 16.7).

The 4-finger breaths rule: MFP should be located 4-finger breaths above the glabella. This is unreliable, as fingers vary in size from person to person.

Leonardo da Vinci's "rule of thirds": Perfect face should be divided into equal thirds with the distance between the chin to the nose, nose to the glabella, and glabella to the hairline all being the same.

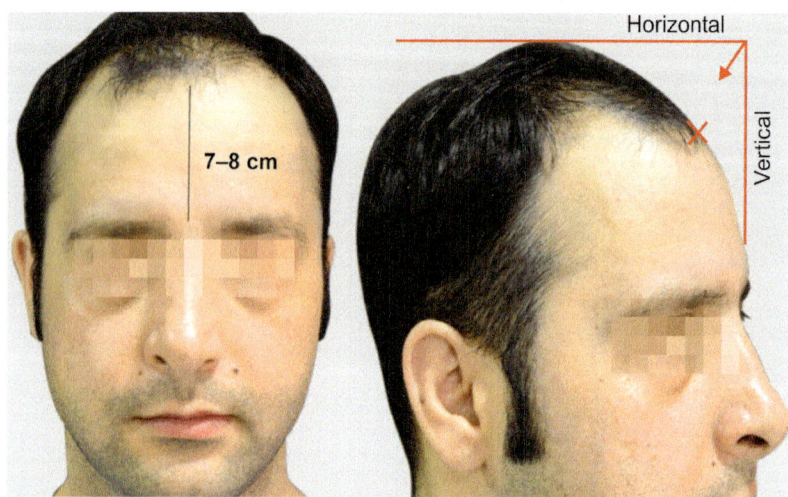

Fig. 16.7: Locating MFP (mid-frontal point)

7 to 10 cm rule: The MFP lies on point drawn somewhere between 7 and 10 cm above the glabella.

Curve of the forehead rule: The forehead takes on a gentle curve as it transitions from the vertical plane of the face to meet the horizontal plane of the scalp. The MFP usually lies somewhere within this curve. A good starting point is a line drawn to this curve from the intersection of these 2 planes. This places the MFP somewhere in the middle of the curve.

B. Mid-pupillary point

Point lateral to the MFP where the hairline begins to bend posteriorly on a line drawn vertically from the pupil. Distance between MFP and labella is measured and the same distance is marked from the mid of eyebrow along the mid-pupillary line.

C. Frontotemporal angle

Locating the frontotemporal angle (FTA) appropriately is the one of the most important and difficult criteria to design a mature good looking hairline (Fig. 16.8). The following guidelines are useful for locating the FTA.

The lateral epicanthus line rule: This rule states the FTA lies on a line drawn vertically from the lateral epicanthus of the eye called the lateral epicanthi line (LEL).

The FTA is located at the point where the LEL intersects the temporal hairline.

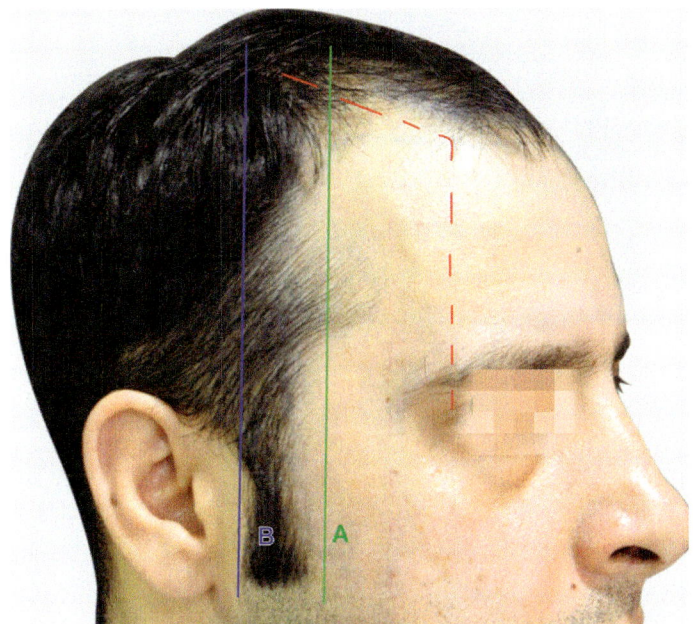

Fig. 16.8: Locating FTA (frontotemporal angle)

Up-sloping line rule: A line drawn from the MFP to the FTA should always slope slightly upward when viewed from the side. It should never slope downward.

Once the locations of the MFP and FTA have been determined, the frontal hairline is created by drawing a gently curving line that connects the MFP to both FTAs. The MPP is an additional landmark that assists in the drawing of this line. The contour of the frontal hairline can range from round, to oval, to bell-shaped. The more conservative a hairline needs to be, the more its shape moves from a rounder shape toward an oval or bell-shaped design.

D. Temporal point (TP)

Before the use of FU grafts, the TP could not be transplanted naturally. Now, with the use of FU grafts, it can be done. However, this is an extremely visible area that is unforgiving to mistakes. It requires a high level of skill and should not be undertaken lightly by novices. A common rule for finding the TP is the intersection of the following 2 lines (Fig. 16.9):

Line 1 is drawn from the tip of the nose, over the center of the pupil.

Line 2 is drawn from the tip of the earlobe to the proposed MFP.

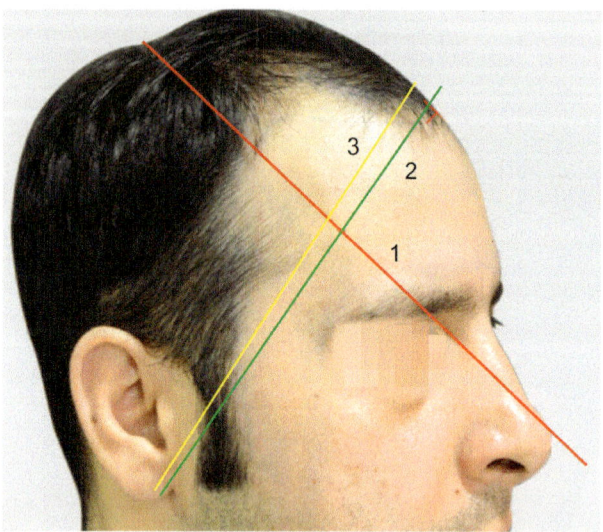

Fig. 16.9: Locating TP (temporal point)

Mimickers of Visual Characteristics of a Normal Hairline

A. Zone identification

The frontal hairline is an area approximately 2 to 3 cm deep that bridges the bald forehead to the hair-bearing scalp. It can be visualized as an extended area that consists of 3 zones: The anterior portion or transition zone (TZ); the posterior portion or defined zone (DZ); and an oval-shaped area in the center of the DZ called the frontal tuft (FT). All 3 zones make their own unique contribution to the overall appearance of the hairline. It is hence imperative that while performing transplant each zone is created as it occurs naturally (Fig. 16.10).

Transition zone (TZ): It consists of the first 0. 5 to 1 cm of the hairline. It should initially appear irregular and illdefined, but gradually takes on more definition and substance as it reaches the DZ. One-hair graft should be used only in the anterior portion of the TZ with a shift toward 2-hair graft in the posterior portion. This helps ensure a natural, softer look.

Defined zone (DZ): It sits directly behind the TZ. In this area, the hairline should develop a higher degree of definition and density. Increasing density in the DZ creates a fuller looking hairline by limiting the distance seen through the TZ. As a benefit, it creates this effect without placing hair directly in the TZ, limiting the chance of creating an unnatural straight or solid appearance. Increasing density in the DZ is a safe and effective way to make the hairline appear thicker.

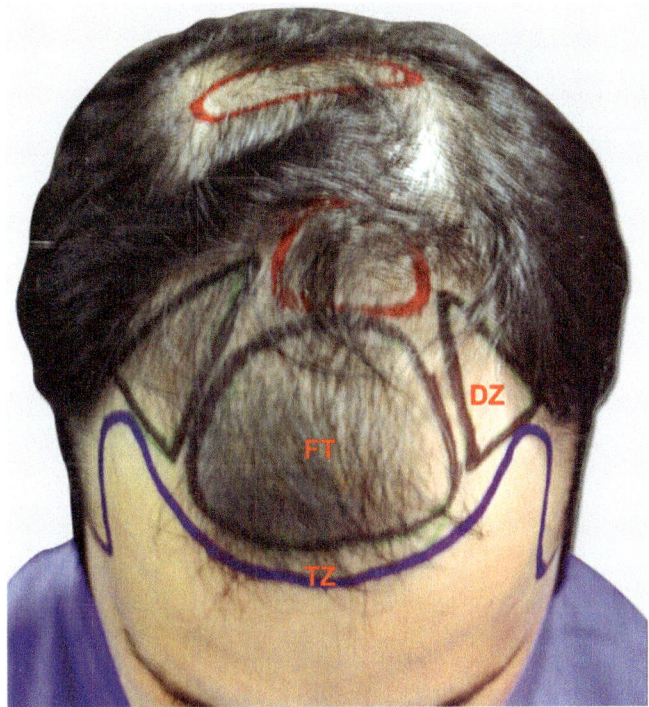

Fig. 16.10: Zone identification

Frontal tuft (FT): The FT is a small but esthetically significant oval-shaped area that overlies the central portion of the DZ. The density in this area should be higher than the rest of the DZ. Creating fullness in this area has a tremendous influence on the overall appearance of fullness.

B. Micro- and macro-irregularities

No natural hairline is absolutely straight. Designing an absolutely straight hairline is one of the most commonly done mistakes by a novice surgeon. The normal hairline has macro- and micro-irregularities (Fig. 16.11). Close examination of the TZ reveals small, intermittent clusters of hairs along its border. These clusters vary in shape and depth but often resemble ill-defined triangles of various sizes. Their existence creates variable and intermittent density along the TZ. This form of irregularity is referred to as micro-irregularity because it is more noticeable viewed close-up than from a distance. If one stands back and looks at a normal hairline from a distance, the path of the anterior border is seen to be more serpentine or curvaceous than linear. This form of irregularity is referred to as macro-irregularity because it is more obvious when one stands back and observes the hairline from a distance.

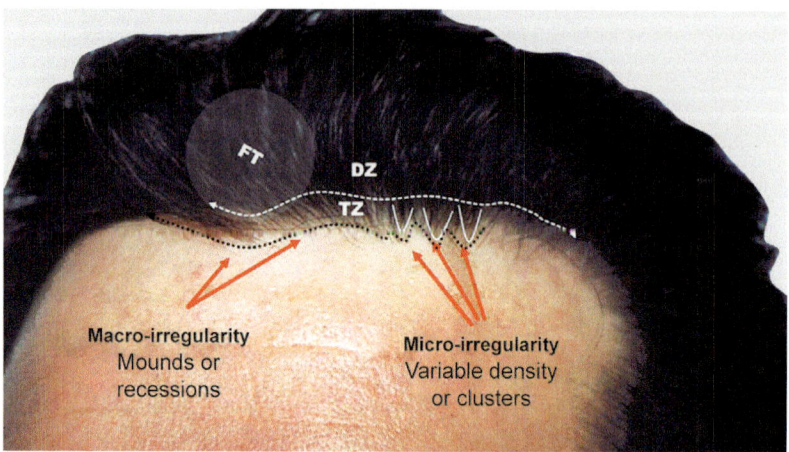

Fig. 16.11: Macro- and micro-irregularities in hairline

C. Angle and directions of implantation

Angle and direction are distinct entities. Angle refers to the degree of elevation that hair has as it exits the scalp. Direction refers to the way hair points (right or left) when leaving the scalp. It is important to pay attention to changes in both angle and direction as one transplants different parts of the hairline (Fig. 16.12).

In the mid scalp, hair usually exits at 30 to 45° and points forward toward the nose. As one reaches the frontal hairline, the angle becomes more acute at 15 to 20, and the direction usually remains pointing forward. On occasion, hair in this area may bend slightly to the left or

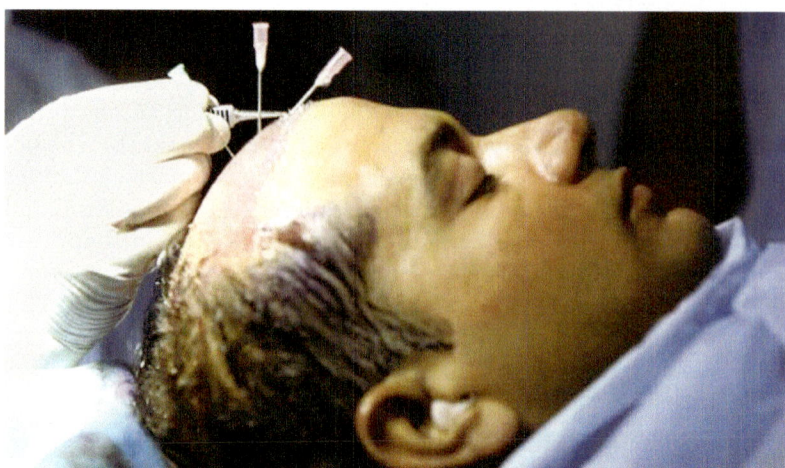

Fig. 16.12: Angles and directions at the time of implantation

right. As one moves laterally along the hairline, the direction remains forward until nearing the FTA. As one reaches and sweeps around the FTA toward the temporal hairline, there is a gradual change in direction from forward to inferior lateral. Simultaneously, a gradual change in angle occurs from approximately 15 in the frontal hairline to almost flat (5–10) in the temporal hairline.

D. Selective distribution of the grafts

Selective distribution is an important tool that helps us mimic the density gradient found in normal hairlines. It is a safer and more powerful tool than increasing incisional density (Fig. 16.13).

The TZ contains only 1-hair graft with a shift to 2-hair graft toward the posterior aspect of this zone. The DZ contains predominantly 2-hair graft. The FT area contains a greater concentration of 3-hair graft. Follicular pairing is a useful tool to use in the FT area if not enough 3-hair graft is found naturally. With follicular pairing, a 1-hair graft and a 2-hair graft are combined to make an artificial 3-hair graft.

Preparation of the Recipient Area (Fig. 16.14)

Recipient area is anesthetized by giving blocks of bilateral supratrochlear and supraorbital nerves. These blocks are usually sufficient to anesthetize the entire frontal area. However, infiltration anesthesia is usually require for temporal area. Tumescence is created in the recipient zone before making the slits which can hold the grafts. It is usually recommend to use only normal saline to create tumescence. Use of adrenaline is usually avoidable. There has been occasional case reports of even skin necrosis on usage of adrenaline. Based on the

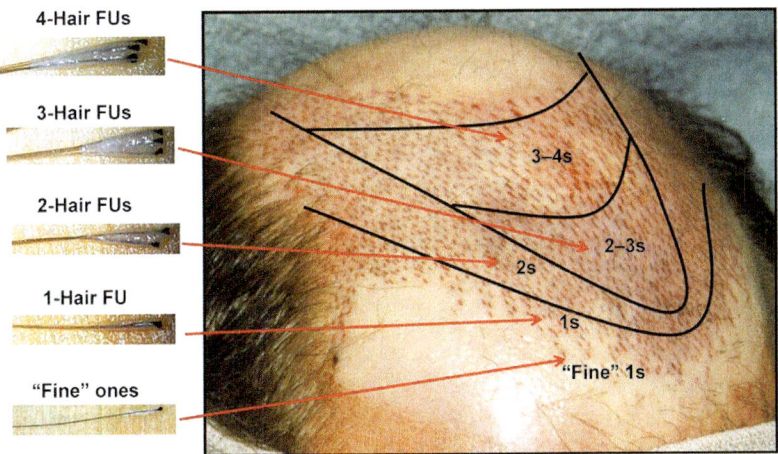

Fig. 16.13: Selective distribution of grafts

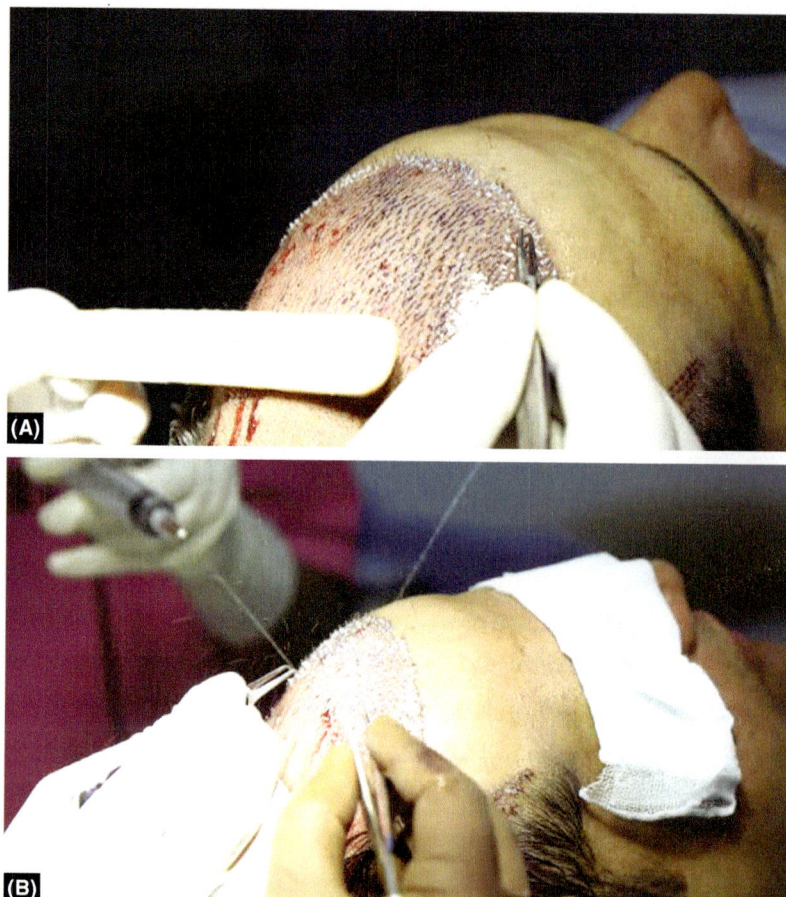

Fig. 16.14A and B: (A) Recipient site preparation and follicle implantation; (B) Implantation done by multiple people so that out of body time is kept to minimum

above guidelines of designing the recipient area, slits are made to place the follicular grafts. During this whole process one should ensure that the grafts are kept wet with cold saline to prolong their survival time. Every effort is made that "out of body" time for each hair follicle remains as less possible and never exceeds 6 hours.

Postoperative Care

Postoperatively patient is given a broadspectrum antibiotic, analgesic, anti-inflammatory. We usually prefer to also prescribe low dose steroids like prednisolone 10 mg once daily for 5 days. This has been shown to decrease postoperative swelling. There is generally no need of any dressing. However, we make the patient wear a head band for

72 hours. This prevents the tumescent fluid in the scalp to descent down to periorbital area which makes the patient and doctor unduly worried.

All these transplanted hair fall from shaft and go through telogen (resting) phase. These hairs start erupting again after 3 months or so and final result is usually only achieved by 8 to 10 months.

ETHICS AND ADVERTISEMENT

Hair transplant surgery is one of the most exploited surgery in terms of who all performing it. There are many examples of non-qualified technicians/dentists/MBBS/ENT surgeons/gynecologist ortho-pedicians and of course dermatologist and plastic surgeons entering this field. Most of their confidence stem from the fact that many (may be 60–70%) of the hair transplanted will grow done by anyone. Moreover, the image of being very lucrative in monetary terms have made many such clinics (who hire untrained/unqualified technicians or doctor) mushroom in every city which are exploiting hair transplant surgery. However, these clinics in equal measure give unsatisfactory results in terms of density creation and hair line designing. Many of their patients suffer from unnatural looking results. This has resulted in bringing the whole concept and science of hair transplant into disrepute.

In India, since their is no stringent "board or authority" which keeps a check on what can be advertised in newspapers, some clinics have started advertising this surgery as "No cut/no scar surgery". This is far from the truth, as explained above, in all techniques of hair transplant scars and cuts are inevitable, however, these are concealed. They also advertise "unlimited follicle transplant". This is also very misleading as their is always a finite number of follicles which can be harvested from the scalp as well as their is a finite number of follicles which can be harvested from any given technique. Many of these clinics also advertise that one technique is better than others, or they use "latest" techniques. This is again far from truth as both the techniques of hair transplant is a must in the armamentarium of a good hair transplant surgeon, as both the techniques have their pros and cons. Ideally choice of technique should based on need and requirements of a particular patient. And surgeons can only offer both the techniques if he/she has skills to execute either of them with equal ease.

CONCLUSION

Hair transplant is very gratifying surgery. If done properly, patients not only get the fresh crop of hairs they always wanted but also get their self-esteem and confidence back. As in any other surgery there is lot of science in the whole procedure. It requires a knowledge of the science and techniques to be a reputable transplant surgeon. One also needs to understand the science for achieving a natural looking hairline to give a esthetically pleasing result. Patients expectations have to be realistic and this can only be made after making them understand the science behind surgery. In these days of Consumer Protection Act and medicolegal issues, it is our duty to educate patients the truth in each surgery and what can/cannot be achieved from a surgery. And lastly we should also make it a point to advertise ethically as unrealistic expectations of patients bring disrepute to the surgery and our profession.

Bibliography

1. ASAPS 2000 Statistics on Cosmetic Surgery. New York, American Society for Aesthetic. Plastic Surgery, 2001.

2. Bernstein RM, Rassman WR. Follicular transplantation, patient evaluation and surgical planning. Dermatol Surg 1997;23:771.

3. Norwood OT. A classification of male pattern baldness. South Med J 1975;68:1359.

4. Shapiro R. Creating a natural hairline in one session using a systemic approach and modern principles of hairline design. Int J Cosm Surg Aesthetic Dermatology 2001;3(2):89–99.

5. Shapiro R. How to use follicular unit transplantation in the hairline and other appropriate areas. In: Unger WP, Shapiro R, editors. Hair transplantation. 4th edition. New York: Marcel Dekker; 2004:454–69.

6. The importance of donor evaluation. In: Unger W, Unger R, Unger M, Shapiro R (eds). Hair Transplantation. 5th edn. New York, NY: Marcel Dekker; 2011:256–260.

7. Unger WP, et al. Estimating the Number of Lifetime Follicular Units: A Survey and Comments of Experienced Hair Transplant Surgeons. Dermatol Surg 2013 May;39(50): 755–60. Aesthet Surg J 2013 Jan;33(1):128–51.

8. Unger W. Hairline zone. In: Unger W, Shapiro R, editors. Hair transplantation. 5th edition. Informa; 2011. p. 133–40 Chapter 6A.

9. Yildiz H, et al. Recipient Site Necrosis After Tumescent Infiltration with Adrenaline in Hair Transplantation. Acta Dermatovenerol Croat 2015 Sep;23(3):233–4.

17

Advanced Hair Restoration

Abhinav Kumar, Pradeep Sethi, Arika Bansal

INTRODUCTION

There is a flurry of advancements in hair transplantation. Refinement in FUE is happening by every hair restoration surgeon, resulting in tremendous improvement in the quality of results. FUE has become the standard method of hair transplantation nowadays. Although in mid-twentieth century hair restoration surgeries reveal a troubling history, the future is filled with great optimism now.

A good hair transplant is evaluated by the naturalness of the end result in terms of hair growth, hairline and density. The follicular unit extraction (FUE) technique has been gaining acceptance among patients and physicians. One of the main drawbacks of FUE is that the grafts are skinny and can be easily damaged during handling in transplantation.

This chapter deals with innovations in FUE surgeries, direct hair implantation which is a modified FUE surgery, various innovation in instruments and methods used in various steps of hair transplantation, ways to overcome various issues and complications which crop up during or after the procedure in a hair transplant patient.

METHODS OF IMPLANTATION

Traditionally there are **three methods** of implantation in FUE surgery:
1. Stick and place method
2. Pre-made recipient sites: Can be made using CTS blades or needles. The graft can be inserted using jeweler's forceps (holding the grafts just below or lateral to the bulb) or can be inserted by dilating the recipient site using a jeweler's forceps.
3. Implanter: Choi, SAVA implanters. Others are implanter pen (Dr Pascal Boudjema), Carousel implanter, Lion implanter, Shiao implanter.
4. Direct hair transplantation: Modification of FUE which combines the creation of pre-made recipient sites and use of implanters.

We hereby discuss our method direct hair transplantation and its advantages over the older method. This method involves the creation of premade slits at the recipient sites, simultaneous extraction and implantation at various body positions with the use of implanters (Table 17.1).

During the past decade, several instruments have been developed for implantation of follicles, most of which involve direct puncture of the scalp with loaded implanter. The rationale behind doing so was to decrease the duration of surgery and reduce the handling of the grafts. Some of the popular implanters include the SAVA implanters, Choi implanter, Lion implanter, KNU implanter, DR TK implanter, the pen and multi-channel implanter. Though these devices are easy to use, they are expensive, their needles have to be replaced frequently due to loss of sharpness and have been associated with popping of graft and graft loss especially when the grafts are placed closed together.

To overcome this problem, Lee et al suggested preparing recipient site with pre-made slits using 23-G needle. Direct hair transplantation technique devised a system with which not only is the graft handling minimal, but the duration of surgery and out of body time are also significantly reduced as all the steps of hair transplant can be performed simultaneously by various members of the team. The advantages of our modification over the other techniques are:

1. Nearly zero mechanical handling of follicular graft.
2. The risk of popping of the adjacent implanted grafts is reduced. The force required to insert the graft into the scalp into the scalp is minimized because of pre-made site.
3. Less number of sharp implanters are required thus cutting the cost of surgery.
4. The physician's time is saved as they can plan the shape of hairline, density, direction and angulations of the implanted grafts. If pre-made sites are not made, the grafts need to be implanted by the physician himself.
5. Another advantage of implanting into pre-made sites is that the graft enters the recipient site without being touched below the epidermal portion thus avoiding the dermal portion and preserving the viability of the graft.
6. Learning curve of surgical assistant implanting the graft is reduced, thus reducing the staff dependence.
7. It is made possible to implant in any position, whether the patient is lying in prone, supine or lateral positions.
8. Simultaneous extraction is also made possible because the implantation continues unabated in spite of the slight vibrational movement of patient's head.
9. Implantation can be done with patient's head in any position.

	Stick and place method	Pre-made recipient sites method	Implanter method	Direct hair transplantation
Performed by	Physician	Physician and assistant	Physician	Physician and assistant
Mechanical handling of the hair root	Present	Present (one hand technique) Less (2 hand technique)	Absent	Absent
Popping risk	High	Less	High	Less
Learning curves for technicians	High	High	High	Less
Cost	Less	Less	High	Lesser than implanter method
Position of patient's head	Supine	Supine	Supine	All positions

Table 17.1: Modifications of FUE surgery

In direct hair transplantation, one can use various types of implanters. Our experience with SAVA implanters has been excellent. It is broad from above, making it easy to introduce the graft into the implanter, called loading. As we move inferiorly, there is a mild constriction which holds the grafts inside the lumen of implanter. The exit of the needle is beveled with a sharp tip to ensure smooth movement into pre-made recipient site (Fig. 17.1).

Other types of implanters include multi-channel implanter in which the density can be determined by the surgeon and we can spare the pre-existing hair in the recipient zone. In the Choi, KNU and Lion implanters, the lumen is closed from the front and the space for loading of is very narrow because there is a plunger which pushes the graft from above. The learning curve to use these implanters is steep and they are difficult to use when hair shafts are short as in most cases (1–1.5 mm).

Magnification: The magnification depends on surgeon's choice, however, a higher magnification of 4X and 5X drastically improves the quality of surgery and the investment made in the loupe is worth every penny as it drastically improves the quality of surgery (Fig. 17.2).

Safe Donor Zone Hair

The safe donor area (SDA) is based on imprecise medical science and it varies from person to person. Unger's definition of SDA remains the gold standard in defining the SDA. Lorenzo defines an unsafe

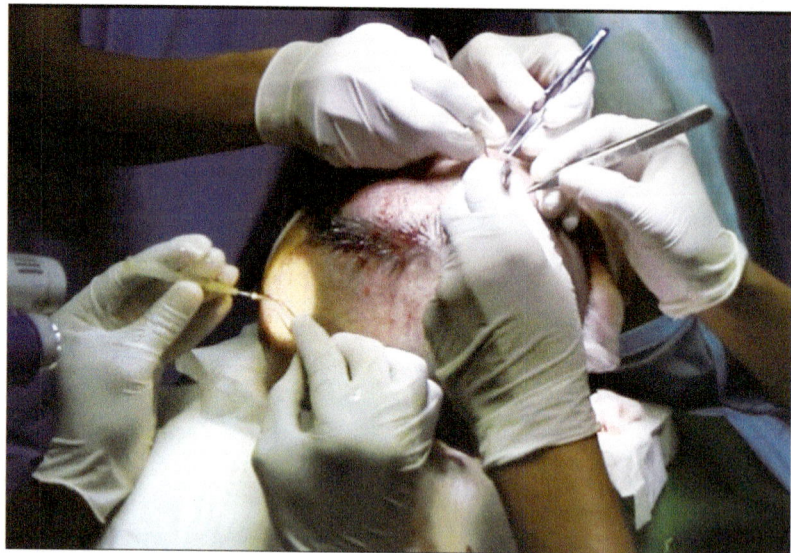

Fig. 17.1: Shows direct hair transplantation with simultaneous extraction and implantation of grafts

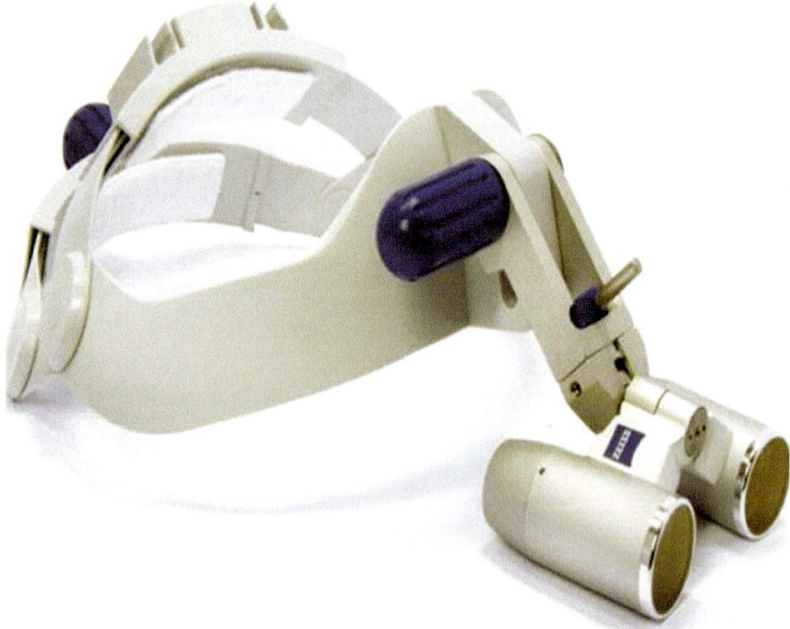

Fig. 17.2: Shows Carl Zeiss loupe used during slit preparation, graft extraction and implantation

donor zone when 15% or more miniaturization is present compared to SDA. For a young surgeon it is always wise to stay within SDA but the SDA can be expanded based upon the patients' individual history, examination of donor region, and estimation of miniaturization and clinical experience of surgeon. A dermatoscopic evaluation tells about the stability of the donor site and degree of miniaturization in donor zone. In large single sessions of FUE surgery, the physician operator usually removes 10% of the follicles outside the SDA. The justification for such approach involves proper candidate selection (patients with late onset of baldness), follicles transplanted on low risk patients with stabilized hair patterns with good donor, lack of family history of advanced baldness and inclusion of patients who are compliant with medications (Boden S in hair transplant 360, 2016).

Points to Consider while Giving Local Anesthesia

The ideal layer for injection of vasoconstrictors is just below the dermis and above the galea. Injecting below the subgaleal layer (needle tip will be felt scrapping the bone) which is relatively avascular increases the risk of periorbital edema due to the fluid tracking inferiorly in the subgaleal plane.

1. The arterial supply to the recipient scalp courses up from below like spokes from rim of a wheel. The nerve supply differs; the supraorbital nerves supply most of the anterior 1/2–2/3rds of the recipient area. These structures exit the skull deep to the eyebrow and run superiorly. Once these nerves are blocked bulk of the frontal recipient site is blocked. The blocking of nerves is easier than hemostasis (since we keep encountering new arteries as we move back in recipient sites).

2. Epinephrine in the scalp: The medication must be placed where larger vessels are (subcutaneous plane) and in a large enough concentration to produce vasoconstriction. Tumescence (0.1% lidocaine and 1:200,000 epinephrine) should be injected 1 to 15 minutes prior and 2–3 cm beyond the boundaries of planned recipient zone (upstream in vessel's path). More concentrated epinephrine (1:50,000) can be injected immediately prior to the recipient site creation in the partially vasoconstricted zones (due to tumescent injection prior to it).

3. Tumescence also helps in separating the galea from the subcutaneous layer and providing extra protection to deeper vessels and galea during surgery.

4. In the donor area, the neurovascular supply runs from inferior to superior, and ring blocks need only be done below the inferior aspect of planned harvest zones.

5. Staging of injections: It is important to not inject anesthesia, epinephrine and tumescence in an area which is not to be operated in the next two hours of surgery to avoid systemic toxicity. This applies to both donor area and recipient sites. Recipient sites need not be infiltrated earlier than 10 to 15 minutes prior to incision creation.

6. Intradermal injections produce wheals and are often painful. Both anesthesia and tumescence are injected best when the needle is advanced. The spreading fluid from needle tip creates a wave in front of the needle tip which pushes the galea away thus helps in keeping the needle in proper plane.

7. The dilution minimizes the risk of side effects if tumescence is injected into the vessels.

8. New recipient site bleeding and pain is often a clue that anesthesia may soon begin to fade and needs top up.

9. If patients complain of frontal headache, the culprit may be excessive pressure on the scalp from elastic gauze bandage placed around the scalp to absorb fluids or incomplete hairline anesthesia. Loosening of bandage, repeating ring block and supraorbital block is recommended.

10. Incomplete recipient site hemostasis is corrected by injecting 1:50,000 epinephrine in normal saline, 2 cm inferior to the hairline and extending through the recipient site. Other method is intradermal tumescence.

11. Incomplete late donor anesthesia can be addressed by reinjecting the anesthesia 2–3 cm inferior to the area of pain.

12. Use of vibrator and contact cooling along with injections for local anesthesia decreases the pain significantly. This occurs because vibration closes the gates of pain pathway to the brain through presynaptic inhibition.

13. Use of bupivacaine has limited use due to its potential cardiac toxicity. The maximum dosage of bupivacaine in adults in 175 mg. Ropivacaine produces less reduction of left ventricular pressure than bupivacaine. Ropivacaine is one of the safest long acting local anesthetics in peripheral nerve blockade and carries the potential to replace bupivacaine in future.

Designing a Male Hairline

This is the most important area of hair restoration. It should be natural and accurately designed. The hairline consists of two parts: Anterior hairline that runs primarily horizontally and temporal hairline that runs vertically and connects hairline with the sideburns.

The hairline can be further divided into "macro hairline" and "micro hairline". It can be imagined as a U-shaped area that is 1 to 3 cm deep and its limit is defined by two lines—the anterior line and the posterior line. The zone in between these two hairlines is filled with hair, with anterior hairline filled with 1-hair FU (3–5 mm deep), while at the posterior hairline, the hair is denser filed with 2 to 3 hairs FU predominantly. This provides a gradual transition from a bare scalp to a more defined (macro) hairline. The "macro hairline "determines the area where true visual density begins.

There are two major considerations while drawing a male hairline: Position (how high the hairline is going to be situated) and shape (bell-shaped versus round). The factors to be kept in mind is the patient's age (a young patient should not have a too low a hairline so as to accommodate future hair loss and to maintain age-appropriate appearance with time and with added consideration for donor depletion with time), donor density (a greater donor density permits a more aggressive hairline) and degree of hair loss already present (a greater degree of hair loss would indicate a more conservative design). The cardinal sin is designing a hairline which will fail to look natural with progression of age, still simply creating a high hairline and playing safe will fail to accomplish the purpose for which the transplantation was done,which is to re-establish the proper frame to the face.

Leonardo Da Vinci conceptualized the youthful face as being divided into equal thirds from trichion (central-anterior point) to the glabella, from glabella to the subnasale and subnasale to the menton. This point of trichion should be considered the absolute lowest for a hairline, but must be adjusted upwards based in age, gender, hair loss progression, donor availability and other factors.

Another rule that helps to establish the lowest centre-anterior point, describes that the lowest acceptable point of a hairline should fall at the intersection of vertical and horizontal plane of the scalp. A line is drawn at 45 degree angle to bisect the horizontal and vertical plane of the scalp. The centre anterior point can be adjusted upwards as deemed appropriate.

After establishing the centre anterior point, the lateral extent of anterior hairline needs to be created (four points, two on each side of centre-anterior point). Starting from the centre point, the hairline goes almost flat across the forehead and then curves back to meet the temporal hairline. The point where the hairline curves from frontal towards temporal hair is referred to as the lateral-anterior point.

The "flat" portion of anterior hairline extends between left and right lateral-anterior points, which are defined by two vertical lines drawn through the mid-pupil. The lateral extent of the hairline terminates at an imaginary vertical line drawn through the lateral canthus of each eye and it is the point where anterior and temporal hairline meets. (frontotemporal point). With 5 points established (one centre-anterior and two lateral anterior and two frontotemporal), the surgeon should stand behind the patient with patient's head tilted back and ensure symmetry of the hairline.

After determining the points of hairline, the shape of hairline needs to be determined. Generally, there are two shapes bell-shaped and round.

The bell-shaped hairline fits a narrower head, conserves graft, and matches the arc of temporal recession. The curve of bell shape transitions from a central convexity to lateral suppressed concavity approximately at the lateral-anterior point (mid-pupil).

The round design is better suited for a wider head with mature, stable temporal hair. The round hairline has a relative convexity maintained throughout. The lateral terminus of the hairline can either end with tail moving backward or with slight flare with towards the temples. In case of hairline ending with tail moving backwards, then the temple can progress in recession backward along this hairline and continue to look natural, however, in case of slight flare towards the temple, the surgeon will need to commit to build the temple hair in future to avoid artificial look with progression of baldness. It should be emphasized that transplantation of anterior temple is tricky and bit difficult for a young surgeon. The difficulty lies in ability to create recipient sites at a very low angle and also that changes direction, which if poorly executed cannot be easily camouflaged (Figs 17.3 to 17.7).

Path D laser assist hairline design device: Dr Damkerng Pathomvanich, hair transplant surgeon from Thailand invented this device for designing symmetrical hairline. Caution must be exercised with regards to laser safety and patients should always be instructed to close their eyes or wear eye protection (Fig. 17.8).

PRINCIPLES FOR RECIPIENT SITE CREATION

Before making all the recipient sites with a needle, the surgeon should initially make 3 to 5 sites with each type of needle at correct depth (by measuring graft length) and ensure that there is good graft-to-site fit (neither sinks nor ride too high above the skin).

There are two principal methods for creating recipient sites: Sagittal and coronal. Sagittal sites are created with edge of the needle facing forward so that a site with anterior–posterior axis is created. Coronal sites are created with edge of needle facing side to side. Two major benefits claimed for sagittal recipient sites are as follows: (1) they point in the direction in which hair is naturally facing, reducing the risk of transection of hair and (2) it is easier to interlock sites making it easier to design pattern.

Coronal sites offer two advantages: (1) They keep the hair angle consistent with the angle of the site because in sagittal site there is a chance that graft will move to a less desirable angle and (2) hence they may offer improved visual density. Different surgeons use this method at different sites, for example, temple may require more coronal sites since hair is sparser there and require low hair angle. Very often sagittal and coronal sites are mixed in hairline to make the hairline look natural and ensure better control of hair direction (Fig. 17.9).

When creating recipient sites, the surgeon should fully understood how hair grows in each region of scalp. The surgeon must be aware of the "angle" and "direction". The angle of a recipient site refers to the anterior–posterior tilt of the site relative to the scalp. The direction refers to the left to right rotation of the recipient site. The surgeon can follow the angle of the vellus hair while slit making and can minimize transections (Table 17.2).

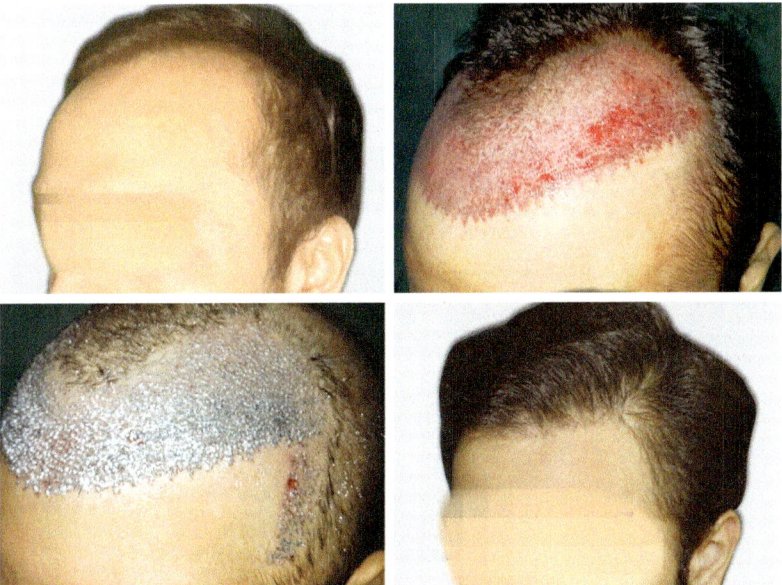

Fig. 17.3: Depicts before, after slit preparation, immediate postoperative and 8 months follow-up pictures of an aesthetically designed hairline in a hair transplant patient (4000 grafts implanted for hairline reconstruction and hair transplantation on frontal region)

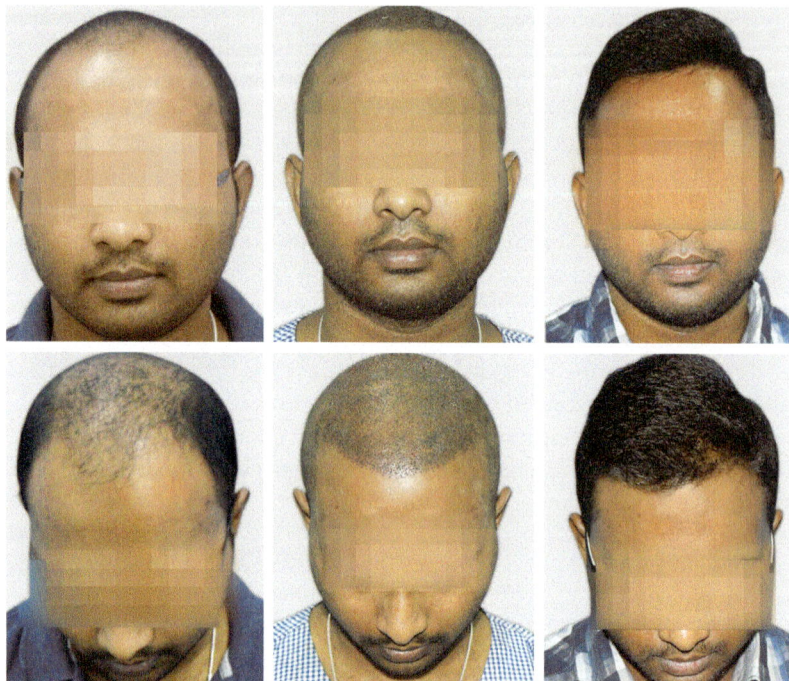

Fig. 17.4: Depicts a preoperative, immediate postoperative and 8 months follow-up pictures of a patient who has undergone hair transplantation (5000 grafts implanted for hairline reconstruction and hair transplantation on frontal region and mid scalp)

Counting incision device: It helps to maintain the count of slits during the recipient site creation. The accurate count by this instrument helps to cut the staff cost and helps in maintaining accurate count of the slits, thus helps in savings for the surgeon as well as patient as he is usually paying per follicle or per graft to the doctor.

POINTS TO CONSIDER WHILE SCORING OF GRAFT

A smaller exit angle potentially increases the trauma to the donor area because a punch directed at a steeper angle creates an elliptical wound that is significantly larger in area than if perpendicular punch is used for the same area. As punch comes in contact with the skin and dissects through it and the dermis, the increased force of friction causes follicular displacement. This displacement of follicle increases the transection rates in hands of a new surgeon. This will increase the graft requirement and potential trauma to the donor sites hampering future FUE surgery. To increase the exit

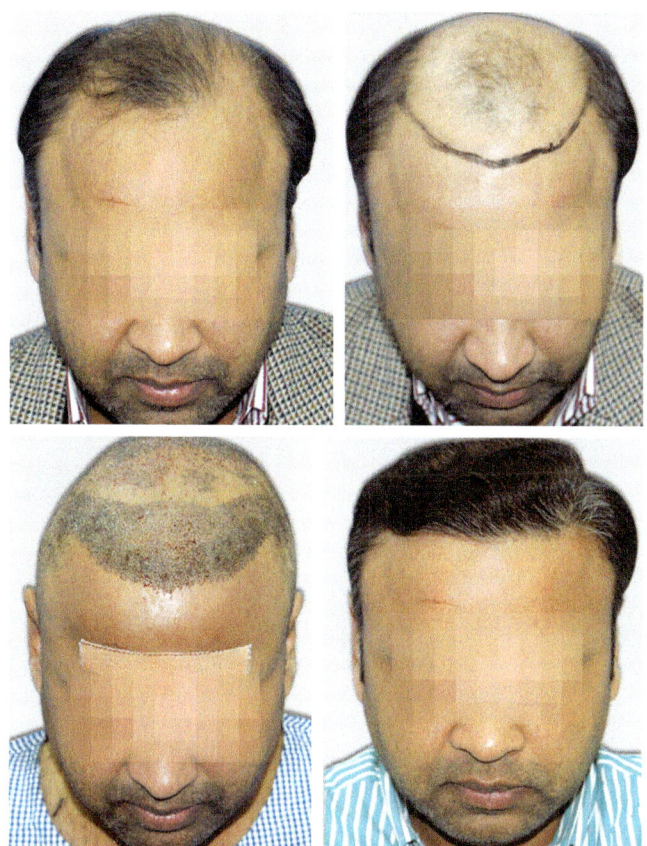

Fig. 17.5: Depicts preoperative, hairline designed, immediate postoperative and 8 months follow-up pictures of a patient following hair transplant surgery (4000 grafts implanted for hairline reconstruction and coverage of frontal region of scalp)

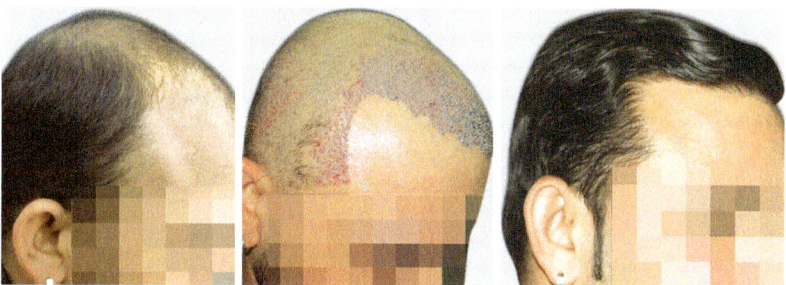

Fig. 17.6: Shows a hair transplantation in the temple region with correct angle, curl and direction (250 grafts implanted on each side for temple region hair transplantation)

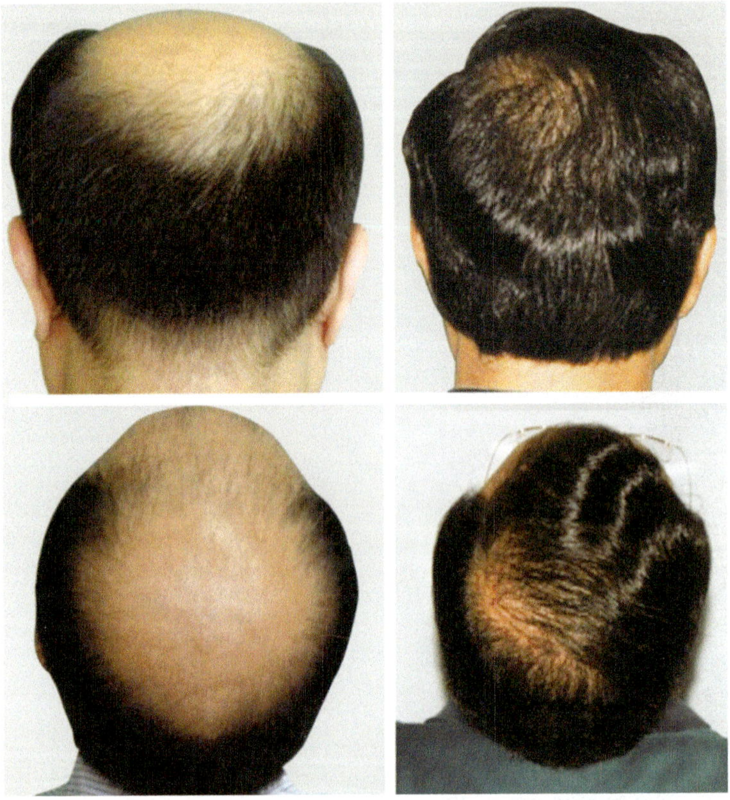

Fig. 17.7: Shows crown reconstruction with hair implantation done at correct angles and correct directions (4000 grafts used in crown reconstruction)

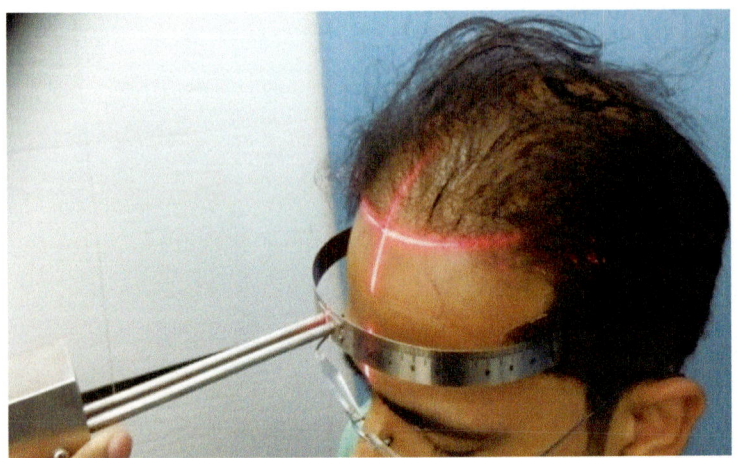

Fig. 17.8: Laser assist hairline design device

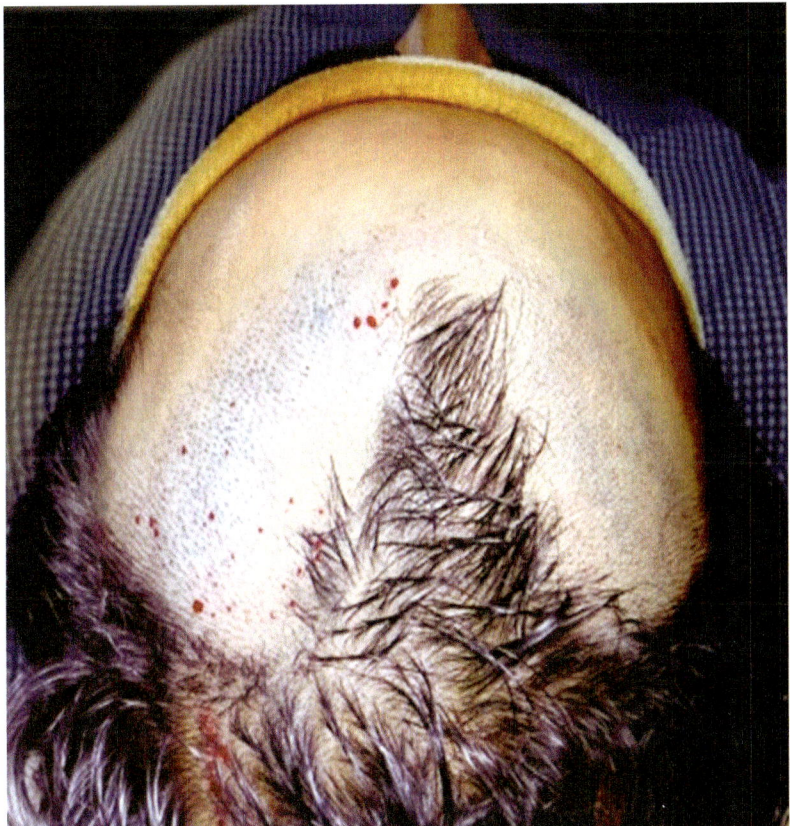

Fig. 17.9: Coronal slits made in the recipient sites except the frontal hairline where sagittal slits were made

Table 17.2: Angles and directions of hair at various sites on scalp		
Location	*Angle*	*Direction*
Anterior hairline	Low (<30 degree)	Anterior
Temporal hairline	Very low (<10 degree)	Follow sweep of temporal hairline
Lateral hump	Medium (<45 degree)	Transition from forward progressing downward
Mid-scalp	Medium (<45 degree)	Anterior
Vertex transition point	Medium (<45 degree)	Slight radial arrangement
Crown	High (45–90 degree)	Whorl
Coronet	Low (<30 degree)	Downward

angle 0.2 to 0.3 ml/square cm of normal saline needs to be injected to make the direction of hair follicle less acute to minimize transection rates (Zontos G, 2014).

Punch Characteristics

1. Optimally one should use the smallest possible punch diameter that will encircle the intact follicle.
2. FUE pioneers such as Dr Cole, Dr Robert, Dr Wolf, Dr Lorenzo and Dr Harrishave developed a consensus that punch sizes between 0.8 to 1 mm leave no noticeable difference in donor site appearance and excellent harvesting rates.
3. Harvesting devices include manual punches, mechanically assisted devices, vacuum assisted extraction devices and automated robotic assisted devices.
4. The cutting edge of follicular extraction punches can be either sharp or blunt. Cole described the characteristics of modern day sharp punches and advocates minimizing the thickness of these punches to reduce adjacent tissue damage. The sharp punch reduces mechanical force and torque that cause mechanical trauma to follicular structures and dermal tissue thus reducing graft transection. Reduced mechanical force also reduces the risk of buried grafts.
5. An ideal sharp punch is a circular punch made of hardened stainless steel with sharp edge on outside and blunt inner surface to protect the follicle.
6. "Serrounded" punch developed by Dr Rassman and Dr Cole and "triple wave" or serrated punch are designed to reduce the cutting surface area thus reducing the friction and axial force required to penetrate the skin.
7. The depth of the incision should be limited to the minimum depth possible to obtain intact follicle without damaging the outer root sheath of hair. Disrupting the attachment of erector pili muscle is generally required. Once muscular attachment is severed the follicle can be removed in total. The punch penetration ranges from 2 to 3 mm. The physician must be aware of the changing harvesting parameters like hair directions, angle, depth of penetration and punch size as he moves from one donor area to other.
8. Often, the narrowest portion of multi-hair follicle is at the surface and surface area of follicle may increase below the surface due to splaying of follicles. Limiting the depth of the punch and carefully removing the follicle using "hand over hand" technique with a fine jeweler's forceps will yield an intact follicle. Using a larger punch may also in preserving the multi-hair follicle. If a portion

of dermal papilla is remained behind, there will be regrowth of the partial follicle.

9. Removal of the scored graft requires use of jeweler's forceps. The physician should keep in mind the bulge region of hair follicle which can be compressed or traumatized while scoring. Foerster and jeweler's forceps should not come in contact with the bulge region during extraction.

10. Curly hairs are prone to transections. Before committing for FUE surgery, a small trial of donor harvesting site is recommended. With very curly hair, it is recommended to use a larger punch (1–1.2 mm) to score the skin superficially. If the transection rates are high it is helpful to use blunt punch. However, using sharp punch with minimal advancement (<2 mm) followed by extremely delicate two-hand removal technique will yield intact graft (Boden S, 2016). Use of hypodermic needle as describe by Dr Poswal for body hair extraction is useful in cutting the subdermal tissue and erector pili muscles.

11. Dr James Harris invented the blunt dissecting punch and methodology of tissue dissection is described as surgically advanced follicular extraction system (SAFE). Blunt punch requires greater physical force, that may damage the follicles and increases the risk of buried grafts but a sharp punch is usually unforgiving in hand of a new surgeon than a blunt punch and results in high transection rates. The theory behind this dissection method is the bunt punch follicular transection by acting as a wedge when dissecting the follicles from attached tissues. The punch and the dissecting technique direct the splayed follicles into the lumen of the punch thus reducing follicular transection. The first step requires a sharp punch to be centered over the exiting hair and skin is cut 0.3 to 0.5 mm depth. The second step involves inserting the blunt punch through the scored skin.

12. Hex punch introduced in 2014 (Lorenzo J), it is a hexagon shaped blunt punch which allows faster donor harvesting or dissection with acceptable transection rates. The points of hex punch induce vibration to the skin that helps to separate the tissues.

13. An increase in punch diameter from 0.8 to 1 mm increases the surface area of scar by 58%, thus size of the punch should be carefully selected.

14. Beard and torso hair vary widely in angle and direction of hair emergence even in same patient. Therefore direction of punch must constantly be adjusted during extraction. The submental beard area and the torso subcutaneous tissue is generally soft and fatty, rather than fibrous, so there is a little popping and require minimal jerk.

INNOVATIONS IN TRANSPLANTATION

Grafts

KD spreader: Invented by Dr Kuldeep Saxena, it is a slit dilator and tissue holding device (personal communication). It is used to give traction in FUE surgery for smooth scoring and graft extraction by exerting a pulling force in opposite direction. It minimizes the risk of decapping and reduces the fatigue of the assistant during surgery (Fig. 17.10).

Suction assisted punch: The only motorized FUE device currently approved in the United States by a French firm MedicaMat. It combines the use of rotator punch system and an internal vacuum. There is limited experience among surgeons but it makes the process extremely fast and is the easiest way to learn FUE. However, suction assisted punch can damage graft as they are susceptible to desiccation. The suction assisted extraction can be stepping stone to manual hand extraction.

Vacuum assisted follicular extraction device (VAFED): Invented by Dr Anil Garg, is a motorized punch attached to the suction device (personal communication). Dissected grafts are extracted directly in storage suction media (personal communication). The dermis is cut up to the sebaceous gland. According to Garg, there are negligible follicular transections, preservation of perifollicular tissue with no buried grafts.

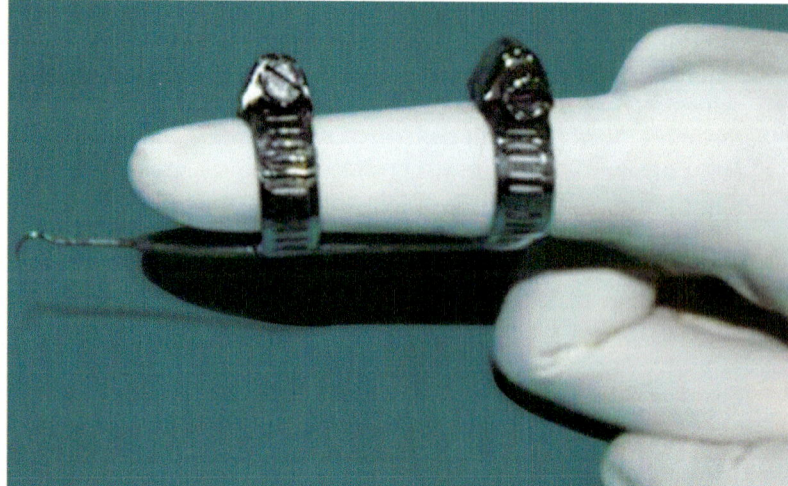

Fig. 17.10: KD spreader developed by Dr Kuldeep Saxena to provide stretch to the skin during the extraction process

Improving Graft Survival

After donor harvesting, the graft is exposed to stress, hypoxia and anaerobic environments. There is production of free radicals which produces cellular damage. When reintroduced into the scalp, graft may suffer from reperfusion injury. HypoThermosol FBS (BioLife Solutions, Bothell, USA) and liposomal ATP (ATPv) are used as holding solutions. HypoThermosol FRS provides a substrate that scavenges free radicals, provides pH buffering, osmotic support, energy substrates and ionic concentrations that balance the intracellular state at low temperature. Liposomal ATP provides hair follicles this vital nucleotide containing an enormous amount of chemical energy.

Use of Implanters

1. Since hair is trimmed short (1–1.5 mm) before extraction, determining the curl of the hair is difficult since orientation is critical while placing hair at temple and crown where angles are more acute. The epidermal cap surface should be parallel to the skin surface to ensure correct orientation and to prevent sinking of graft.

2. All bulbs should be enclosed within the implanter to prevent bending of bulb while insertion before unloading. Graft must be held by epidermal cap and forceps must slide through the slit to guide the graft into the implanter.

3. Before physician makes all the sites, a few test sites must be made to ensure implanter properly fit inside the sites to avoid popping or sinking of the graft.

4. The problem of popping can be avoided by placing a graft and then skipping to other sites 8 to 10 slits away. One should place graft in a row from one side to the middle and then repeating the sequence until the row is complete. If more than one staff is placing the graft avoid close proximity among grafts.

5. If the frontal hairline is going to be implanted, the 1 hair graft is to be loaded first followed by two-hair graft (with 19G implanter).

6. Implanter pen: It has been invented by Dr Pascal Boudjema of France and the effort required during loading of graft is minimized by this pen.

7. Choi implanter: This implanter has a plunger. The needle is inserted into the graft and plunger is pressed to insert the graft.

Avoiding Poor Outcomes

Careful attention to donor-harvesting management is critical to achieving aesthetic cosmetic outcomes in a donor region. Too aggressive harvesting will result in unaesthetic appearance of donor site. A young surgeon should focus on transplanting greater number of grafts with low transection rates and reasonable harvesting rates. The concentrated focus for harvesting in young surgeons can result in loss of appreciation of aesthetics in the occipital and temporoparietal regions.

Dr Jose Lorenzo advocates leaving partially transected follicles to be left at the donor sites by using small punches. This partially transected follicle will eventually grow into complete follicle in the donor regions. Others advocate leaving behind melanin containing follicles from complex follicular groupings thus decreasing donor site hypopigmentation.

The ideal appearance of donor site is a pattern of random distribution without evidence of excessive thinning or density loss to donor region. The young surgeon should avoid exclusively harvesting from occipital region of the scalp as it results in thinned out occipital region. Attempt should be made to harvest randomly and uniformly from the entire SDA. The potential of retrograde alopecia developing from the nape of the neck upward must also be taken into consideration.

Donor site hypopigmentation does not occur in all cases but can occur in some patients. Proper consent regarding such cosmetic outcome must be taken.

Role of Bioenhancement Technology

Our experience with platelet-rich plasma (PRP) therapy in surgery hair transplant recipients helps in minimizing the post-transplantation hair loss and achieving the desired result in a relatively short time as compared to those not receiving PRP. Similarly, Acell Matristem Micromatrix (AMM), and liposomal ATP have helped in more consistent results, healthy hair growth, a shorter and improved recovery period and earlier onset of growth of transplanted hair. These bioenhancement techniques can never overcome bad technique.

Automated FUE

ARTAS system (AS) for FUE is a computer controlled robotic device that employs a one or two-camera system for its acquisition of information about the hair and algorithms to compute details such as hair angles, directions, and follicular unit density. The dissection mechanism is a two-punch system, an inner sharp needle and an outer blunt tipped coring punch, which separates the follicular group from the skin. Patient preparation begins with shaving of hair to a length of 1.5–2 mm in length. The interaction of the mechanical system and the skin requires a device called skin tensioner which has small pins on each four sides and it stretches the skin for punching. After anesthesia, skin tensioner is placed in the selected dissection or harvesting region and moves the dissection mechanism into position. The system automatically moves to the lower left hand corner of the grid and starts the process of punching with a command from the operator. After dissection, the staff removes the grafts that still remain in the scalp and ready the patient for recipient site creation. The primary advantage with ARTAS is in the terms of graft per hour produced and the consistency of the quality of graft generated (Fig. 17.11).

Piloscopy

Invented by Dr Carlos Wesley piloscopy is also called Pilofocus Carlos hair transplantation technique. The piloscope is a handheld device that allows for removal of the subcutaneous portion of target hair follicle without traumatizing the skin surface overlying each selected follicle. The four essential components of the piloscope are (1) the subdermal arm comprised of a coring cannula and clipping edges, (2) the handheld control paddles, (3) the monitor on which target follicle can be visualized, (4) the graft-storage container.

An entry port is created by introducing a scalpel into the scalp surface at a perpendicular plane and advancing it deeply to the level of galea aponeurotica. Through this 1.4 cm long entry port, the tissue dissection device is inserted into the subcutaneous plane and, using side to side sweeping motion, performs blunt dissection within the subcutaneous level just deep to the bed of overlying hair follicle bulbs.

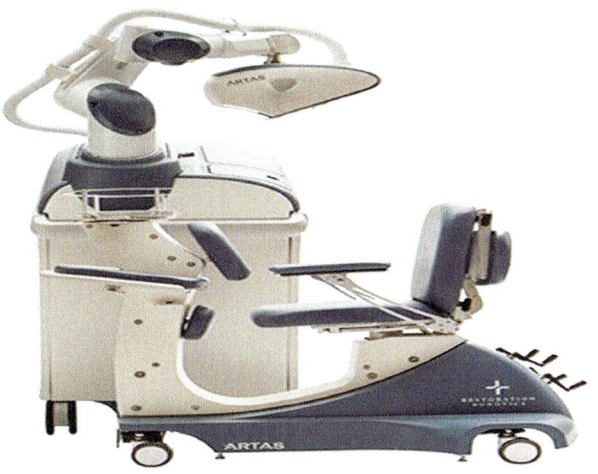

Fig. 17.11: ARTAS machine (robotic hair transplant)

The resultant cavity dissected lies entirely within the safe donor area. Insertion of subdermal arm of the piloscope occurs through the entry port and external body of piloscope move in tandem. The subdermal arm contains dull rotating cannula capable of coring around stem cells enriched segments of the desired follicle and clipping off the hair shaft of the target follicle at its most superficial level just below the skin surface. The piloscope is currently being used in clinical trials to verify the safety and efficacy.

CONCLUSION

Hair transplant is a rapidly advancing field with modifications in surgery. Its an art and science combined into one as doctor has to imagine the results of his surgery at the time of starting of surgery. The imagination of doctor should meet the patients' expectation when the regrowth of transplanted hair occurs. One who plans to do hair transplant should put his heart into this field for achieving excellence.

The authors are coming up with a pictorial book and a textbook on hair transplantation.

Bibliography

1. Boden S, Kenneth W. Motorized FUE with sharp punch. In: Lam M, Jr Williams KL. *Hair Transplant*. 1st edition. Jaypee Brothers Medical Publishers 2016;360(4):241–307.

2. Boden S. FUE Donor evaluation and surgical planning. In: Lam M, Jr Williams KL. *Hair Transplant*. 1st edition. Jaypee Brothers Medical Publishers 2016;360(4):109–19.

3. Caroli S, Pathomvanich D, Amonpattatana K, Kumar A: Current status of hair restoration surgery. Int Surg 2011;96(4):345–51.

4. Cole Jp. An analysis of follicular punches, mechanics, and dynamics in follicular unit extraction. Facial Plast Surg Clin North Am 2013;21:437–47.

5. Cole JP. CID-Counting incision device [Internet] United States. Cole instruments. [2017 February 27]. Available from: https://www.coleinstruments.com/surgical-instruments/hair-transplant/cid-counting-incision-device-details.

6. Eliott Vance. Scalp anaesthesia and hemostasis for FUE. In: Lam M, Jr Williams KL. *Hair Transplant*. 1st edition. Jaypee Brother Medical Publishers 2016;360(4):95–97.

7. Eliyahu R. Path D laser assist hairline design device—a new product [Internet] United States. Cole instruments. 2013 July 18 [2017 february 27]. Available from: https://www.coleinstruments.com/path-d-laser-assist-hairline-design-new-product.

8. Harris JA. Automated FUE. In: Lam M, Jr Williams K. *Hair Transplant*. 1st edition. Jaypee Brothers Medical Publishers 2016;360(4):309–25

9. Harris JA. New methodology and instrumentation for follicular unit extraction: lower follicle transection rates and expanded patient candidacy. Dermatol Surg 2006;32(1):56–61.

10. Harris JA. Follicular unit extraction. Facial Plast Surg Clin North Am 2013; 21(3):75–384.

11. Lam M Samuel. *Hair Transplant*. 2nd edition. Jaypee Brothers Medical Publishers 2016;360(1):67–166.

12. Lardner T. Improving Graft Survival: Graft placement and the use of implanters.In: Lam M, Jr Williams K. *Hair Transplant*. 1st edition. Jaypee Brothers Medical Publishers 2016;360(4):151–63.

13. Lee DY, Choi YL, Kim MG, Kim JA, Lee KJ, Park JH, Cho HJ, Yang JM, Sim WY. The combined use of needle with hair transplanter for hair recipient sites. Dermatol Surg 2007;33(1):128–29.

14. Lee DY, Lee JH, Yang JM, Lee ES. New instrument for hair transplant: multichannel hair transplanter. Dermatol Surg 2005;31(3):379.

15. Lee W, Lee S, Na G, Kim M, Kim J. Survival rate according to grafted density of Korean one-hair follicular units with a hair transplant implanter: Experience with four patients. Dermatol Surg 2006;32(6):815–18.

16. Lorenzo J. Manual FUE. In: Lam M, Jr Williams KL. *Hair Transplant*. 1st edition. Jaypee Brothers Medical Publishers; 2016;360(4):238–39.

17. Poswal A. Expanding needle concept for better extraction of body hair grafts. Indian J Dermatol 2013;58(3):240.

18. Rassman W, Berstein R. Follicular unit extraction: minimally invasive surgery for hair transplantation. Dermatol Surg 2002;28:720–8.

19. Rose PT. Hair restoration surgery: challenges and solutions. Clin Cosmet investing Dermatol 2015;8:361–370.

20. Sethi P, Bansal A. Direct hair transplantation: a modified follicular unit extraction technique. J Cuta Aesthet Surg 2013;6(2):100–5.

21. Vories M. Suction-assisted FUE. In: Lam M, Jr Williams KL. *Hair Transplant*. 1st edition. Jaypee Brothers Medical Publishers 2016;360(4):299–307.

22. Wesley CK. Piloscopy. In: Lam M, Jr Williams K. *Hair Transplant*. 1st edition. Jaypee Brothers Medical Publishers; 2016;360(4):454–64.

23. Zontos G, Rose P, Nikiforidis G. A mathematical proof of how the outgrowth angle of hair follicles influences the injury to the donor area in FUE harvesting. Dermatol Surg 2014;40(10):1147–50.

24. Zontos G. The physics of follicular unit extraction. In: Lam M, Jr Williams KL. Hair Transplant. 1st edition. Jaypee Brothers Medical Publishers 2016; 360(4):47–57.

18

Hirsutism

Kabir Sardana, Deep Dutta, Sidharth Tandon

INTRODUCTION

Hirsutism is defined as androgen-dependent excessive male-pattern hair growth in women. Hirsutism must be distinguished from hypertrichosis, the term used to describe the excessive growth of androgen-independent hair which is vellus, prominent in nonsexual areas, and most commonly familial or caused by metabolic disorders (for example, thyroid disturbances, anorexia nervosa) or medications (for example, phenytoin, minoxidil, or cyclosporine).

In adult Caucasian and Afro-American women, hirsutism has traditionally been defined by a total score of 8 or more on the scale proposed by Ferriman and Gallwey (FGS) (Fig. 18.1). However, it must be highlighted that in clinical practice, we often do come across individuals who have concerns of excessive body/facial hair and their FGS score is less than 8. These patients often have dark terminal hair limited to a few areas of the face or the body (such as the upper lip and chin areas). It has been suggested that FGS, scores ≥2 to 3 in Han Chinese and Thai women may be considered as clinically significant in contrast to ≥9 to 10 in Mediterranean, Hispanic, and Middle Eastern women. Females from Mediterranean area often present with facial hirsutism and 9% of Caucasian females are also hirsute.

Hirsutism, acne, and pattern balding are variably expressed cutaneous manifestations of androgen excess. Some hyperandrogenic patients have hirsutism or acne alone, others both (Fig. 18.2), yet others neither ("cryptic hyperandrogenemia"). Either male- or female-pattern (diffuse) balding can be the sole manifestation of hyperandrogenism. Moderately severe hirsutism or cystic acne is even more likely to be hyperandrogenic. However, the amount of sexual hair and sebaceous gland development seems to depend as much upon the factors determining sensitivity of the skin to androgens as it is dependent upon the serum androgen level itself.

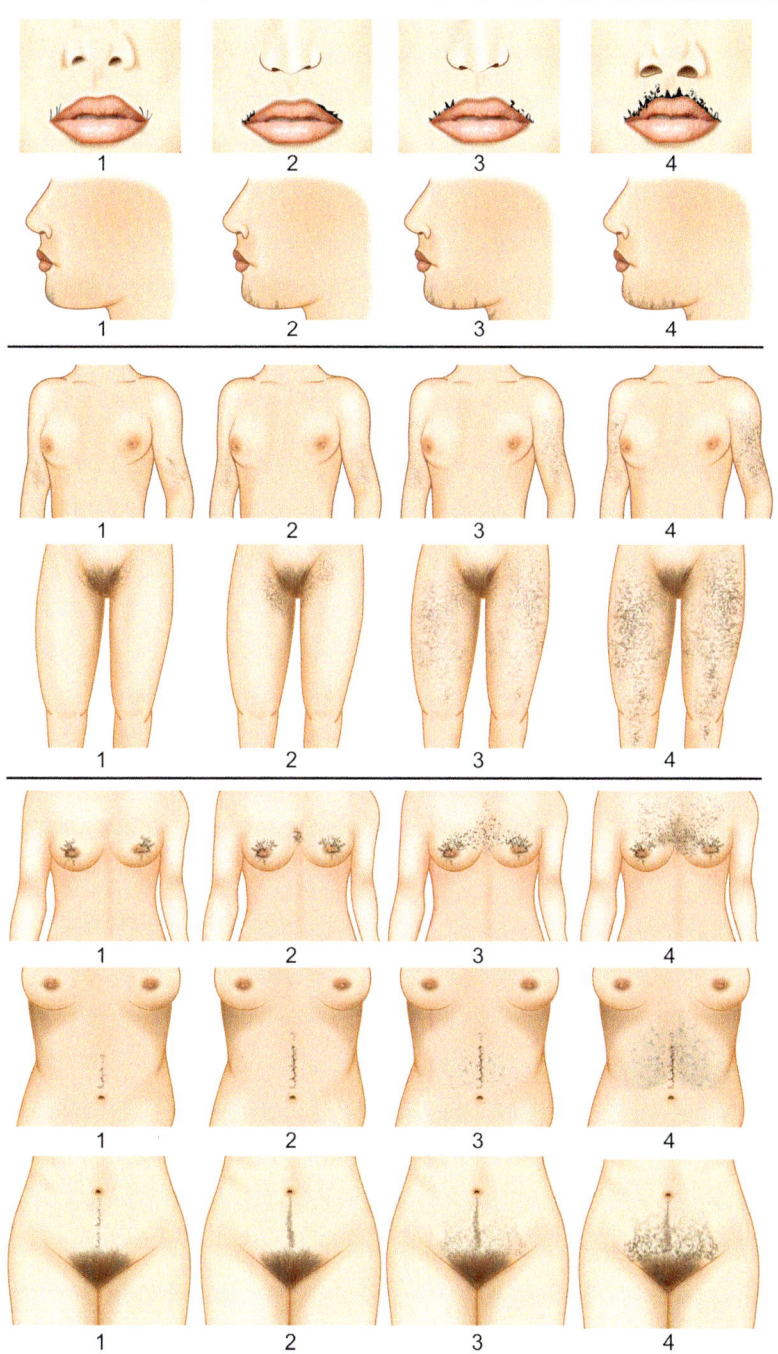

Fig. 18.1A

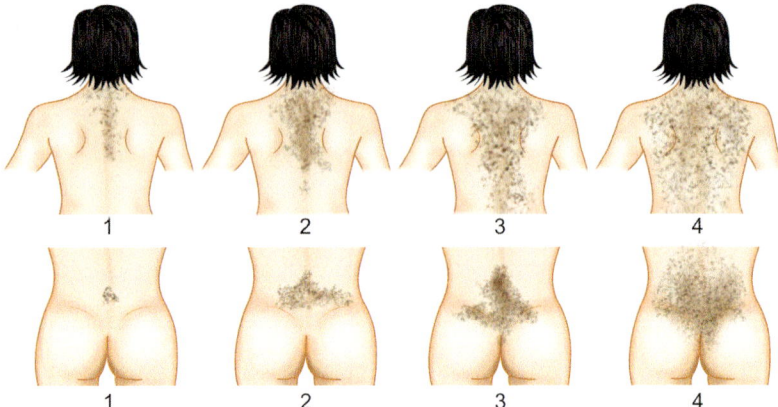

Fig. 18.1 A and B: Modified Ferriman-Gallwey score (mF6): Nine body regions are evaluated for their degree of hair growth from 1 to 4. A total score >8 is a sign for hirsutism

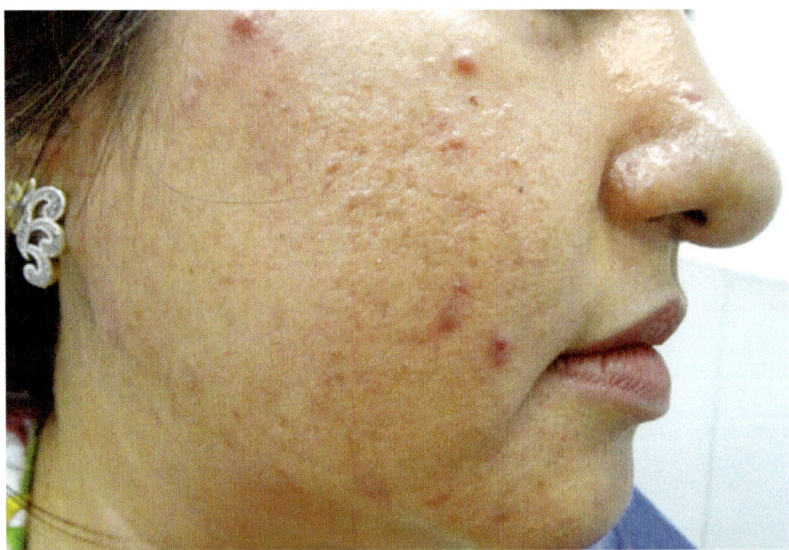

Fig. 18.2: A 42-year-old female with mild hirsutism and acne with a distinct involvement of the jaw line, a diagnostic sign of a hormonal dysfunction. Here she had a raised free androgen index

The spectrum ranges from women whose skin seems "hypersensitive" to normal blood-free androgen levels; this seems to account for "idiopathic" hirsutism and acne. At the other ends of the spectrum are women whose skin is relatively insensitive to androgens; this seems to account for the so-called "cryptic" hyperandrogenemia (hyperandrogenism without skin manifestations).

ANDROGEN ORIGIN AND PATHWAYS (Fig. 18.3)

Testosterone which is circulating in the blood is either converted to DHT by 5α-reductase activity of the target tissue or it is converted to estradiol in an intracrine fashion by the aromatase activity of the target tissue. Testosterone itself is thought to be a biologically active androgen and among the natural C19 steroids, DHT is a biologically active potent androgen which acts through the androgen receptors of target tissues. It has been seen that the effect of testosterone at different body sites is also different as the dermal papilla cells of beard secrete autocrine growth factors like IGF-1 in response to testosterone which causes enlargement of hair follicle, paradoxically investigations performed on dermal papilla from balding scalp of stump-tailed macaque show that testosterone inhibited the growth of hair follicle.

Testosterone in reproductive-age women is produced by two major mechanisms: Direct secretion by the ovary, which accounts for roughly one-third of testosterone production, and conversion of the precursor androstenedione to testosterone in the peripheral (extragonadal) tissues, which accounts for two-thirds of testosterone production (Fig. 18.3). These peripheral tissues include the skin and adipose tissue. Testosterone binds to its nuclear androgen receptors to exert its biologic effects.Testosterone is also converted to a more potent steroid, DHT, to exert full androgenic effects on certain target tissues such as hair follicles and external genitalia. The protein products of two genes (5α-reductase type 1 and type 2) exhibit this enzymatic activity. DHT is necessary for hair growth and virilization. Androgen action in target tissues is determined at least in part by the level of local 5α-reductase activity and the androgen receptor content. Polymorphisms and skewed X-inactivation of the androgen receptor have been variably invoked as determinants of sensitivity to androgen.

Androgen receptors mediate androgenic action in critical target tissues. Local enzymes other than 5α-reductase (e.g. aromatase, oxidative 17β-HSD) also regulate androgen action by metabolizing testosterone, to the androgenically inactive androstenedione or to a potent estrogen estradiol, in the target tissues. There appears to be a balance between potent androgen action when DHT is formed and reduction of androgenicity when inactive C19 steroids or estradiol is formed from testosterone in target tissues and other extragonadal tissues. Plasma or urinary *3α-androstanediol glucuronide*, a metabolite of DHT, has been touted as a marker of sensitivity of the hair follicle to androgen and is probably of great value in cases of cutaneous hyperandrogenism (Lobo et al, 1987).

Over 96% of the plasma testosterone and structurally related 17β-hydroxysteroids circulate in plasma bound to carrier proteins, with only a small fraction remaining free. Sex hormone binding globulin

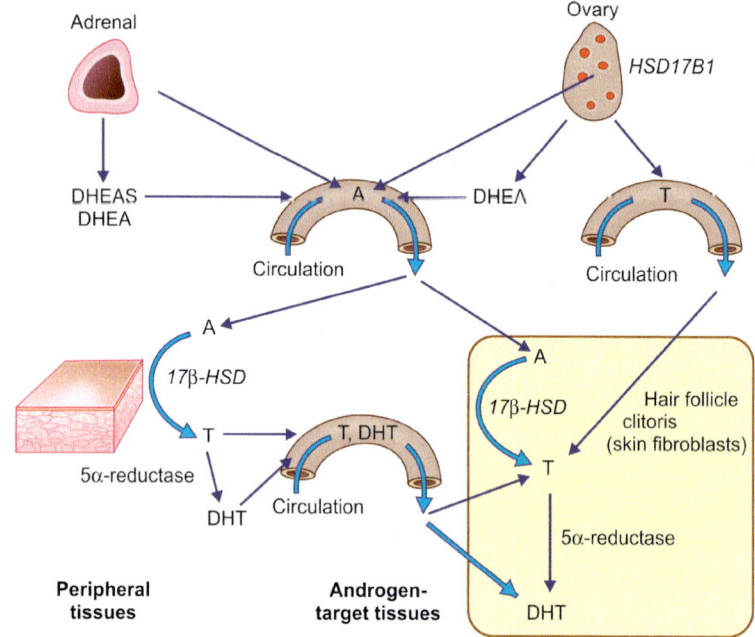

Fig. 18.3: Androgen origin and pathways in women. About 20 to 30% of testosterone (T) is secreted by the ovary. The rest is accounted for by the conversion of circulating androstenedione (A) to T in various peripheral tissues. Both the adrenal and the ovary contribute to circulating A directly or indirectly, T may also be formed locally in androgen target tissues. T is converted to the biologically potent androgen dihydrotestosterone (DHT) within the target tissues and cells. For example, local conversion of T to DHT by 5α-reductase activity. The enzyme activity of 17β-HSD in peripheral tissues may be conferred by protein products of several genes with overlapping functions; DHEAS dehydroepiandrosterone sulfate; 17β-HSD, 17β-hydroxysteroid dehydrogenase.

(*SHBG*) and albumin are the principal sex steroid-binding proteins in plasma. Although there has been interest in the possibility that albumin-bound testosterone is bioactive, most evidence suggests that it is only the free steroid intermediate that is bioavailable. Due to its high binding affinity for testosterone, SHBG concentration is the major determinant of the fraction of testosterone binding to plasma albumin and determines the fraction remaining free, which is biologically active in blood. SHBG levels are increased by estrogens and thyroid hormone excess; serum concentrations are decreased in hyperandrogenic, obese, hyperinsulinemic, or chronic inflammatory states. A simpler test is the free androgen index (FAI; discussed below) which is calculated as (Nestler et al, 1991).

FAI = total testosterone (nmol/L) × 100/sex hormone-binding globulin (SHBG) (nmol/L)

Androstenedione, the direct precursor of testosterone, is produced in the ovary and the adrenal. The C19 steroids DHEAS and DHEA of adrenal origin and DHEA of ovarian origin indirectly contribute to testosterone formation by first being converted to androstenedione, which is subsequently converted to testosterone (*see* Fig. 18.3). DHEA, DHEAS, and androstenedione are biologically inert steroids that serve as precursors for testosterone or estrone production. Up to 20 mg of DHEAS is produced daily, compared with only 3 mg of androstenedione and 8 mg of DHEA per day. The conversion rate of circulating androstenedione to testosterone in extragonadal tissues is about 5% in both men and women.

Serum 17-hydroxyprogesterone, like serum testosterone and androstenedione, may arise from either the adrenal glands or ovaries.

ETIOLOGY OF ANDROGEN EXCESS

A list of prevalent disorders associated with androgen excess is listed in Table 18.1. The term extraovarian steroid formation is used synonymously with extraglandular, extragonadal, or peripheral steroid formation.

Overall, the prevalence of androgen-excess disorders was found to be as follows: 72.1% for PCOS (anovulatory patients, 56.6%; mildly affected ovulatory patients, 15.5%); 15.8% for idiopathic

Table 18.1: Causes of androgen excess in females	
Ovarian	Polycystic ovary syndrome (PCOS)
	Hyperthecosis (a severe PCOS variant)
	Ovarian tumor (e.g. Sertoli-Leydig cell tumor)
Adrenal	Nonclassic congenital adrenal hyperplasia
	Cushing's syndrome
	Glucocorticoid resistance
	Adrenal tumor (e.g. adenoma, carcinoma)
Specific conditions of pregnancy	Luteoma of pregnancy
	Hyperreactio-luteinalis
	Aromatase deficiency in fetus
Other	Hyperprolactinemia, hypothyroidism
	Medications (danazol, testosterone, anabolizing agents)
	Idiopathic hirsutism (normal serum testosterone in an ovulatory woman)
	Idiopathic hyperandrogenism (patients who do not fall into any of the other categories listed)
	Hepatic hirsutism
	Hirsutism due to peripheral failure

hyperandrogenism; 7.6% for idiopathic hirsutism; 4.3% for 21-hydroxylase-deficient non-classic congenital adrenal hyperplasia; and 0.2% for androgen-secreting tumors (Carmine et al, 2006).

In most hyperandrogenic disorders, androgen originates from more than one source. For example, testosterone secretion is somewhat increased from the ovary in PCOS, but the bulk of testosterone comes from extraovarian conversion of significantly elevated circulating androstenedione of ovarian origin to testosterone. Patients with PCOS also show increased adrenal output of DHEAS, which (after peripheral conversion to DHEA that is further converted to androstenedione) contributes indirectly to extraovarian testosterone formation. An overview of PCOS is given in Box 18.1.

If androgen excess is associated with primary amenorrhea, abnormal *in utero* sexual differentiation should be strongly suspected.

A now common cause in urban patients is exogenous androgen use. These include supplements and injections given in gyms, but these are not revealed on blood tests.

Constitutional Hirsutism

It can be of 4 types; *Peripheral, ovarian, adrenal* and *idiopathic*. Of these probably *obesity* is an underdiagnosed cause.

Idiopathic (constitutional) hirsutism is characterized by excessive hair growth in the absence of excessive circulating androgen levels in ovulatory women, and it occurs more frequently in certain ethnic populations, particularly in women of Mediterranean ancestry. It is defined as hirsutism in conjunction with regular menstrual cycles and normal levels of serum testosterone. Idiopathic hirsutism is not associated with any signs of virilization. Its cause is not understood completely. It has been proposed that women with idiopathic hirsutism have significantly increased cutaneous 5α-reductase activity, but this association has not been confirmed. It is also unclear whether either of the 5α-reductase isoenzymes (type 1 or 2) is predominant in the development of idiopathic hirsutism.

Obesity may account for most cases of idiopathic hyperandrogenism and may mimic PCOS in some cases. In a large series of PCOS patients who met NIH diagnostic criteria in the idiopathic hyperandrogenemia subset most were obese (Rosenfield et al, 2011). These patients were characterized by mild hyperandrogenemia, and most had normal-size ovaries and normal LH and AMH levels. Adipose tissue is a major site for the formation of testosterone from the circulating precursor androstenedione. Thus, obesity is accompanied both by increased testosterone production and suppressed SHBG. Gonadotropins are suppressed in obesity, in part from increased clearance, possibly partly

Box 18.1: Snapshot of PCOS

Clinical features

- Oligo-/amenorrhoea (70%)
- Hirsutism (66%)
- 25% of patients also suffer from acne or male pattern alopecia. Virilization is not a feature of PCOS
- There is often a family history of hirsutism or irregular periods (<1% of hirsute patients have non-classic congenital adrenal hyperplasia)
- Slower onset of hirsutism
- Obesity (50%)
- Acanthosis nigricans may be found in 1–3% of insulin-resistant patients with PCOS
- Infertility (30%). PCOS accounts for 75% cases of anovulatory infertility

Symptoms often begin around puberty, after weight gain, or after stopping the oral contraceptive pill, but can present at any time

Investigations

Testosterone concentration

Performed primarily as a screen for hyperandrogenism. Normal serum testosterone level in females is <0.4 ng/ml. Any value between 0.4 and 0.9 ng/ml is considered to be borderline hyperandrogenism. Any value more than 0.9 ng/ml is diagnostic of definitive biochemical hyperandrogenism. Testosterone values >2 ng/ml is highly predictive of underlying androgen secreting tumors, or hyperthecosis

However, it must be realized that in PCOS, serum androgen concentrations may not always reflect the degree of hirsutism because of variable androgen receptor sensitivity

SHBG

Low in 50% of patients with PCOS, owing to the hyperinsulinemic state, with a consequent increase in circulating free androgens

(Contd.)

Free androgen index	FAI = 100 × total testosterone/SHBG
Anti-müllerian hormone (AMH)	Reliable and more sensitive than USG
Pelvic ultrasound (US)	Ultrasound criteria for PCO defined >12 follicles between 2 and 9 mm in diameter or ovarian volume >10 cm (Rotterdam Criteria)
	US is sensitive but not specific (occurs in CAH and Cushing). Usually trans-vaginal but transabdominal possible in experienced hands
	Measurement of endometrial thickness is of major importance in the diagnosis of endometrial hyperplasia in the presence of anovulation. Transvaginal US will also identify 90% of ovarian virilizing tumours

Associated endocrinopathy

Serum prolactin	Up to 100 ng/ml in 30%
17OH progesterone (17OHP)	Hyperprolactinemia is a cause of secondary PCOS and is often associated with hyperandrogenism
DHEAS and androstenedione	Morning serum 17OHP, preferably done on the day 2 to day 3 of the menstrual cycle is a good screening test to rule out non-classical congenital adrenal hyperplasia (NCCAH). Baseline 17OHP <2 ng/ml rules out NCCAH, whereas >8 ng/ml is diagnostic of NCCAH. For patients having values between 2 and 8 ng/ml, one needs to measure 1 hour post 250 µg ACTH serum 17OHP, if being >10 ng/ml is diagnostic of NCCAH, and being less than or equal to 10 ng/ml rules out NCCAH
	Useful in determining the origin of hyperandrogenism. DHEAS is primarily of adrenal origin, where as andro-stenedione is primarily ovarian in origin. Differential elevation is seen in different androgen secreting tumors

related to abnormal estrogen metabolism. Estrone formation from androstenedione is increased, and estradiol metabolism is diverted to active rather than inactive metabolites.

The presence of oligo-ovulation or anovulation in hirsute women after exclusion of related disorders (e.g. hypothyroidism, hyperprolactinemia, nonclassic adrenal hyperplasia) is consistent with the diagnosis of PCOS. Thyroid dysfunction and hyperprolactinemia should be excluded by the measurements of serum thyroxine, thyroid stimulating hormone (TSH) and prolactin. The follicular phase basal 17-hydroxyprogesterone level should be measured to exclude 21-hydroxylase deficient, nonclassic adrenal hyperplasia. The use of exogenous androgens should also be excluded. In summary, the diagnosis of idiopathic hirsutism is one of exclusion (Fig. 18.4). A depictive flowchart is detailed in Fig. 18.5.

DIAGNOSIS OF HYPERANDROGENISM

There are numerous protocols for testing patients but we will focus on a practical, cost effective and evidence-based protocol, which takes into consideration assay sensitivity. It must be mentioned that in *most* cases of hirsutism most of the tests may be normal and the patient may represent merely end organ hypersensitivity. Hyperandrogenemia must be considered in women with hirsutism or moderately severe acne vulgaris, anovulatory symptoms, or central obesity. An approach is given in Fig. 18.4.

Whom to Assess?

1. Most women with *focal hirsutism* and *regular menses* who have no other evidence to suggest an underlying cause have a very low likelihood of excess androgen production and do not require an endocrine workup. Similarly, women with isolated mild hirsutism (score 8 to 15) are unlikely to have a medical disorder that would change management. However, in women with symptomatic hirsutism of any degree, or acne that is poorly responsive to topical treatment, androgen levels should be assessed.

2. *Rapid* development or progression of hirsutism, progression despite therapy, or evidence of virilization (such as clitoromegaly, increasing muscularity, deepening of the voice, or balding) increase the likelihood of an androgen secreting *neoplasm*. However, tumors producing only moderate amounts of androgen have indolent progression of sign and symptoms. Very high levels of total testosterone (>200 ng/dl [6.94 nmol/liter]) or of dehydro-epiandrosterone sulfate (more than 700 μg/dl [19 μmol/liter]) heighten the likelihood of an underlying ovarian or adrenal

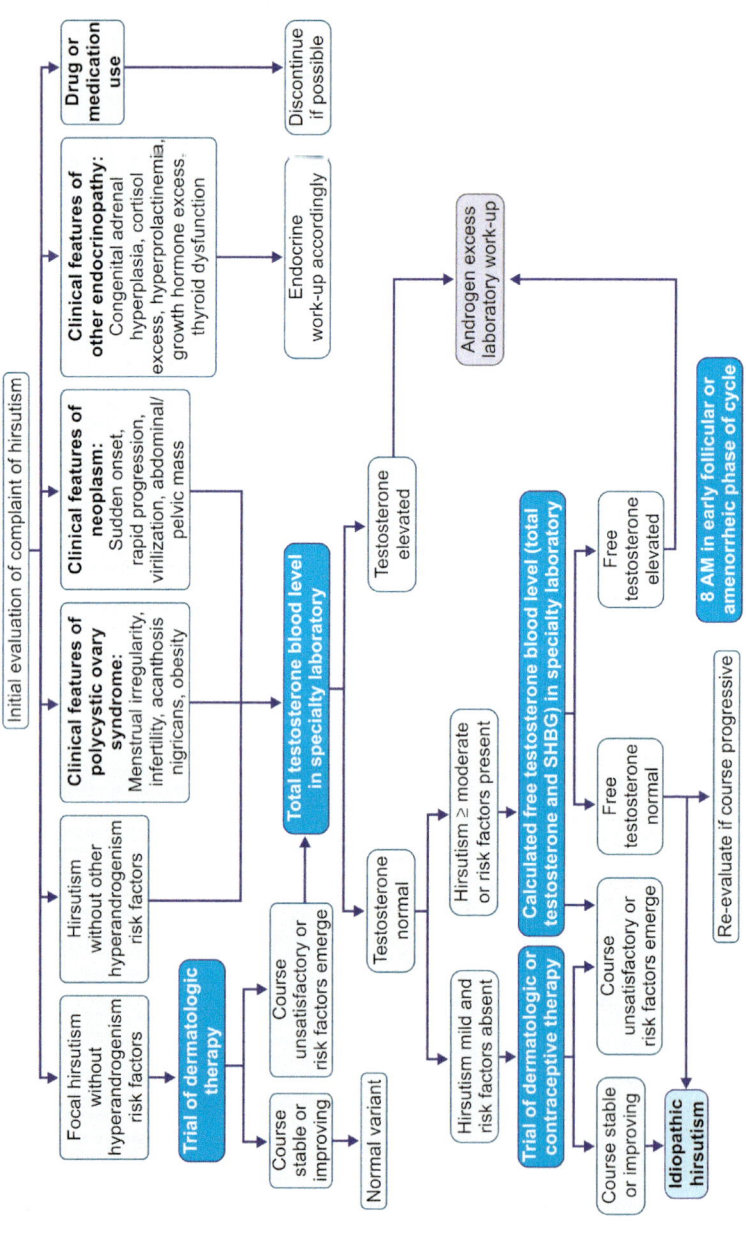

Fig. 18.4: A diagnostic approach to hirsutism

neoplasm. However, such high levels do not always indicate an androgen-secreting neoplasm, and lesser elevations may occur with androgen-secreting tumors (Waggoner et al, 1999). If a neoplasm is suspected, a vaginal probe pelvic ultrasound should be done. If no ovarian tumor is identified, further imaging studies (e.g. abdominal computed tomography for an adrenal neoplasm) may be warranted. Ovarian hyperthecosis, a severe variant of PCOS, also gives rise to severe androgen excess that may progress rapidly, especially at the time of expected puberty.

3. Testing for hyperandrogenemia is suggested if there is other evidence of PCOS or endocrinopathies that cause hyperandrogenism, even in the absence of hirsutism or other cutaneous hyperandrogenic manifestations. Most important is an abnormal degree of menstrual irregularity (e.g. missing more than 3 to 4 periods per year), excessive anovulatory ("dysfunctional") uterine bleeding, or infertility.

4. Central or intractable *obesity* should raise a suspicion for hyperandrogenism, especially if it is associated with acanthosis nigricans, suggesting insulin resistance, as should diabetes or metabolic syndrome in the patient or primary relatives.

5. High risk for *nonclassic* CAH is posed by a positive family history or ethnicity.

6. Clinical findings that best discriminate for *Cushing's* syndrome in adults are easy bruising, facial plethora, proximal muscle weakness, and abdominal striae.

7. About 1 to 2% of hirsute women without galactorrhea have idiopathic hyperprolactinemia. Acromegaly is suggested by the coarsening of facial features or by hand enlargement.

8. Androgen excess emerging at the time of puberty may be indicative of PCOS or nonclassic adrenal hyperplasia.

Laboratory Tests

An overview of the tests employed is detailed in Table 18.2 and discussed here.

1. **Testosterone:** The purpose of measuring serum testosterone is to establish the presence of circulating androgen excess and to detect extremely high values that may originate from an androgen-secreting neoplasm. It circulates in three forms; that which is bound to sex hormone-binding globulin (SHBG), the portion not bound to SHBG but loosely associated with albumin, and the fraction not bound by SHBG or albumin (i.e. free or dialyzable testosterone). The blood testosterone that is available to diffuse into target tissues

Table 18.2: A cost effective approach to testing females with androgen excess

Initial testing

Total testosterone	Normal up to 40 ng/dl; borderline hyperandrogenism (40–90 ng/dl; definitive biochemical hyperandrogenism >90 ng/dl	>166 mg/dl: Investigate for other cause >200 ng/dl: Tumors
FAI	Free androgen index test [FAI = total testosterone (nmol/L) × 100 /sex hormone-binding globulin (SHBG) (nmol/ L)]	FAI >5 = hyperandrogenemia
Prolactin	Normal 2–29 ng/ml	25–150 ng/ml: Drugs (H2 receptor blockers, proton pump inhibitors, domperidone, levosulpride, tricyclic antidepressants, selective serotonin reuptake inhibitors), PCOS, hypothyroidism >200: Prolactinomas; drug induced hyperprolactinemia less likely
TSH	Hypothyroidism can reduce SHBG levels and can mimic PCOS	

Testing based on other features and values of initial testing

17-hydroxyprogesterone (8:00 am) ACTH stimulation test	Value below 170 to 200 ng/dl excludes nonclassic CAH with about 95% specificity	>800 ng/dl—diagnostic 200–800 ng/dl are considered increased but not diagnostic of nonclassic adrenal hyperplasia Disease-free women and patients with PCOS may also have basal levels of 17-hydroxyprogesterone in this indeterminate range Here an ACTH stimulation test should be used to

(Contd.)

Table 18.2: A cost effective approach to testing females with androgen excess (*Contd.*)

Testing based on other features and values of initial testing

		distinguish non-classic adrenal hyperplasia from PCOS. A rise of the 17-hydroxyprogesterone level to at least 1000 ng/dl 60 minutes after intravenous injection of ACTH has been considered diagnostic of nonclassic adrenal hyperplasia
Cortisol	A normal morning cortisol (7–9 am) is helpful in ruling out exogenous Cushing syndrome. Overnight dexamethasone suppression test is a reliable easy to do screening test for endogenous Cushing syndrome	
DHEAS	Adrenal source of androgens	>800 µg/dl, tumors
Imaging of ovaries/adrenals	To diagnose PCOS and tumors	Transvaginal ultrasonography, abdominal ultrasonography, CT, MRI

includes the free and albumin-bound fractions and is referred to as bioavailable or non-SHBG-bound testosterone. The remainder is tightly bound to the protein SHBG. SHBG is one of the primary regulators that determine the amounts of circulating bound and bioavailable testosterone available to act on target tissues. Conditions that decrease SHBG binding (e.g. androgen excess, obesity, acromegaly, hypothyroidism, liver disease) also increase bioavailable testosterone, augmenting the effect of testosterone. SHBG also regulates the circulating amounts of bioavailable estradiol by binding a significant fraction of circulating estradiol. Conditions that decrease SHBG levels give rise to increased bioavailable (non-SHBG-bound) estradiol.

The measurement of non-SHBG-bound (bioavailable) forms of testosterone has been advocated for states of androgen excess to detect more accurately subtle forms of hirsutism. Although the diagnostic yield of this measurement is superior to that of total serum testosterone, the correlation between total and non-SHBG-bound testosterone is excellent, so that bioavailable testosterone can usually be predicted from the total testosterone level (Schwartz U).

The normal serum levels of androgens, especially free testosterone determined by radioimmunoassay (RIA), vary from laboratory to laboratory. A group of investigators compared serum-free testosterone levels measured by equilibrium dialysis with those measured by direct RIA and with those calculated from the free androgen index (100 × testosterone/SHBG), a simple index that correlates with the free testosterone level (Miller KK). They concluded that as there is wide variation in lab values of free testosterone, FAI is a useful tool for assessing androgen excess and is a practical and useful measure. But if a reliable method for measuring serum free or bioavailable testosterone is readily available, cost is not an issue, and it would facilitate patient management, this would be a more reasonable choice for initial testing than total testosterone. As of today, equilibrium dialysis for free testosterone assay is *not* available in India for routine clinical use. Even in the developed countries equilibrium dialysis for free testosterone is available mainly in the larger endocrine hospitals and research centers. Hence, assay reliability (CLIA/RIA) and costs limits the use of free testosterone in routine clinical practice in India.

Measuring the levels of all C19 steroids is not clinically necessary for most patients presenting with androgen excess. The most useful initial test is a serum total testosterone level. An abnormal level in the presence of hirsutism or virilization may be associated with PCOS, hyperthecosis, nonclassic adrenal hyperplasia, or an androgen-secreting neoplasm. Most androgen-secreting tumors are of ovarian origin. The likelihood of a neoplasm correlates roughly with increasing testosterone levels (Fig. 18.5).

2. The following tests may be added on the basis of the clinical presentation:
   a. Serum 17-hydroxyprogesterone (i.e. nonclassic adrenal hyperplasia)
   b. Serum prolactin and TSH (i.e. mild androgen excess associated with hyperprolactinemia)
   c. Serum DHEAS (i.e. adrenal tumors). The level of DHEAS can be informative, however, it is increased in approximately 15% of women who have normal levels of total and free testosterone. A mildly elevated level in a woman with a normal-free testosterone

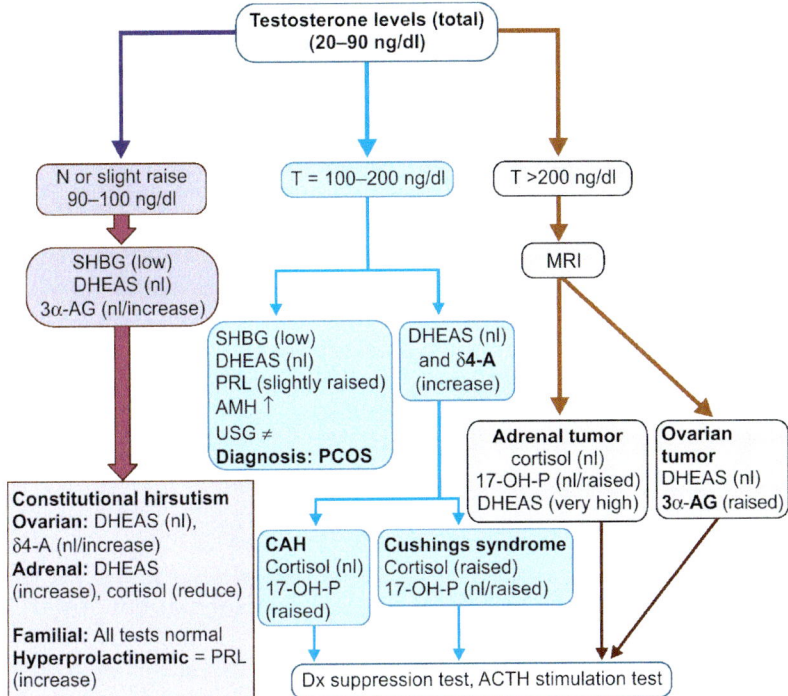

Fig. 18.5: Algorithm for diagnosis of hirsutism using testosterone levels as the guiding principle (17-OH: 17-OH progesterone, δ4-A: δ4-androstenedione, 3α-AG: 3α-androstanediol glucuronide, ACTH: Adrenocorticotropic hormone, CORT: Cortisol, DHEAS: Dehydroepiandrosterone sulfate, Dx: Dexamethasone, NMR: Nuclear magnetic resonance, PCOS: Polycystic ovary syndrome, PRL: Prolactinemia, PSA: Prostate-specific antigen, SHBG: Sex hormone binding globulin, US: Ultrasound, nl: Normal)

    level is unlikely to be clinically relevant aside from being associated with acne.

d. AMH: A measure of follicular reserve, is elevated in PCOS, has good sensitivity, but relatively poor specificity in diagnosing PCOS. Again it is a costly test, not routinely available, and assay reliability remains an issue in India. A pilot study by Sardana K et al have though found a good sensitivity and specificity with a cut off value of 3.6 ng/ml being predictive of PCOM.

e. Imaging of ovaries and adrenals (i.e. PCOS and steroid-secreting tumors).

    For testing the minimum pause in hormonal contraception has to be 2 months. The measurements should be taken between 08.00 and 09.00 hours, on days 4 to 10 of the menstrual cycle in regularly cycling women, the time for which norms are standardized.

Laboratory Testing to Aid the Differential Diagnosis of Androgen Excess

Initially a detailed *history* which should look for any clinical signs, which may orientate our initial diagnosis (a clinical impression of acromegaly, Cushing's features, physical virilization, menstrual alterations, infertility, hypertension, galactorrhea, etc.), and then start the laboratory evaluation. A detailed *testing protocol* is detailed in Fig. 18.5 and Table 18.2, though some tests maybe excluded due to cost considerations. Representative case scenarios are detailed in Figs 18.6 and 18.7, though many may not have marked changes and are possibly due to end organ hyperresponsiveness.

An ideal testing protocol entails ordering levels of *testosterone*, free testosterone (if the laboratory is reliable), 5α-DHT, *DHEAS*, 17β-hydroxyprogesterone, *prolactin*, δ4-androstenedione, *SHBG*, and 3α-androstanediol glucuronide, a metabolite of 5α-DHT. To make this more cost effective, the 5α-DHT, δ4-androstenedione and 3α-androstanediol glucuronide can be done away with as they are costly tests.

Cortisol levels will be normal in CAH and adrenal tumors, and increased in Cushing syndrome. If CAH is a possibility, the levels of 17-hydroxyprogesterone before and after an "ACTH stimulation test" may be investigated. When cutaneous signs of Cushing's syndrome are present, 24-hour urinary-free cortisol and creatinine excretion must be determined, and the overnight "dexamethasone (Dx) suppression test" can also be performed. With this test we can observe: (1) CAH: The Dx test causes a previously increased 17-hydroxyprogesterone level and a previously normal cortisol level to decrease; (2) Cushing syndrome: The Dx test does not change a previously normal or slightly increased 17-hydroxyprogesterone level, or a previously increased cortisol level; (3) adrenal tumors: 17-hydroxyprogesterone that was also normal or slightly increased does not change after a Dx test, and cortisol that was normal decreases after the Dx test.

LH, FSH and the LH:FSH ratios were considered useful for PCOS but this ratio is not always reliable (as discussed above) and the AMH is a better test. Given the prevalence of impaired glucose tolerance in PCOS, and its consequent morbidity, all women with PCOS must be screened for type 2 diabetes mellitus. Serum triglycerides, total cholesterol, and HDLs must be also screened because dyslipidemia is predictive of associated cardiac morbidity. When HAIRAN syndrome is suspected, insulin serum levels must also be determined. When evaluating PCOS patients, ultrasound examination of the ovaries should be performed, and as these patients usually carry excess weight, obesity can be assessed using the BMI. Also the "waist-to-hip ratio"

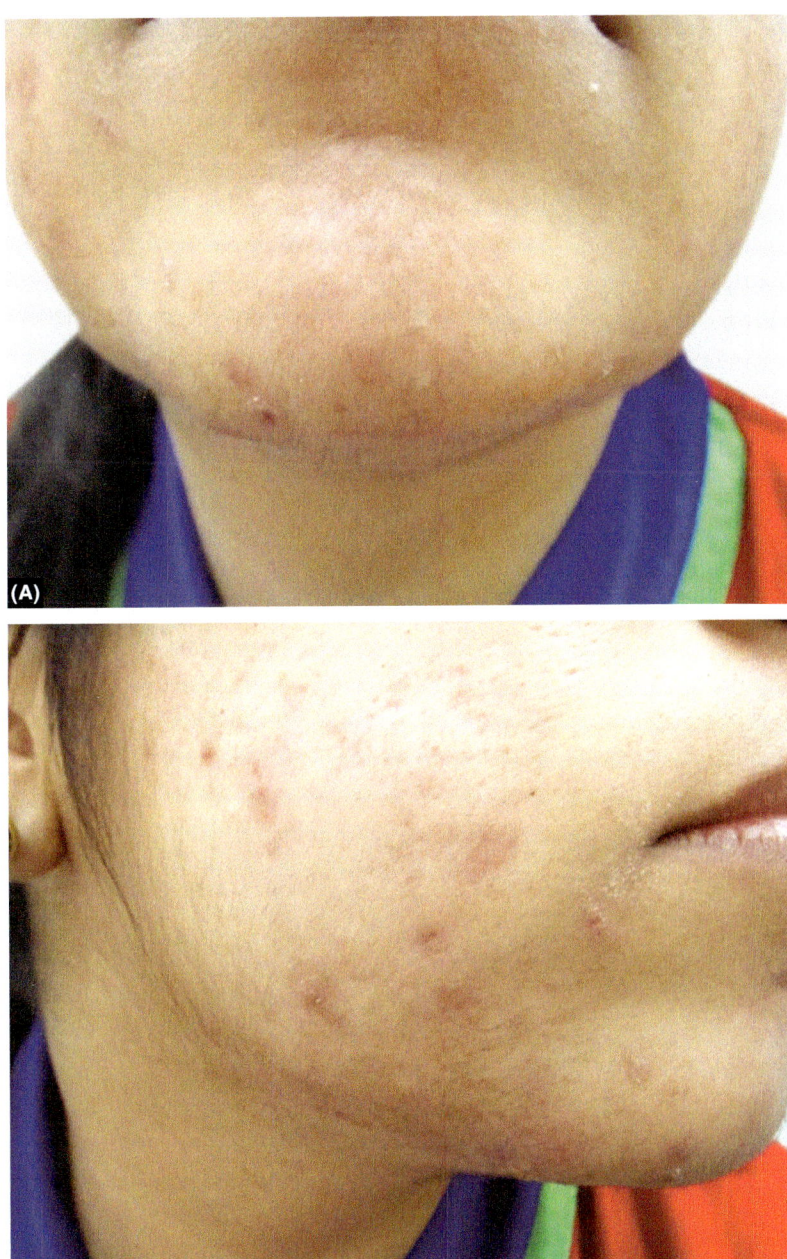

Fig. 18.6A and B: A case of a 26-year-old girl with persistent acne and hirsutism. Her androgen index was 11.1, with a testosterone of 64 ng/dl and SHBG of 11 nmol/L with a AMH of 7. A case of PCOS, she was initiated on OCP, EE/DRSP (24/4)

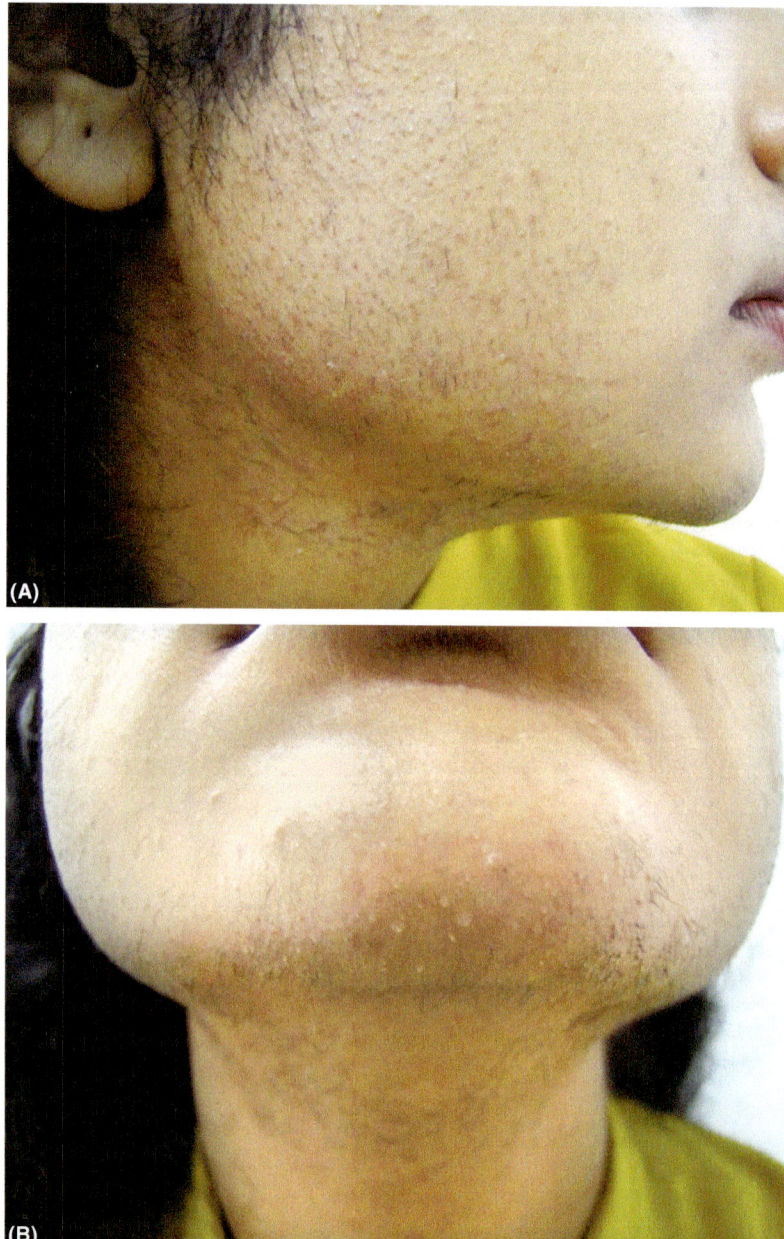

Fig. 18.7A and B: This patient had a raised testosterone (104 ng/dl), low SHBG (11 nmol/L) , raised AMH: 7.3, high DHEAS: 615 μg/dl and a borderline high 17-OH-P: 2.10 ng/ml. The raised borderline 17-OH-P and the DHEAS can be seen in case of PCOS. She was put on OCP plus anti-acne therapy

must be evaluated to determine the fat distribution. In cases of clear obesity, transvaginal ultrasound must be used. When tumors are suspected magnetic resonance imaging (MRI) and ultrasound may be necessary.

TREATMENT OF HIRSUTISM

Therapy for androgen excess should be directed toward its specific cause and suppression of abnormal androgen secretion. Specific treatments for hirsutism and virilization are indicated for ovarian and adrenal tumors, hyperthecosis, Cushing's syndrome, and adrenal hyperplasia.

Neoplasms warrant surgical intervention while suppression with a GnRH analogue may be tried initially for ovarian *hyperthecosis*. However, bilateral oophorectomy is ultimately necessary to control androgen excess arising from hyperthecosis in most patients. For *Cushing's syndrome*, treatment correlates with the source of hypercortisolism. For *nonclassic adrenal hyperplasia*, glucocorticoid replacement is needed but it is an accepted view that the glucocorticoid effect on hirsutism of nonclassic CAH appears to be modest (Spritzer P et al). When treating androgen excess associated with nonclassic adrenal hyperplasia, an antiandrogen (e.g. spironolactone) in combination with an oral contraceptive or a glucocorticoid may be used. Another option is to combine oral contraceptive plus spironolactone.

The general treatment of androgen excess is directed towards the prevention of abnormal hair growth and virilization. For practical purposes, the same approach is used for androgen excess associated with idiopathic hirsutism, PCOS, and nonclassic adrenal hyperplasia. The existing hair follicles and manifestations of virilization remain and hence terminal hair should be removed by mechanical methods (e.g. electrolysis) at least 3 *months* after androgen suppression is achieved. Thus, it is important to point out the laser hair reduction should follow medical therapy.

The principles of systemic therapy revolve around:

1. Suppression of ovarian androgen production
2. Alteration of binding of androgens to their serum binding proteins
3. Impairment of the peripheral conversion of androgen precursors to active androgen
4. Inhibition of androgen action at the target tissue level.

With all medical treatments, there appears to be an inverse association between efficacy and body mass index. The other cosmetic measures including lasers are not the focus of this chapter and are an essential ancillary aspect of treatment.

Importantly the principles of therapy given above can be safely extended to acne, specially in persistent acne in females with a hormonal dysfunction. The choice of therapy should be based on the degree of hirsutism, potential underlying hormonal disorders, the impact on the individual's quality of life, and the desired degree of unwanted hair reduction. An overview of the different agents is given in Table 18.3 and is discussed in the text that follows.

Lifestyle Modification

In obese adolescent women with PCOS, lifestyle modification (i.e. diet with a 500 kcal/day deficit and exercise 30 min/day) alone resulted in a 59% reduction in the testosterone/SHBG ratio, with a 122% increase in SHBG (Hoeger K). Needless to say this forms an extremely important part of management, though as is the experience of most clinicians, it is difficult to achieve in most patients.

Medical Therapy

Eflornithine

Eflornithine is an irreversible inhibitor of ornithine decarboxylase. This enzyme catalyzes the conversion of ornithine to polyamines, which are involved in the regulation of cell growth and differentiation in several tissues. The enzyme is modulated by androgens and takes part in the physiology of hair growth, regulating the proliferation of matrix cells in the hair follicle. Studies have indicated that blockade of this enzyme activity in hair follicles slows hair growth. Though it is effective, hair growth returns to pretreatment rates within a few weeks after stopping treatment. Mild irritation and folliculitis may affect the skin with treatment.

Table 18.3: Overview of medical therapies for hirsutism				
Systemic treatments	Combined oral contraceptives	Antiandrogens	Insulin-lowering drugs	Steroids
	EE 35 µg/ CPA 2 mg	Spironolactone, cyproterone acetate, finasteride, flutamide	Metformin Thiazoli-dinediones	Dexametha-sone
Topical treatments	Eflornithine hydrochloride	Finasteride		

Oral Contraceptives (OCPs)

Oral contraceptives reduce circulating testosterone and androgen precursors by multiple mechanisms including:
a. Suppression of LH
b. Stimulation of SHBG levels
c. Decrease circulating androgen in patients with PCOS
d. Have an additive effect with other antiandrogens.

The estrogenic component of OCP plays the main role in suppression of LH androgen levels, increasing SHBG levels and lowering the free fraction of serum testosterone. It also decreases DHEAS levels, perhaps by reducing ACTH levels (Wild RA). The dose of EE required to suppress sebum is much higher (100 µg) and is rarely administered (Palitz L). It is advisable to use an oral contraceptive containing 30 or 35 µg of ethinyl estradiol to achieve effective suppression of LH (Aziz R, 2002).

The progestins used in combination with EE should ideally be those that have low androgenic potential and include norgestimate, desogestrel and cyproterone which is anti-androgenic. Drospirenone, a progestational analogue of spironolactone, has both anti-androgenic and anti-mineralo-corticoid activities and is this author's preferred drug. Importantly OCP carry about a fourfold increased risk for venous thromboembolism in first-time users; this risk decreases with duration of use and decreasing estrogen dose, but is less than that of pregnancy (Jick SS).

The OCP, EE 35 µg/CPA 2 mg is the only OCP approved by the European Medicines Agency (EMA) for the treatment of hirsutism in premenopausal women. There is no difference between the oral 0.03 mg ethinyl estradiol/3 mg drospirenone 21/7 regimen or 0.02 mg ethinyl estradiol/3 mg drospirenone 24/4 regimen, for 6 months, with moderate to severe hirsutism. The choice of these two regimens revolves around the dose of estrogen which dictates breakthrough bleeding, headaches, weight gain and cycle control.

Assessment of adequacy of ovarian suppression can be made at the end of the *third week* after starting treatment; by this time, ovarian androgen suppression is complete. A meta-analysis showed that treatment with oral contraceptives for *6 months* reduced Ferriman-Gallwey scores of hirsutism by an average of 27% (Koulouri). The use of, drospirenone (3 mg) based OCP is considered by many to a better option as it has a diuretic effect and helps in addition to loose weight, but this has a potential risk of thromboembolism (discussed above). The effect on acne can be expected to be maximal in 1 to *2 months*. OCP therapy is FDA-approved for the treatment of acne and improves it by 50 to 100% (Lemay AY). Thus, this can help treat the two disorders concomitantly (Fig. 18.8).

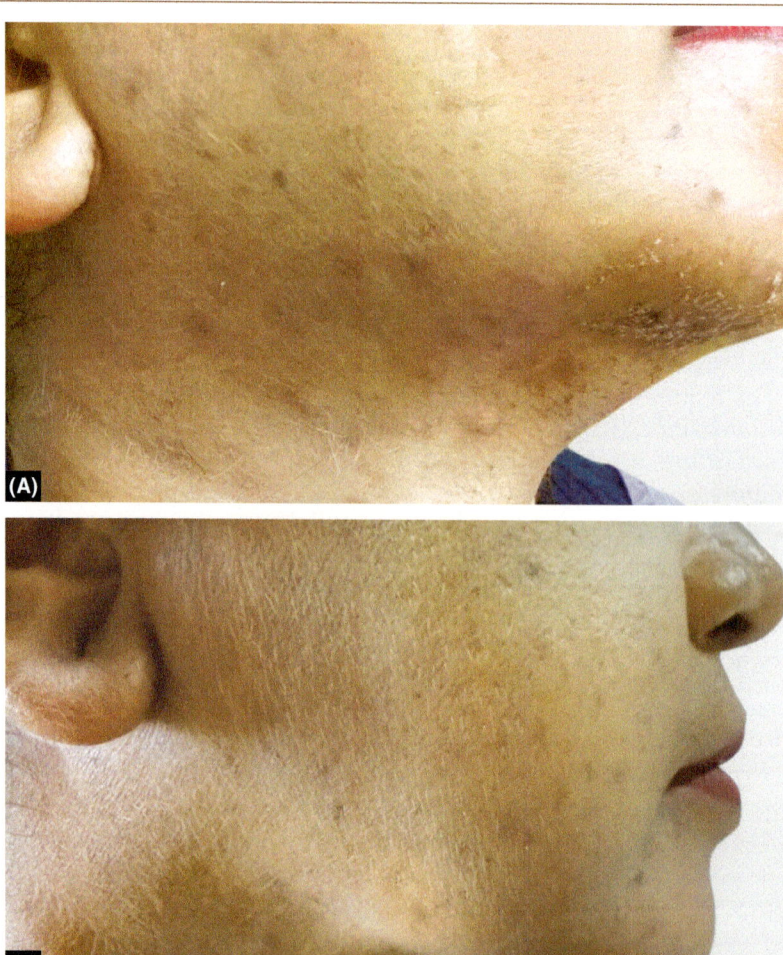

Fig. 18.8A and B: This 42-year-old female had persistent acne and except for a raised androgen index with a low SHBG, all other tests were normal. She was initiated on OCP (DRSP/EE) with isotretinoin 1 mgh/kg /day. After 2 months her acne resolved and at 6 months there was a marked reduction in her hirsutism. The marked improvement in her complexion is attributed to the benefits of estrogens and isotretinoin, though the patient was made to believe that the superficial peels helped the integument

GnRH Agonists

Chronic administration of GnRH agonist suppresses pituitary-ovarian function, thus inhibiting both ovarian androgen and estrogen secretion. Uncontrolled trials of GnRH agonists in ovarian hyperandrogenism have reported significant reduction in the Ferriman-Gallwey score.

Because of the reduction of serum estrogen levels and the concomitant reduction in bone mineral density with GnRH agonist therapy, an agonist should always be combined with estrogen–progestin combination.GnRH agonist therapy may be most useful in women with severe forms of ovarian hyperandrogenemia such as ovarian hyperthecosis, but the effect on hirsutism appears to be modest (Martin KA).

Spironolactone

This drug is one of the safest antiandrogens and if combined with OCP can prove to be effective for most cases of hirsutism, specially those associated with PCOS or idiopathic hirsutism.

Mode of action: Apart from inhibiting steroidogenesis and acting as an androgen antagonist, spironolactone has a significant effect in inhibiting 5α-reductase activity (Lobo RA,1985).

Basic experimental and several clinical studies have confirmed the efficacy of spironolactone for hyperandrogenism and suggest that the principal effect is related to its ability to block peripheral androgen production and action.

Dose: Doses of spironolactone vary from 50 to 400 mg daily. Although doses of 100 mg/day usually are effective for the treatment of hirsutism, higher doses (200 to 300 mg/day) may be preferable in extremely hirsute or markedly obese women.

The initial dose is 100 mg/day, gradually increasing it by increments of 25 mg/day every 3 months up to 200 mg/day on the basis of the response. Adjustments in dose should be made only after 3 to 6 months, as with other antiandrogens, to account for the slow changes in the hair cycle.

If there are complaints of menstrual irregularity with spironolactone; a lower dose can be used or the drug can be combined with oral contraceptive. Effective contraception should always be provided in women taking spironolactone. Increased diuresis, breast tenderness, and abdominal discomfort are other frequently reported mild side effects of spironolactone, at least with high doses (200 mg).

Summary: It is always instructive to compare various drug therapies, and such studies are uncommon. A 6-month randomized, double-blind, placebo-controlled comparative study including spironolactone, flutamide, or finasteride as active drugs (Moghetti), found a 12% reduction in hair shaft diameter and a 41% reduction in the hirsutism score in women receiving spironolactone. These changes were statistically significant as compared to placebo. Interestingly, the improvements observed with spironolactone were similar to those seen with flutamide or finasteride. Thus, this drug can be used in most cases and is better than most other drugs in this disorder.

Treatment with spironolactone for 6 *months* reduces Ferriman-Gallwey scores of hirsutism by an average of **38.4%**. Because spironolactone acts through mechanisms different from those of oral contraceptives, overall effectiveness is improved by combining these two medications in patients with hirsutism, including those with PCOS, idiopathic hirsutism, or nonclassic adrenal hyperplasia.

Cyproterone Acetate

Cyproterone acetate is a 17-hydroxyprogesterone acetate derivative with strong progestagenic properties.

MOA: Cyproterone acetate acts as an antiandrogen by competing with DHT and testosterone for binding to the androgen receptor. There is also some evidence that cyproterone acetate and ethinyl estradiol in combination can inhibit 5α-reductase activity in skin.

Dose: The drug usually is administered daily in doses of 50 to 100 mg on days 5 through 15 of the treatment cycle. Because of its slow metabolism, it is administered early in the treatment cycle; when ethinyl estradiol is added, it is usually administered in 50 μg doses on days 5 through 26. This regimen is needed for menstrual control and is usually referred to as the reverse sequential regimen. Cyproterone acetate in doses of 50 to 100 mg/day, combined with ethinyl estradiol at 30 to 35 μg/day, is *as effective* as the combination of spironolactone (100 mg/day) and an oral contraceptive in the treatment of hirsutism (Aziz R, 2000).

The use of the OCP where a smaller dose (2 mg), is used in daily combination with 50 or 35 μg of ethinyl estradiol is ideal for a milder form of hyperandrogenism.

Finasteride

Finasteride inhibits 5α-reductase activity and can be used in the treatment of hirsutism (Rittmaster et al). Increased 5α-reductase activity in the skin is considered to be the major pathogenetic mechanism of "idiopathic" hirsutism (i.e. excessive hair growth occurring in the absence of increased serum androgens and with ovulatory cycles). Selective enzyme inhibition has been proposed as a rational medical approach to this condition. In the skin, the type 1 isoenzyme of 5α-reductase appears to be primarily expressed; the importance of the type 2 isoenzyme in hair growth is still unclear. However, the isoenzyme selectivity of finasteride is not absolute at therapeutic doses.

Dose: At a dose of 5 mg/day, a significant improvement of hirsutism is observed after 6 months of therapy, without significant side effects. In hirsute women, the decline in circulating DHT levels is small and cannot be used to monitor therapy. Although this treatment regimen increases testosterone levels, SHBG levels remain unaffected (Rittmaster RS).

Though finasteride is less effective than spironolactone with respect to the reduction of hirsutism in women, but finasteride at a dose of 5 mg/day has a favorable tolerance and minor side effects (Castello R). A meta-analysis showed that finasteride treatment for 6 months reduced Ferriman-Gallwey scores of hirsutism by an average of 20.3% (Koulouri O). Interestingly a combination of spironolactone and finasteride was found to be better than spironolactone alone, highlighting the role of 5α-reductase in hirsutism (Kelesimur et al, 2004). Studies assessing finasteride efficacy in women with hirsutism consistently indicated positive results, without noticeable side effects. Finasteride has been used in a dose of 5 mg/day in most published trials, although similar effects on skin androgens were found with 1 mg.

As a large proportion of patients is adolescents, a recent study (Tartagni MV) examined the dosimetry and found that in both cases of PCOS and idiopathic hirsutism, a low-dose of finasteride, given in a dose of 2.5 mg every 3 days, reduces the hirsutism score and this can be a safe, cheap and effective option in this age group (Tertagni et al, 2014).

Flutamide

Flutamide is a nonsteroidal drug, considered a "pure" antiandrogen in that it seems to act only at the androgen receptor as a competitive antagonist (Simard et al). It has been shown to be effective in the treatment of hirsutism. The mean Ferriman-Gallwey score is reduced by **41.3%** (Koulouri O).

Dose: Flutamide has been administered to hirsute women in doses ranging from 62.5 to 750 mg/day.

A large 20 year analysis of flutamide 125 or 250 mg/day alone with OCP found significant improvements in hirsutism scores after 6 months of treatment with a maximum effect at 12 months that was maintained during all the therapy time. But the side effects can be a deterrent with up to 24.1% patients being affected, leading to a withdrawal of the medication (Castelo-Branco et al). Thus, though this drug is probably the most effective, it remains a third-line option.

Summary: Some studies reported that this drug might have favorable effects on visceral fat and on the lipid profile in patients with PCOS.

These effects are of great interest in subjects who frequently show abdominal obesity, insulin resistance, and multiple metabolic abnormalities.

Flutamide does not interfere with ovulation and is generally well tolerated. The only common complaint of patients given flutamide is dry skin, attributable to reduced sebum production. Liver toxicity is an uncommon, but potentially severe, risk with this drug.

Metformin and Thiazolidinediones

Most studies conducted during the past decade have suggested that treatment with metformin (1500 to 2700 mg/day) for 6 months significantly reduces hirsutism as assessed by the Ferriman-Gallwey scoring system (Koulouri O).

But our view is that these drugs are highly overated as most studies have shown only modest reductions in hirsutism scores (average, 19.1%). In obese adolescent women with PCOS, metformin in combination with lifestyle modification (i.e. diet with a 500 kcal/day deficit and exercise 30 min/day) and oral contraceptives reduced the total testosterone level and waist circumference (Hoeger K).

A better option is the thiazolidinediones (4 mg/day of rosiglitazone or 30 mg/day of pioglitazone), which reduced Ferriman-Gallwey scores significantly (Koulouri O). These studies suggested that insulin sensitizing agents may be used in the treatment of hirsutism, especially for women who do not wish to use other oral agents.

Comparative studies

A Cochrane review of metformin versus oral contraceptives in PCOS evaluated 4 randomized controlled trials and reported no evidence of a difference in effect between COC and metformin on hirsutism. The dose of metformin was 500 mg three times daily in one trial and 500 mg twice daily for the first 3 months increasing to 1,000 mg twice daily for the next 3 months. The COC type was EE 35 µg/CA 2 mg in all trials.

A recent study has compared low-dose PioFluMet with EE-CA in adolescents with androgen excess and without pregnancy risk (Ibáñez L). The latter combination contains a low-dose combination of pioglitazone (7.5 mg/day), flutamide (62.5 mg/day), and metformin (850 mg/day) (PioFluMet). The PioFluMet was found to be comparable to EE-CA in terms of androgen suppression but was better in improving other parameters, including insulinemia; circulating cholesterol, triglycerides, C-reactive protein, high molecular-weight adiponectin, leptin, and follistatin; carotid intima-media thickness; lean mass; and on abdominal, visceral, and hepatic fat (Ibanez et al).

SUMMARY AND CONCLUSION

1. In clinical practice and in reference to the most common cause of hirsutism (PCOS) treatment is with a combination of two agents, one that suppresses the ovary (e.g. an oral contraceptive) and another that suppresses the extraovarian (peripheral) action of androgens (e.g. spironolactone). A similar choice can be used for cases of idiopathic hirsutism. The safest combination seems to be EE/DRSP + spironolactone. Another useful combination is spironolactone 100 mg + finasteride 5 mg.

2. For women with only minor complaints of hirsutism, the use of an oral contraceptive alone may be an appropriate first approach.

3. Moderate lifestyle modification (i.e. diet with a 500 kcal/day deficit and 30 min/day of exercise) should be a part of hirsutism management in obese patients.

4. Because the growth phase of body hairs lasts 3 to 6 months, a response should not be expected before 6 months after onset of treatment. Most patients with PCOS and idiopathic hirsutism respond to this strategy within 1 year. Patients should be encouraged to continue treatment for at least 2 years.

5. The best and most practical reproducible method of monitoring therapy is pictures of the face and selected midline body areas before and during therapy.

6. Suppression of androgen production and action inhibits only new hair growth. Existing coarse hair should be removed mechanically. Plucking, waxing, and shaving are ineffective for hair removal and cause irritation, folliculitis, and ingrown hairs. Electrolysis is still the gold standard but laser epilation has supplanted this in recent times.

An overview of therapeutic option is given in Box 18.2.

Box 18.2: Therapeutic interventions of hirsutism

Cause	Teatment
Idiopathic (constitutional)	Aldactone/finasteride or combination
Ovarian/PCOS	OCP + Aldactone
Adrenal cause	Low dose evening steroid*
Obesity	Lifestyle modification
	DRSP based OCP
	Metformin/pioglitazone

*Some experts believe that OCPs are good for NCCAH.

Bibliography

1. Azziz R, Carmina E, Sawaya ME. Idiopathic hirsutism. Endocr Rev 2000; 21:347–62.

2. Bardin CW, Lipsett MB. Testosterone and androstenedione blood production rates in normal women and women with idiopathic hirsutism or polycystic ovaries. J Clin Invest 1967;46:891–902.

3. Carmina E, Rosato F, Janni A, et al. Extensive clinical experience: relative prevalence of different androgen excess disorders in 950 women referred because of clinical hyperandrogenism. J Clin Endocrinol Metab 2006;91: 2–6.

4. Castello R, Tosi F, Perrone F, et al. Outcome of long-term treatment with the 5α-reductase inhibitor finasteride in idiopathic hirsutism: clinical and hormonal effects during a 1-year course of therapy and 1-year follow-up. Fertil Steril 1996;66:734–40.

5. Castelo-Branco C, Hernández-Angeles C, Alvarez-Olivares L, BalaschJ. Long-term satisfaction and tolerability with low-dose flutamide: a 20-year surveillance study on 120 hyperandrogenic women. Gynecol Endocrinol 2016 Sep;32(9):723–27.

6. Derksen J, Nagesser SK, Meinders AE, et al. Identification of virilizing adrenal tumors in hirsute women. N Engl J Med 1994;331:968–73.

7. Gambineri A, Pelusi C, Genghini S, et al. Effect of flutamide and metformin administered alone or in combination in dieting obese women with polycystic ovary syndrome. Clin Endocrinol (Oxf) 2004;60:241–49.

8. Hoeger K, Davidson K, Kochman L, et al. The impact of metformin, oral contraceptives, and lifestyle modification on polycystic ovary syndrome in obese adolescent women in two randomized, placebo-controlled clinical trials. J Clin Endocrinol Metab 2008;93:4299–306.

9. Ibáñez L, Diaz M, Sebastiani G, Sánchez-Infantes D, Salvador C, Lopez-Bermejo A, de Zegher F. Treatment of androgen excess in adolescent girls: ethinylestradiol cyproterone acetate versus low-dose pioglitazone flutamide metformin. J Clin Endocrinol Metab 2011 Nov;96(11):3361–6.

10. Jick SS, Hernandez RK. Risk of non-fatal venous thouromboembolism in women using oral contraceptives containing drospirenone compared with women using oral contraceptives containing levonorgestrel: case control study using the United States claims data. BMJ 2011;342. d2151.

11. Keletimur F, Everest H, Unlühizarci K, Bayram F, Sahin Y. A comparison between spironolactone and spironolactone plus finasteride in the treatment of hirsutism. Eur J Endocrinol 2004 Mar;150(3):351–4.

12. Koulouri O, Conway GS. A systematic review of commonly used medical treatments for hirsutism in women. Clin Endocrinol (Oxf) 2008;68:800–5.

13. Lemay A, Dewailly SD, Grenier R, Huard J. Attenuation of mild hyperandrogenic activity in postpubertal acne by a triphasic oral contraceptive containing low doses of ethynyl estradiol and D, L-norgestrel. J Clin Endocrinol Metab 1990;71:8–14.

14. Lobo R, Paul W, Gentzsschein E, et al. Production of 3α-androstanediol glucuronide in human genital skin. J Clin Endocrinol Metab 1987;65:711.

15. Lobo RA, Shoupe D, Serafini P, et al. The effects of two doses of spironolactone on serum androgens and anagen hair in hirsute women. Fertil Steril 1985;43:200–5.

16. Mahendroo MS, Russell DW. Male and female isoenzymes of steroid 5α-reductase. Rev Reprod 1999;4:179–83.

17. Martin KA, Chang RJ, Ehrmann DA, et al. Evaluation and treatment of hirsutism in premenopausal women: an Endocrine Society Clinical Practice Guideline. J Clin Endocrin Metab 2008;93:1105–20.

18. Marynick SP, Chakmakjian ZH, McCaffree DL, Herndon Jr JH. Androgen excess in cystic acne. N Engl J Med 1983;308: 981–86.

19. Miller KK, Rosner W, Lee H, et al. Measurement of free testosterone in normal women and women with androgen deficiency: comparison of methods. J Clin Endocrinol Metab 2004;89:525–33.

20. Moghetti P, Tosi F, Tosti A, et al. Comparison of spironolactone, flutamide and finasteride efficacy in the treatment of hirsutism: a randomized, double-blind, placebo-controlled trial. J Clin Endocrinol Metab2000;85:89–94.

21. Nestler J, Powers L, Matt D, et al. A direct effect of hyperinsulinemia on serum sex hormone-binding globulin levels in obese women with the polycystic ovary syndrome. J Clin Endocrinol Metab 991;72:83–89.

22. Palitz L. Estrogen–progestin in the control of acne in girls. Clin Med. 1968;75:43–54.

23. Rittmaster RS. Finasteride. N Engl J Med. 1994;330:120–125.

24. Rosenfield RL, Moll GW. The role of proteins in the distribution of plasma androgens and estradiol. In: Molinatti G, Martini L, James V, eds. Androgenization in women. New York: Raven Press; 1983:25–45.

25. Rosenfield RL, Mortensen M, Wroblewski K, et al. Determination of the source of androgen excess in functionally atypical polycystic ovary syndrome by a short dexamethasone androgen-suppression test and a low-dose ACTH test. Hum Reprod 2011;26:3138–46.

26. Rosenfield RL. Clinical practice. Hirsutism. [Comment in: N Engl J Med. 2006;354(14):1533–35; author reply 1533–35]. N Engl J Med. 2005;353: 2578–88.

27. Sardana K, Singh C, Narang I, Bansal S, Garg VK. The role of antimüllerian hormone in the hormonal workup of women with persistent acne. J Cosmet Dermatol 2016 Dec;15(4):343–49.

28. Schwartz U, Moltz L, Brotherton J, et al. The diagnostic value of plasma free testosterone in non-tumorous and tumorous hyperandrogenism. Fertil Steril 1983;40:66–72.

29. Simard J, Luthy I, Guay J, Belanger A, Labrie F. Characteristics of interaction of the antiandrogen flutamide with the androgen receptor in various target tissues. Mol Cell Endocrinol 1986;44:261–70.

30. Simo R, Barbosa-Desongles A, Lecube A, Hernandez C, Selva DM. Potential role of tumor necrosis factor-α in downregulating sex hormone-binding globulin. Diabetes 2012;61:372–82.

31. Spritzer P, Billaud L, Thalabard JC, et al. Cyproterone acetate versus hydrocortisone treatment in late-onset adrenal hyperplasia. J Clin Endocrinol Metab 1990;70:642–46.

32. Tartagni MV, Alrasheed H, Damiani GR, Montagnani M, De Salvia MA, De Pergola G, Tartagni M, Loverro G. Intermittent low-dose finasteride administration is effective for treatment of hirsutism in adolescent girls: a pilot study. J Pediatr Adolesc Gynecol 2014 Jun;27(3):161–5.

33. Waggoner W, Boots LR, Azziz R. Total testosterone and DHEAS levels as predictors of androgen-secreting neoplasms: a populational study. Gynecol Endocrinol 1999;13:394–400.

34. Wild RA, Umstot ES, Andersen RN, Givens JR. Adrenal function in hirsutism. Effect of an oral contraceptive. J Clin Endocrinol Metab 1982;54:676–81.

35. Wong IL, Morris RS, Chang L, et al. A prospective randomized trial comparing finasteride to spironolactone in the treatment of hirsute women. J Clin Endocrinol Metab 1995;80:233–38.

Books

Shlomo Melmed, Kenneth S. Polonsky, P. Reed Larsen, Henry M. Kronenberg, Williams Textbook of Endocrinology. 12th Edition. Elseiver, 2011.

J. Larry Jameson, Robert G. Dunlop, Leslie J De Groot, David M. de Kretser, Linda C. Giudice, Ashley B. Grossman, ShlomoMelmed, John T. Potts, Gordon C. Weir, Endocrinology: Adult and Pediatric, Volume II. 7th Edition. Elseiver.

Selected Bibliography

1. Andrew G. Messenger, Rodney D. Sinclair, Paul Farrant and David A.R. de Berker. Acquired Disorders of Hair. **Rook's Textbook of Dermatology, Ninth Edition**. Edited by Christopher Griffiths, Jonathan Barker, Tanya Bleiker, Robert Chalmers and Daniel Creamer. 2016 John Wiley & Sons, Ltd.

2. Blume-Peytavi U, Tosti A, Whiting DA, et al (eds): **Hair Growth and Disorders**. Berlin, Springer, 2008.

3. **Hair Loss** in **Diagnosis and Management of Skin Disorders** by Kabir Sardana. Diagnosis & Management of Skin Disorders: An Evidence-Based Approach, 1/e.: Lippincott Williams & Wilkins, 2015.

4. **Hair Replacement Surgery:** Textbook and Atlas, Springer-Verlag, Berlin, Heidelberg, 1996.

5. Ioannides D, Tosti A (eds): **Alopecias: Practical Evaluation and Management**. Curr Probl Dermatol. Basel, Karger, 2015.

6. Jennifer Marsh, John Gray, Antonella Tosti. **Healthy Hair.** ©Springer International Publishing, Switzerland, 2015.

7. Jerry Shapiro and Nina Otberg. **Hair Loss and Restoration**, Second Edition, English 2015. CRC Press, Taylor & Francis Group. © 2015 by Taylor & Francis Group, LLC.

8. Ralph M. Trüeb. **The Difficult Hair Loss Patient**. Guide to Successful Management of Alopecia and Related Conditions. ©Springer International Publishing, Switzerland, 2015.

9. Rodney Sinclair and Vicky Jolliffe. **Fast Facts: Disorders of the Hair and Scalp**, 2nd edn, Published in 2013, Health Press.

10. Zoe Diana Draelos. **Hair Care An Illustrated Dermatologic Handbook**. CRC Press, 2004.

Index

A

Acell matristem micromatrix (AMM) 384
Acetyl tetrapeptide-3 90, 340
Acne 56
Acne keloidalis nuchae (AKN)/folliculitis keloidalis nuchae 170
Acne necrotica (varioliformis) 172
Acquired
 generalized hypertrichosis 201
 localized hypertrichosis 203
Acrodermatitis enteropathica 335
Acromegaly 79
ACTH stimulation test 404
Acute diffuse 243
Acute diffuse and total alopecia 243
Acute TE 70
Adalimumab 145
Aderans 313
Adipose-derived stem cells 312
Aging 254
Alfatradiol 235
Alopecia areata 8, 105
Alopecia areata incognita 243
Alopecia mucinosa 140
α-estradiol 50
α-tocopherol (vitamin E) 328
Amino acids 339
Anagen 4
Androgen receptor 42, 305
Androgen receptor (AR) inhibitors 308
Androgenetic alopecia 214
Androgens 54
3α-androstanediol 54
Androstanediol glucuronide 391
Androstenedione 54, 391, 393
Angiofibrotic streamers 48

Anisotrichosis 19
Antagonists 314
Anthralin 123, 135
Antimalarials 149
Anti-müllerian hormone (AMH) 55, 397
Antinuclear antibody 148
Antioxidants 339
Antipsychotics 296
Anxiolytics 287
Apremilast 130
Arnica montana 341
Aromatase 55, 391
Atrichia congenita (congenital atrichia) 187
Auber's line 257
Automated FUE 384
Azathioprine 151
Azoles 272

B

Benzodiazepines 287
Bhringraj 341
Bifonazole 273
Bimatoprost 51, 62, 224
Biochanin 90
Biochanin A 340
Bioenhancement 384
Biopsy 142
Biotin 52, 259, 329, 335
Biotinyl tripepdide-1 340
Bitemporal recession 56
Black cohosh 52
Black dot 207
Black dots 16
Blue-gray dots 16
Bone morphogenic protein 6 73
Botulinum toxin 68
Brauer's nevus 188

Bromocriptine 64
Brotzu lotion 318
Bulb 1

C

Cabergoline 64
Caffeine 50
Calcineurin inhibitors 274
Calcipotriol 135
Calcium pantothenate 259
Camouflage 159
Canities 200, 255
Cannabinoids 284
Capixyl™ 340
Carboxylase 335
Cardiospermum halicacabum 282
Casts 150
Catagen 4
Central centrifugal cicatricial alopecia 140
CG210TM 62
Chamomile (*Matricaria chamomilla*) 282
Chaste berry 52
Chédiak-Higashi syndrome 182
Christmas tree 56
Chronic cutaneous lupus erythematosus 140
Chronic diffuse telogen hair loss 70
Chronic telogen effluvium 70, 81, 214
Cicatricial (scarring) alopecias 8, 140
Ciclopirox 273
Cinnamidopropyltrimonium chloride 260
Ciprofloxacin 145, 168
Circle hairs 19
Clarithromycin 168
Classic pseudopelade (Brocq) 140
Clindamycin 145
Clomipramine 243
Coal tar 274
Coenzyme Q10 259
Cognitive therapy 288
Coiled hairs 19
Comma hairs 19

Comma shaped 20
Congenital hypertrichosis lanuginosa 201
Congenital hypotrichia/atrichia 183
Contact immunotherapy 124
Copper 259
Corkscrew 20
Corkscrew hairs 20
Cortex 5
Cortexolone 17α-propionate 308
Corticosteroids 125, 149
Cradle cap 263
Cryptic hyperandrogenemia 388
Cushing's syndrome 392
Cuticle 5
Cyanocobalamin 329
Cyclophosphamide 151
Cyclosporine 145
CYP complex 90
Cyproterone acetate 65, 66, 228, 412

D

Dandruff 263
Dapsone 149, 166
Decalvans 145
Defined zone 360
Dehydroepiandrosterone sulfate 391
Delayed
    anagen release 71
    telogen release 71
Delusions of parasitosis (Ekbom's syndrome) 296
Demodex 280
Dermoscopy 14
Dexamethasone 126
Dexamethasone (Dx) suppression test 404
DHEAS 54
Dihydrotestosterone (DHT) 391
5α-dihydrotestosterone 54
Dinitrochlorobenzene 124
Diode 103
Diphenylcyclopropenone 124

Direct hair implant (DHI) 350
Direct hair transplantation 367
Discoid lupus erythematosus 146
Dissecting cellulitis 140, 145
Disturbances 56
Doll hair 19
Dong quai 52
Doxepin 287
Doxycycline 145, 163
D-panthenol 308
Dronabinol 243, 294
Drospirenone 65, 409
Dutasteride 52, 65, 226, 305

E
Ebling 219
Eclipta alba extract 341
Ectodermal dysplasias 183
Eflornithine 408
Eflornithine hydrochloride 103
EGF 5
Electrolysis 415
Elejalde syndrome 182
Emblica officianalis 341
Epidermal growth factors 312
Epiluminescence microscopy 14
Epithelial strand 7
Equilibrium dialysis 402
Erectile dysfunction 51
Erosive pustular dermatoses 140
Essential fatty acids (EFA) 338
17β-estradiol 235
Estradiol 55
Etanercept 145
Excimer laser 125, 244
Exclamation mark hairs 19
Exogen 4
Exogen/teloptosis 213

F
Factitial dermatitis of the scalp 288
FAGA.M 54
False unicorn 52
Faun tail 201

Favus 176, 208
Female androgenetic alopecia of male
    pattern (FAGA.M) 219
Female pattern hair loss 54, 214
Ferriman and Gallwey 388
Ferritin 79, 328, 333
FGF-5 5
FGF-7 310
Finasteride 63, 227, 305, 412
Finasteride 0.05% gel 62
Flame hair 20
Fluconazole 276
Fluridil 235
Flutamide 65, 68, 231, 413
Foam 61
FOL-005 320
Folate 80
Folic acid 89, 329, 338
Follica 312
Follicle stem cells 7
Follicular
    hair units (FHU) 1
    keratotic 16
    unit extraction (FUE) 350
    units 346
    unit transplant (FUT) 350
Folliculitis 145
    decalvans 140, 165
Folliculitis (acne)
    keloidalis 140
    necrotica 140
Follicum 320
Follistatin 312
Fractional erbium 233
Free androgen 89
    index 89, 392
Friar tuck 239
Frontal
    fibrosing alopecia 140, 243
    tuft 361
Frontotemporal angle 358
Fulvestrant 235
Fusidic acid 167

G

Gene reawakening 312
Genetic testing 206
Genotrichoses 181
GnRH agonists 410
Graft 376
Graham Little syndrome 140
Graham Little-Piccardi-Lassueur
    syndrome 157
Green tea polyphenols 259
Grey patch 208
Griscelli syndrome 182
Growth factor 305

H

Hair
    collar 201
    dyes 74
    pluck test 70
    powder 20
    pull test 60
    transplantation 68
    tufting 19
Hair follicle stem cells 73, 310
Hair restoration 53, 346
    surgery 159
Hair shaft 5
    disorders 188
HAIRAN 404
Hairline 355
Hallermann-Streiff 187
Hamamelis virginiana 282
Hamilton 347
Hand-held trichoscopes 35
Headington's classification 214
Heartseed 282
Heartseed (*Cardiospermum halicaca-
    bum*) 282
Hedgehog 335
Henley 5
Hepcidin 333
HGF 310
Hibiscus 341
Hirsutism 56, 388

Histogen 318
HoVert 143
Huxley 5
Hydroxychloroquine 145
Hyperadrenocorticism 79
Hyperandrogenemia 54
Hyperprolactinemia 79, 392
Hyperthecosis 392
Hyperthyroidism 79
Hypertrichosis 61, 200
Hypoparathyroidism 79
Hypopituitarism 79
Hypothyroidism 79, 392
Hypotrichosis simplex 183
Hypoxia inducible transcription factor 1
    (HIF1) 62

I

IGF-1 310
Immediate
    anagen release 71
    telogen release 71
Immunotherapy 136
Implanter 367
Infliximab 145
Infundibulum 1
Inner root sheath 5
Interface dermatitis 162
Iron 79, 328, 329
Isotretinoin 145, 276
Isthmus 1
Itraconzaole 275

J

JAK-STAT 235
Janus kinase (JAK) receptors 106

K

Kenogen 4, 213
Keratin 6 73
Keratosis follicularis spinulosa decal-
    vans 140
Kerion 176, 207
Ketoconazole 50, 52, 62, 272, 276
KROX20 316

L

Lanugo 3
Laser 52
  hair removal 168
Lasers 103
Latanoprost 51, 62, 314
Lateral epicanthus line rule 358
LH:FSH ratio 404
Lichen planopilaris 140
Light therapy 52
Liposomal ATP 384
Lithium gluconate 274
L-lysine 328, 339
L-methionine 259
Localized
  congenital alopecia 188
  hypertrichosis 201
  hypotrichosis 183
Low level laser 230
Ludwig 216
  stage 58

M

Macro hairline 373
Malassezia 263
male-pattern alopecia 3
Marie Unna hereditary hypotrichosis 186
Matricaria chamomilla 282
Matrikines 340
Matrix 5
MC1-R 259
Medulla 5
Melatonin 50, 52, 259
Melitane 259
Menopause 237
Menstrual 56
Menthol 287
Mesenchymal stem cells (MSCs) 312
Metformin 414
Methotrexate 127, 136, 151
Methoxypsoralen 125
Metronidazole 274
Micro hairline 373

Micro-irregularities 361
Microneedling 235
Mid-frontal point (MFP) 357
Miniaturization 39, 52, 214
Minocycline 163
Minoxidil 48
Modified wash test 221
Molecular replacement therapy 274
Monilethrix 191
Morphea 178
Mucin 148
Mycophenolate mofetil 151

N

N-acetylcysteine 243, 294
Nanoparticles 306
Nd:YAG 103, 172
Neurotic excoriations of the scalp 286
Nevoid hypertrichosis 203
Nexos disease 193
Niacin 329, 338
Nitric oxide 315
NK-1 receptor inhibitors 284
NKG2D 105
No difference 338
Nonclassic congenital adrenal hyperplasia 392
North American Virginian witch-hazel (Hamamelis virginiana) 282
Norwood 347
Norwood-Hamilton classification 42

O

Obsessive–compulsive disease 290
Olanzapine 243
Olsen 216
Ophiasis 108
Ophiasis inversus (sisapho) 108
Oral contraceptives 409
Oxidative stress 255

P

Pantothenic acid 329
Para-aminobenzoic acid 259
Pediculosis capitis 209

Peony (*Paeonia lactiflora*) 282
Perifolliculitis capitis abscedens et
    suffodiens 169
Periodic acid–Schiff 143
Peripilar
    casts 16
    sign 19, 45
Permethrin 209
PGF$_2$ 314
Phosphodiesterase 130
Photochemotherapy 125
Phototrichogram 86
Phytoestrogens 259
Piebaldism 199
Pili annulati 194
Pili torti 194
Piloscopy 385
Pimecrolimus 274
PioFluMet 414
Pioglitazone 145, 414
Pitting 112
Pityriasis amiantacea 267
Pityrosporum 264
Platelet derived 73
Platelet derived growth factor-β 73
Platelet-rich plasma 53, 68, 233, 314
Polarizing 16
Poliosis 198
Polycystic ovarian syndrome 217
Polycystic ovary syndrome (PCOS)
    392
Polygenic 55
Polytrichia 19
Postpartum telogen effluvium 235
Prednisolone 126, 149
Premature canities 255
Procapil™ 340
17OH progesterone (17OHP) 396
Prolactin 55, 402
Promac® 336
Propylene glycol 48
Prostaglandin
    analogs 62, 224, 314
    D2 314

Proteins 339
Pseudofolliculitis barbae 94
Pseudopelade of Brocq 160
Psychogenic 285
    pseudoeffluvium 73
Punch 380
PUVA 125, 136
Pyridoxine 308, 329

R
Rain 320
Red
    clover 52
    dots 17
    scalp disease 279
5α-reductase 54, 391
    inhibitors 304
Reetha 341
RepliCel 313, 316
Reticular 111
Retinoids 50, 149
Reverse sequential 412
Riboflavin 329
Rifampicin 145, 166
Rosacea-like dermatosis 279
Rosiglitazone 145, 414
Rotterdam criteria 397
Roxithromycin 315
Ruxolitinib 128

S
Safe donor area 348
SAHA (seborrhea, acne, hirsutism,
    androgenetic alopecia) 63
SAHA syndrome 218
Sapindus trifoliatus 341
Saw palmetto 52, 341
Scalp
    biopsy 86
    burnout 279
Scutula 176
Seasonal 245
    moulting 9
Seborrhea 282

Seborrheic dermatitis 263
Sebostasis 282
60-second hair count 84
Secondary
   syphilis 80
   vellus hair 45
Selective serotonin reuptake inhibitors
   243, 287
Selenium 259, 329, 337
   sulfide 273
Senescent alopecia 258
Serums 340
Setipiprant 321
Sex hormone binding globulin (SHBG)
   391
Short anagen phase 71
Silvery grey hair syndromes 182
Skin surface microscopy 14
SM04554 320
Spironolactone 63, 66, 229, 411
Squaric acid dibutylester 124
Standardized wash test 83
Staphylococcus aureus 165
Statins 131
Stem cell 305
   activation 310
Stem cells 235
Stemoxydine® 62
Substance P 9, 283
Sulfasalazine 136
Suprabulbar area 1
Sycosis barbae 98
Systemic lupus erythematosus 80

T

Tacrolimus 274
Tea tree oil 273
Telogen 4
   effluvium 54, 214
   gravidarum 74, 235
Teloptosis 76
Temporal point 359
Terbinafine 275
Terminal 3

Terminal to vellus 45, 60
Testosterone 54, 391
Tetracycline 163, 283
Thalidomide 149, 159
Thiazolidinediones 414
Tinea capitis 207
Tocotrienols 336
Tofacitinib 128
Tonsure 239
Total alopecia 243
Traction alopecia 173, 244
Transferrin 89
Transforming growth factor β_2 73
Transit-amplifying
   cells 5
   daughter cells 7
Transition zone 360
Transmembrane protein with EGF-like
   and follistatin-like domains 1 73
Traumatic
   alopecia 284
   folliculitis 99
Travoprost 62
Tretinoin 50
Triamcinolone acetonide 159
Trichoclasis 191
Trichodaganomania 296
Trichodynia 283
Trichogram 14
Trichomalacia 292
Trichomegaly 201
Trichophytic 350
Trichoptilosis 20
Trichorhinophalangeal syndrome 186
Trichorrhexis
   invaginata 190
   nodosa 189
Trichoschisis 190
Trichoscopic trichogram 82
Trichoscopy 14
Trichoteiromania 296
Trichotemnomania 294
Trichothiodystrophy 196

Trichotillomania 174, 238, 289
Trichotillosis 238, 289
Tufted folliculitis 165
Tulip hair 20
Type II 5α-reductase 51

U

Ultrasound 397
Ultraviolet B 172
Uncombable hair syndrome 194
Ustekinumab 130, 151

V

V sign 20
Valproic acid 311
VEGF 310
Vellus 3
Vellus-like hair 3
Vertex transition point 378
Video dermatoscopes 35
Virilization 56
Vitamin 329
Vitamin A 338

Vitamin D 79, 337
Vitamin D$_3$ 315
Vitamin E 336
Vitamin H 335
Vitamins 341

W

Weathering 258
White dots 17
Wickham's striae 150
Wnt 235
Wnt7a 311
Wnt/β-catenin 310
     pathway 9
Woolly hair disease 193

Y

Yellow dots 16, 45

Z

Zigzag shaped hairs 20
Zinc 79, 166, 329, 335
Zinc pyrithione 273

24